Advances in Public Health and Healthcare Management for Chronic Care

Advances in Public Health and Healthcare Management for Chronic Care

Guest Editors

Fabio Petrelli
Giovanni Cangelosi

MDPI

Basel • Beijing • Wuhan • Barcelona • Belgrade • Novi Sad • Cluj • Manchester

Guest Editors
Fabio Petrelli
School of Pharmacy
Polo Medicina Sperimentale e Sanità Pubblica "Stefania Scuri"
Camerino
Italy

Giovanni Cangelosi
Units of Diabetology
ASUR Marche
Fermo
Italy

Editorial Office
MDPI AG
Grosspeteranlage 5
4052 Basel, Switzerland

This is a reprint of the Special Issue, published open access by the journal *Medicina* (ISSN 1648-9144), freely accessible at: https://www.mdpi.com/journal/medicina/special_issues/T89149M66O.

For citation purposes, cite each article independently as indicated on the article page online and as indicated below:

Lastname, A.A.; Lastname, B.B. Article Title. *Journal Name* **Year**, *Volume Number*, Page Range.

ISBN 978-3-7258-5949-8 (Hbk)
ISBN 978-3-7258-5950-4 (PDF)
https://doi.org/10.3390/books978-3-7258-5950-4

Contents

About the Editors

Fabio Petrelli

Fabio Petrelli is Associate Professor of Hygiene at the School of Pharmacy, Experimental Medicine, and Public Health "Stefania Scuri" at the University of Camerino. His academic and research activity focuses on key areas of public health, including type 2 diabetes, obesity, nutrition, drug therapy, supplements, enteral nutrition, nursing management, health organization, and community-based nursing care. He has a strong interdisciplinary approach, integrating medical, nutritional, and organizational perspectives.

Prof. Petrelli began his academic career as a confirmed researcher in Hygiene and Public Health at the University of Camerino in 2002. In 2022, he was appointed Associate Professor and continues to contribute significantly to teaching, mentoring, and research. He currently serves as PhD Supervisor for the "One Health" curriculum within the Life and Health Sciences doctoral program at the University of Camerino.

As of August 2025, his scholarly work includes 118 publications indexed in Scopus, with over 1,300 citations and an h-index of 21, reflecting his leadership and impact in the field of public health and health sciences.

Giovanni Cangelosi

Giovanni Cangelosi is currently a PhD student in the One Health – Life Science curriculum at the SAS – International School of Advanced Studies, University of Camerino. With a multidisciplinary academic background, Dr. Cangelosi holds multiple master's degrees in Lifestyle Medicine (University of Eastern Piedmont), Legal and Forensic Aspects in Healthcare (Unipegaso), Nursing and Obstetric Sciences (Uniupo), and Management and Coordination of Healthcare Professions (Unitelma). His foundational training began with a University Diploma and a Bachelor's Degree in Nursing Sciences from the University of Modena and Reggio Emilia.

His research interests span diabetes, chronic care, nursing science, public health, and healthcare management. He has authored 48 publications indexed in Scopus, with over 200 citations and an h-index of 12 (as of August 18, 2025), reflecting his growing impact in the scientific community.

Dr. Cangelosi's professional and academic trajectory reflects a strong commitment to improving health care systems and advancing the integration of clinical practice with research and education, particularly within the field of chronic care and nursing.

Full affiliation:

Fabio Petrelli and Giovanni Cangelosi

School of Pharmacy, Experimental Medicine and "Stefani Scuri" Public Health Department, University of Camerino, Camerino, Italy

Preface

This Special Issue Reprint "Advances in Public Health and Health Care Management for Chronic Care" focuses on the management of chronic diseases, with particular attention to the implementation of innovative and personalized care models. The included contributions provide an overview of practical and evidence-based approaches aimed at improving both clinical outcomes and patients' quality of life.

The main objective is to highlight the importance of placing the patient at the center of care, promoting strategies that enhance patient and community satisfaction, optimize clinical results, and support medical and nursing practice.

This Reprint serves as a valuable resource for researchers, healthcare professionals, and decision-makers interested in understanding emerging trends in chronic disease management and implementing patient-centered innovative practices.

Fabio Petrelli and Giovanni Cangelosi
Guest Editors

medicina

MDPI

Editorial

Editorial for Special Issue "Advances in Public Health and Healthcare Management for Chronic Care"

Fabio Petrelli * and Giovanni Cangelosi *

School of Pharmacy, Experimental Medicine and "Stefania Scuri" Public Health Department, University of Camerino, Via Madonna delle Carceri 9, 62032 Camerino, Italy
* Correspondence: fabio.petrelli@unicam.it (F.P.); giovanni01.cangelosi@unicam.it (G.C.)

The management of chronic diseases represents one of the foremost challenges for contemporary healthcare systems, demanding increasingly innovative approaches and multidimensional strategies to improve outcomes for patients, families, and their communities [1]. This Special Issue, entitled "Advances in Public Health and Healthcare Management for Chronic Care," brings together original studies and reviews that offer fresh perspectives on epidemiology, clinical management, and organizational models, thereby reinforcing the value of an integrated and multidisciplinary vision of chronic conditions.

Among the original contributions, Al-Dayan [2] analyzed the distribution of hemoglobin-related disorders, underscoring the strategic role of systematic screening and genetic counseling in identifying at-risk groups. Gitto et al. [3] investigated the application of artificial neural networks to distinguish between idiopathic normal pressure hydrocephalus and Alzheimer's dementia, highlighting the potential of advanced technologies to enhance diagnostic accuracy. Park et al. [4] examined adiposity trends among peri- and postmenopausal women, while, in a complementary study, Park et al. [5] analyzed sales patterns of osteoporosis medications, offering valuable insights for health policy and resource allocation.

Borze Ursu et al. [6] assessed the effects of home-based relaxation compared with standard care in patients with fibromyalgia, reporting significant improvements in physiological parameters and suggesting complementary strategies for symptom management. Alruwaili [7] explored knowledge levels and therapeutic adherence among hypertensive patients, identifying key behavioral and educational determinants. Matsugaki et al. [8] investigated the relationship between a cancer diagnosis and the intention to leave the workforce in older individuals, shedding light on the broader social and occupational implications of chronic disease.

The second section of this Special Issue features reviews, beginning with the scoping review by Cangelosi et al. [9], which examined barriers and facilitators to the implementation of artificial intelligence in diabetes management from the perspective of healthcare professionals, emphasizing both the opportunities and challenges of digital innovation. Azzellino et al. [10] analyzed organizational models and the role of family and community nurses in the management of chronic conditions, underscoring the importance of integrated approaches.

The two systematic reviews by Karibayeva et al. [11,12] addressed vitamin D deficiency in Kazakhstan, focusing, respectively, on pediatric and adult populations. Considering both groups provides complementary evidence on the prevalence of a widespread condition, highlighting the importance of preventive strategies across the life course.

Taken together, the contributions included in this Special Issue illustrate the inherent complexity of chronic care, spanning epidemiological, clinical, social, and organizational dimensions. They also underscore the potential of innovative methodologies and interdisciplinary approaches to enhance patient outcomes and overall health system performance. Ultimately, this collection reinforces the vision of chronic care as a domain where clinical, technological, and organizational innovation converge in the pursuit of the most effective and personalized strategies for individuals, communities, and populations, with a strong emphasis on prevention [13].

Author Contributions: Conceptualization, F.P. and G.C.; methodology, F.P. and G.C.; validation, F.P. and G.C.; writing—original draft preparation, F.P. and G.C.; writing—review and editing, F.P. and G.C.; visualization, F.P. and G.C. All authors have read and agreed to the published version of the manuscript.

Conflicts of Interest: The authors declare no conflicts of interest.

References

1. Petrelli, F.; Cangelosi, G.; Nittari, G.; Pantanetti, P.; Debernardi, G.; Scuri, S.; Sagaro, G.G.; Nguyen, C.T.T.; Grappasonni, I. Chronic Care Model in Italy: A Narrative Review of the Literature. *Prim. Health Care Res. Dev.* **2021**, *22*, e32. [CrossRef]
2. Al-Dayan, N. Distribution of Hemoglobinopathy Disorders in Al-Kharj Province Based on Data from the Premarital Screening and Genetic Counseling Program. *Medicina* **2025**, *61*, 1458. [CrossRef] [PubMed]
3. Gitto, L.; Mento, C.; Massini, G.; Buscema, P.M.; Raffa, G.; Germanò, A.F.; Quattropani, M.C.A. Using Artificial Neural Network Models (ANNs) to Identify Patients with Idiopathic Normal Pressure Hydrocephalus (INPH) and Alzheimer Dementia (AD): Clinical Psychological Features and Differential Diagnosis. *Medicina* **2025**, *61*, 1332. [CrossRef]
4. Park, J.Y.; Park, H.M.; Chung, Y.J.; Kim, M.R.; Hwang, K.J.; Song, J.Y. Age-Related Trends in Dual-Energy X-Ray Absorptiometry-Measured Adiposity and Their Clinical Relevance: A Multicenter Cross-Sectional Study of Korean Peri- and Postmenopausal Women. *Medicina* **2025**, *61*, 1301. [CrossRef]
5. Park, J.Y.; Chung, Y.J.; Kim, M.R.; Song, J.Y. Five-Year Sales Trends of Osteoporosis Medications in Korea: A Market Analysis Based on IMS Health Sales Audit Data (2018–2023). *Medicina* **2025**, *61*, 805. [CrossRef] [PubMed]
6. Borze Ursu, T.F.; Pallag, A.; Tarcău, E.; Ciobanu, D.I.; Andronie-Cioară, F.L.; Nistor-Cseppento, C.D.; Ciavoi, G.; Mureșan, M. The Impact of Standard Care Versus Intrinsic Relaxation at Home on Physiological Parameters in Patients with Fibromyalgia: A Comparative Cohort Study from Romania. *Medicina* **2025**, *61*, 285. [CrossRef] [PubMed]
7. Alruwaili, B.F. Evaluation of Hypertension-Related Knowledge, Medication Adherence, and Associated Factors among Hypertensive Patients in the Aljouf Region, Saudi Arabia: A Cross-Sectional Study. *Medicina* **2024**, *60*, 1822. [CrossRef] [PubMed]
8. Matsugaki, R.; Matsuda, S.; Ogami, A. Relationship between Cancer and Intention to Leave Work among Older Workers: A Cross-Sectional Internet-Based Study. *Medicina* **2024**, *60*, 1506. [CrossRef] [PubMed]
9. Cangelosi, G.; Conti, A.; Caggianelli, G.; Panella, M.; Petrelli, F.; Mancin, S.; Ratti, M.; Masini, A. Barriers and Facilitators to Artificial Intelligence Implementation in Diabetes Management from Healthcare Workers' Perspective: A Scoping Review. *Medicina* **2025**, *61*, 1403. [CrossRef] [PubMed]
10. Azzellino, G.; Vagnarelli, P.; Passamonti, M.; Mengoli, L.; Ginaldi, L.; De Martinis, M. Integrated Hospital-Territory Organizational Models and the Role of Family and Community Nurses in the Management of Chronic Conditions: A Scoping Review. *Medicina* **2025**, *61*, 1175. [CrossRef] [PubMed]
11. Karibayeva, I.; Bilibayeva, G.; Iglikova, A.; Yerzhanova, A.; Alekesheva, R.; Maxudova, M.; Ussebayeva, N. Vitamin D Deficiency in Kazakhstani Children: Insights from a Systematic Review and Meta-Analysis. *Medicina* **2025**, *61*, 428. [CrossRef] [PubMed]
12. Karibayeva, I.; Bilibayeva, G.; Yerzhanova, A.; Alekesheva, R.; Iglikova, A.; Maxudova, M.; Ussebayeva, N. Prevalence of Vitamin D Deficiency among Adults in Kazakhstan: A Systematic Review and Meta-Analysis. *Medicina* **2024**, *60*, 2043. [CrossRef] [PubMed]
13. D'Alleva, A.; Leigheb, F.; Rinaldi, C.; Di Stanislao, F.; Vanhaecht, K.; De Ridder, D.; Bruyneel, L.; Cangelosi, G.; Panella, M. Achieving Quadruple Aim Goals through Clinical Networks: A Systematic Review. *J. Healthc. Qual. Res.* **2019**, *34*, 29–39. [CrossRef] [PubMed]

medicina

MDPI

Article

Distribution of Hemoglobinopathy Disorders in Al-Kharj Province Based on Data from the Premarital Screening and Genetic Counseling Program

Noura Al-Dayan

Medical Laboratory, Applied Medical Sciences, Prince Sattam Bin Abdulaziz University, Al-Kharj 16278, Saudi Arabia; n.aldayan@psau.edu.sa

Abstract: *Background and Objectives*: Hemoglobinopathies are genetic disorders of hemoglobin and are among the most common inherited diseases. The prevalence rates of sickle cell disease and thalassemia in Saudi Arabia are higher than those in other countries in the Middle East. Saudi Arabia has launched many prevention programs such as a premarital screening program, genetic counseling programs, and neonatal screening in order to reduce the incidence of genetic diseases. The former program includes the most common genetic diseases: sickle cell disease and thalassemia. Many studies conducted since the premarital program started have reported a decrease in the prevalence of sickle cell disease and thalassemia. However, all studies focus on large cities, including their subdivisions, but there is a lack of studies on subdivisions specifically. *Materials and Methods*: The aim of this study was to assess the prevalence, 5-year time trend, and distribution of β-thalassemia and sickle cell traits in Al-Kharj province using the data of the PMSGC program during the period from January 2017 to February 2021. *Results*: A total of 21,150 individuals were screened, and 508 were diagnosed with sickle cell disease and thalassemia. Also, we showed that thalassemia was more prevalent than sickle cell disease (66% and 34%, respectively), and there was an increase in β-thalassemia and α-thalassemia. *Conclusions*: Riyadh city's prevalence rate of β-thalassemia was reported as 7 per 1000, while the current study found a prevalence rate of 5.6 per 1000 in Al-Kharj, which suggests a possible increase as a result of population growth in Al-Kharj province as part of Riyadh city. This study recommends further improvement in preventive measures in high-risk regions, as well as enhanced community awareness, to provide the highest rate of reduction for disorders.

Keywords: premarital screening and genetic counseling program; sickle cell disease; α-thalassemia; β-thalassemia; premarital screening

1. Introduction

Hemoglobinopathies are genetic disorders in the synthesis of hemoglobin and are among the most common inherited diseases [1]. Global estimates indicate that approximately 300,000–400,000 infants are diagnosed yearly with hemoglobin disorders [2,3]. Thalassemia and sickle cell disease (SCD) are autosomal recessive hemoglobinopathy disorders that have received significant attention from the global public health community because of their impact on increasing mortality and morbidity among affected individuals [4,5]. Thalassemia is further broken down into thalassemia major and thalassemia intermedia. These types of thalassemia require intensive care, resulting in a major disease burden. In general, individuals become clinically asymptomatic in the case of the β-thalassemia (β-thal) trait, which is also known as thalassemia minor [1].

 https://doi.org/10.3390/medicina61081458

In Saudi Arabia, the prevalence of consanguineous marriages is high, contributing to the propagation of hemoglobinopathies and further leading to ongoing health challenges in the Kingdom. Consanguineous marriages in Saudi Arabia are susceptible to genetic disorders that may be inherited by their offspring [2]. Saudi Arabia has the highest prevalence rates of β-thalassemia and SCD compared to other Middle Eastern countries (0.05–4.50%) [6]. The general statistics organization reported that Saudi Arabia has a high prevalence of thalassemia and sickle cell disease, with an estimated prevalence of 1.5–17% for β-thalassemia and SCD, respectively [3,4]. Preventive screening programs have been adopted in many countries, including Middle Eastern countries, to reduce the prevalence of β-thalassemia and SCD, such as the premarital screening program and genetic counseling (PMSGC), neonatal screening, and pre-implantation genetic diagnosis [7]. In 2001, Saudi Arabia started a program known as the premarital screening program (PMS) to lower the burden of hemoglobinopathy disorders and infectious diseases. The hemoglobinopathy included β-thalassemia and SCD, and infectious diseases included human immunodeficiency (HIV) and hepatitis B and C. However, this program became mandatory in 2004 for both Saudi and non-Saudi couples prior to marriage [5–8].

National studies conducted in Saudi Arabia have shown a minor decline in the prevalence of SCD, but there are inconsistent reports on the prevalence of β-thalassemia [1,8]. Studies have demonstrated that the highest incidence was in the eastern region (19.5%), followed by Qunfudah (15.8%), Jazan (7.8%), Al-Hasa (3.1%), and Riyadh (0.15%) [9]. Surprisingly, α-thalassemia was not included in all centers of PMS, as the most commonly reported was α-3.7, which is not considered a risky mutation [10]. However, α-thalassemia has been reported to be highly prevalent in the northern and eastern regions, ranging from 0.4% to 5.9%, respectively, and it is co-inherited with sickle cell disease and β-thalassemia [11,12]. Moreover, a 2022 study reported that the α-thalassemia trait had the highest frequency in Makkah city (6.3%) during premarital screening [13]. Alhuthali et al. (2023) [14] identified seven α-thalassemia mutations that might have a large effect on increased mortality and morbidity.

In general, researchers have identified a marked decrease in the number of risky marriages and have predicted a considerable reduction in the genetic disease burden in Saudi Arabia in recent years as a result of premarital genetic counseling (PMSGC) [8]. The PMSGC program has been one of the strongest tools for reducing genetic diseases by identifying risk factors, providing vaccinations, and offering genetic consulting. Although Riyadh city was reported to have the lowest prevalence rates of β-thalassemia, α-thalassemia, and SCD, there is a population increase in Riyadh city which will increase the prevalence rate [9,10].

Al-Saeed et al. [7] performed a study in Saudi Arabia on hemoglobinopathy disorders and included a total of 13 cities in the Kingdom; however, Al-Kharj province was not covered separately. According to the Saudi census of 2022, Al-Kharj has a population of 373,177, which is the largest province population in the capital city; however, the prevalence of hemoglobinopathy disorders has not yet been recorded for Al-Kharj province. This study aims to evaluate the prevalence of hemoglobinopathy in Al-Kharj province over five years and identify the distribution of the disease among males and females. The findings of this study could shed light on the increased incidence, highlighting the need for further improvement in disease prevention efforts and health promotion. In addition, it could help evaluate the effectiveness of genetic counseling programs in achieving a massive reduction in disease burden.

2. Materials and Methods

2.1. Sample and Population

The current study is a retrospective study that included all samples received at PMS government centers located in Al-Kharj. The samples were collected from individuals, aged 16–55 years, for hemoglobinopathy, HIV, and hepatitis B and C testing. Computerized data were obtained from centers through a digital platform network utilized by health authorities, including the Ministry of Health (MOH), for disease surveillance, reporting, and data collection. The present study only used data uploaded through the network by centers over a five-year period, from January 2017 to February 2021. A total of 21,150 samples were accepted by government centers based on the clinical capacity for hemoglobinopathy and infectious disease testing included in PMS.

2.2. Premarital Screening Program and Genetic Counseling Program (PMSGC)

The PMSGC program is supported by an extensive network spanning 13 administrative districts and 131 Ministry of Health Centers throughout Saudi Arabia. PMSGS targets couples pursuing marriage certificates as a prerequisite for screening. The PMS staff gather demographic information, draw blood samples containing the ethylenediaminetetraacetic acid [EDTA] anticoagulant, and offer educational materials that explain the program. Blood samples were used for complete blood count (CBC) (DxH 600, Beckman Coulter, Brea, CA, USA), peripheral blood film analyses, reticulocyte counts, high-performance liquid chromatography (HPLC) (Bio-Rad Variant II, Hercules, CA, USA), hemoglobin electrophoresis (Interlab, Roma, Italy), sickling tests using sodium dithionite and serum ferritin, and virus tests for hepatitis B, HIV, and hepatitis C.

The hemoglobinopathy test results sort individuals from potential couples into healthy, carriers, and affected cases with regard to the genetic make-up of sickle cell disease and/or thalassemia. A safe marriage was declared when both partners or at least one of them was healthy. An at-risk marriage was declared when both partners were carriers or cases (one was a case and the other was a carrier) of sickle cell disease and/or thalassemia. Couples with safe marriage test results were issued instant compatibility certificates, whereas at-risk couples were asked to attend personal genetic counseling meetings before issuing incompatibility certificates. Further, molecular genetic testing was performed by sending the samples to the MOH reference laboratory, which uploads the results to the center pool.

2.3. Hemoglobin Electrophoresis Analysis

Hemoglobin electrophoresis samples were examined to detect aberrant hemoglobin bands using capillary electrophoresis, HPLC, or a combination of both. Diagnosis of the β-thalassemia trait is indicated when an individual exhibits a Mean Corpuscular Volume (MCV) of <80 fL and Mean Corpuscular Hemoglobin (MCH) of <27 pg, alongside a hemoglobin A2 level over 3.2%. HPLC tests were conducted regardless of the normal CBC results. Diagnosis of α-thalassemia is indicated when the MCV is <80 fL or hypothermia, the MCH is <26 pg, or both, in the absence of iron deficiency anemia. The couple's results were interpreted based on standard laboratory diagnostic protocols that were approved by the MOH specifically for the program [15].

2.4. Statistical Analysis

Statistical analysis of the PMSGC data was performed using PRISM 10.4.2 and Microsoft Excel 2007, including the analysis of prevalence trends and prevalence rates. Statistical tests included descriptive data as mean and SD for both males and females. In addition, statistical analysis was performed to calculate the percentage of sickle cell anemia and thalassemia.

3. Results

3.1. *Details of Hemoglobinopathy Disorders*

The overall study population consisted of 21,150 individuals who attended the PM-SCG centers in Al-Kharj province from January 2017 to February 2021. The mean age of the 508 participants was 30.0 + 12.0. Among the 21,150 participants, hemoglobinopathy disorders were confirmed in 2.4% of cases (n = 508), with 1.57% (n = 333) diagnosed as thalassemia and 0.82% (n = 157) as SCD. Also, in terms of gender distribution, 49% were males and 51% were females, with no statistically significant difference between males and females (p = 0.01). Table 1 shows the gender distribution of hemoglobinopathy disorders. It is clear that females were predominant in thalassemia (51.1%) and in SCD (51%); in contrast, males were the minority in both conditions, with 48.1% and 49.1%, respectively.

Table 1. Gender distribution among individuals diagnosed with hemoglobinopathy disorders.

Gender	Thalassemia Trait	SCD	Hemoglobinopathy Disorders
Males	163 (48.9%)	86 (49.1%)	249 (49%)
Females	170 (51.1%)	89 (50.9%)	259 (51%)

3.1.1. Thalassemia Analysis

Among the total participants, 1.57% were confirmed as having thalassemia traits, of whom 49% were male and 51% were female. Among males, 22.7% of the individuals were under 18 years of age, while 20.75% were aged between 18 and 25 years. The demographics of individuals aged 26 to 35 constituted 18.4%, while those aged 36 to 45 represented 19.63%. The demographics of individuals aged 46–55 years were confirmed to represent 17.06% of the total population. The distribution of females was as follows: 21.18% were under 18 years, 20% were between 18 and 25 years, and 21.76% fell within the 26 to 35 years age range. The percentages of women aged 36–45 and 46–55 were determined to be 20% and 17.06%, respectively. In this study, among the selected individuals of both genders, 21.9% were under 18 years of age, 20.1% fell within the 18–25 and 26–35 age range, 19.8% were aged 36–45, and 18% were within the 46–55 age range. The majority of thalassemia traits were identified in individuals under 18 years of age, encompassing both men and women, as well as a mixed population. In females, thalassemia was notably higher in the age group of 26–35 years at 21.7%, compared to 21.2% in those under 18 years. Table 2 provides the percentages and prevalence of the thalassemia traits observed across different age groups. A two-way ANOVA showed a significant association ($p < 0.0001$) between the male and female groups. Further analysis was conducted to examine thalassemia prevalence.

Table 2. Age group distribution for males and females diagnosed with Thalassemia traits.

Gender	Total Cases	<18 Years	18–25 Years	26–35 Years	36–45 Years	46–55 Years
Males	163 (100%)	37 (22.70%)	33 (20.75%)	30 (18.40%)	32 (19.63%)	31 (19.02%)
Females	170 (100%)	36 (21.18%)	34 (20%)	37 (21.76%)	34 (20%)	29 (17.06%)

3.1.2. Screening of Thalassemia

This study diagnosed 333 patients with thalassemia, further dividing them into α- and β-thalassemia groups. α-thalassemia accounted for 64.3% of cases, while β-thalassemia represented 35.7%. This study was conducted over a period of five years, i.e., from January 2017 to February 2021. Table 3 shows the prevalence of both α- and β-thalassemia over a period of five years along with a graph representation, which is displayed in Figure 1. The prevalence of α-thalassemia was recorded to be 18.7%, 20.1%, 27.6%, 27.1%, and 6.5%, respectively, between 2017 and 2021, while β-thalassemia prevalence was found to be

17.6%, 19.3%, 24.4%, 25.2%, and 13.4%, respectively. The highest recorded prevalence of α- and β-thalassemia was documented in 2019 and 2020, respectively.

Table 3. Positive results confirmed for α- and β-thalassemia traits during the period of 2017–2021.

Year	α-Thalassemia Trait (n = 214)	β-Thalassemia Trait (n = 119)
2017	40 (18.7%)	21 (17.6%)
2018	43 (20.1%)	23 (19.3%)
2019	59 (27.6%)	29 (24.4%)
2020	58 (27.1%)	30 (25.2%)
2021	14 (6.5%)	16 (13.4%)

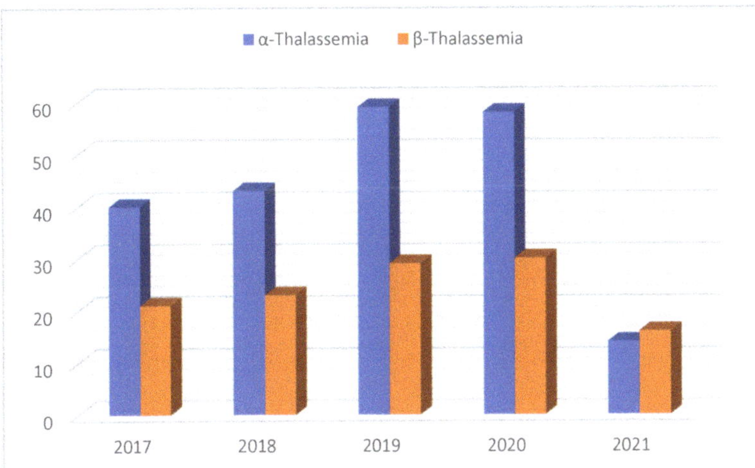

Figure 1. Trends of α- and β-thalassemia traits from 2017 to 2021.

3.2. Prevalence Rate of SCD

In this study, 175 patients were diagnosed with SCD over a duration of five years in Al-Kharj province. The proportion of males and females with SCD was 49.1% and 50.9%, respectively. The analysis was conducted based on age-wise criteria for both males and females. Among men, 9.7% of the participants were younger than 18 years old, 10.3% were 18 to 25 years old, 13.1% were 26 to 35 years old, 8.6% were 36 to 45 years old, and 7.4% were 46 to 55 years old. Among women, 11.4% were younger than 18 years old, 14.9% were 18 to 25 years old, 7.4% were 26 to 35 years old, 10.3% were 36 to 45 years old, and 6.9% were 46 to 55 years old. The highest prevalence of SCD was observed in males aged 26–35 years (13.1%) and in females aged 18–25 years (14.9%). The details are listed in Table 4.

Table 4. Distribution of age groups among male and female individuals diagnosed with SCD.

Gender	<18 Years	18–25 Years	26–35 Years	36–45 Years	46–55 Years
Males	17 (9.7%)	18 (10.3%)	23 (13.1%)	15 (8.6%)	13 (7.4%)
Females	20 (11.4%)	26 (14.9%)	13 (7.4%)	18 (10.3%)	12 (6.9%)

3.3. Prevalence of SCD Between 2017 and 2021

Table 5 confirms the documented prevalence of SCD between the years 2017 and 2021 in Al-Kharj city. The prevalence of SCD was found to be 18.9%, 20%, 21.7%, 25.7%, and 13.7%, respectively, in the years 2017 to 2021. However, the highest prevalence of SCD was 21.7% in 2019.

Table 5. Year-wise SCD prevalence in Al-Kharj province from 2017 to 2021.

Year-Wise	Diagnosis of Sickle Cell Traits (n = 175)
2017	33 (18.9%)
2018	35 (20.0%)
2019	38 (21.7%)
2020	45 (25.7%)
2021	24 (13.7%)

3.4. Prevalence Rate in Hemoglobinopathy Disorders

Overall, the prevalence rate estimated for α-thalassemia in the study population over the 5-year period was 10 per 1000, and the prevalence rate for β-thalassemia was 5.6 per 1000. In addition, the prevalence rate of SCD was estimated to be 8 per 1000 among the 21,150 people examined. Details are shown in Table 6. Among the 21,150 subjects, 23.6% of the participants were recruited between 2017 and 2020, but only 5.4% were enrolled in 2021. The prevalence of thalassemia (α and β) was 12.2%, 13.2%, 17.6%, and 26%, and in SCDs, it was 6.6%, 7%, 7.6%, 9%, and 20%, respectively.

Table 6. Prevalence rates of α-/β-thalassemia and SCD in Al-Kharj province between 2017 and 2021.

	Population Screened	α-Thalassemia	β-Thalassemia	
Year	Total Participants (n = 21,150)	Positive Subjects (n = 119)	Confirmed Subjects (n = 214)	PR
2017	5000 (23.6%)	40 (18.7%)	21 (17.6%)	12.20%
2018	5000 (23.6%)	43 (20.1%)	23 (19.3%)	13.20%
2019	5000 (23.6%)	59 (27.6%)	29 (24.4%)	17.60%
2020	5000 (23.6%)	58 (27.1%)	30 (25.2%)	17.60%
2021	1150 (5.4%)	14 (6.5%)	16 (13.4%)	26%

4. Discussion

In Saudi Arabia, hemoglobinopathies are considered the most prevalent disorders, although their prevalence varies among cities in the Kingdom. Variations in thalassemia and SCD rates can be attributed to multiple factors, including genetic and environmental factors, along with cultural aspects and diseases in the families. Hemoglobin disorders are common monogenic disorders worldwide, in which α-thalassemia, β-thalassemia, SCD, and hemoglobin-E diseases are considered to be more prevalent. All genetic disorders associated with hemoglobin are referred to as hemoglobinopathies and recognized as single-gene disorders [9]. The rate of consanguineous marriage in Saudi Arabia was documented to be high at approximately 56%, which indicates that genetic diseases are common [10].

Saudi Arabia initiated the concept of a premarital screening program, also known as the Healthy Marriage program, in 2001, and it was strictly implemented in 2004. The MOH started and planned this program to identify genetic risks (β-thalassemia and SCDs) and reduce the risk of infectious diseases (HIV and hepatitis B and C) among Saudi couples before marriage. Screening for these diseases can help prevent infectious diseases, identify their prevalence in couples before marriage, and promote a healthier life for their offspring. α-thalassemia was not included in most of the PMS [12]. In Saudi Arabia, the most important issue in marriages is consanguinity, which has a powerful impact on marrying within the family. With the help of genetic counselors, Saudi couples benefit from the PMS program's knowledge and importance. Finally, after the PMS certificate is issued, it allows them to proceed with their marriage [6,11,12].

The PMS program is mainly beneficial for documenting genetic disorders, particularly in Saudi couples with high rates of consanguineous marriages. Autosomal recessive disorders such as thalassemia and SCDs are prevalent in Saudi Arabia. Abnormalities in thalassemia and SCDs will lead to anemia and organ damage, as well as other complications, and there are many risks affecting offspring when both parents are carriers of these mutations, further compounded by the disadvantages of consanguineous unions [13,14].

The prevalence of hemoglobinopathies in Saudi Arabia varies from city to city. The study by Alsaeed et al. [7] established the highest prevalence of β-thalassemia in Jazan (32%), followed by the eastern region (23.7%), Makkah (14.4%), and Al-Baha (13.2%). Furthermore, the distribution of confirmed cases was as follows: 8.1% in Madina, 7.6% in the Northern Border, 7% in Riyadh, 6.7% in Asir, 6.3% in Tabuk, 4% in Qasim, 3.3% in Hail, 2.9% in Al-Jouf, and 2.4% in Najran [7]. An updated study in the southern region has confirmed a prevalence of 7% in hemoglobinopathies [15]. Another study from Jeddah has documented hemoglobinopathy screening results, reporting a 7.2% prevalence of β-thalassemia and 9.4% for SCD [16]. A recent study in Riyadh city has documented an SCD prevalence of 4.7% and a β-thalassemia prevalence of 1.2% [17]. All previous studies in PMS have focused on β-thalassemia and SCD, and only a few mention α-thalassemia [11]. Moustafa et al. [13] have reported the highest frequency of α-thalassemia in Makkah city, with a PR of around 6.3%. Molecular screening and identification of α-thalassemia contribute to prenatal diagnosis and realistic genetic counseling in regions at risk for thalassemia, yet these services are not available at most MOH centers [12].

A significant occurrence of hemoglobinopathies has been recorded in Saudi Arabia among the GCC nations, followed by Oman, which exhibits a notable prevalence of the sickle cell trait. In contrast, the UAE, Qatar, and Bahrain demonstrate a lower frequency of these conditions [17].

The aim of this study was to screen the PMS in Al-Kharj city. Overall, 21,150 individuals participated in this study over a duration of five years, between 2017 and 2021. The study results confirmed that 2.4% of the participants had hemoglobinopathy disorders, in which 1.57% were confirmed for thalassemia and 0.82% for SCDs. The prevalence of hemoglobinopathies was reported to be low in the central region of Saudi Arabia when compared to other regions in the Kingdom. Studies have focused on β-thalassemia and SCDs, with none of the meta-analysis studies recording α-thalassemia because it is considered not risky [18]. A few studies have demonstrated that α-thalassemia mutations are distributed around Saudi Arabia, and some of these are high-risk and might have a large impact on increased mortality and need more attention [14]. A limitation of the current study is the lack of molecular identification for α-thalassemia.

5. Conclusions

This study confirms a hemoglobinopathy prevalence of 1.57% in Al-Kharj city. This is the first documented study in the Kingdom, and future studies are recommended to investigate the prevalence and genetic mutations of hemoglobinopathies in detail in Al-Kharj city.

Funding: This study is supported via funding from Prince Sattam bin Abdulaziz University, project number PSAU/2025/03/34450.

Institutional Review Board Statement: The study was conducted according to the guidelines of the Declaration of Helsinki, and approved by the Institutional Review Board of Deanship of research and graduate studies from Prince Sattam bin Abdulaziz University, Kharj, in Saudi Arabia (IRB No: SCBR-376/2024, date of approval 15 December 2024).

Informed Consent Statement: Informed consent form was received from all the participants involved in this study.

Data Availability Statement: The original contributions presented in this study are included in the article. Further inquiries can be directed to the corresponding author.

Conflicts of Interest: The author declares no conflicts of interest.

Abbreviations

The following abbreviations are used in this manuscript:

PMSGC	Premarital Screening and Genetic Counseling Program
SCD	sickle cell disease
PMS	premarital screening program
HIV	human immunodeficiency
HPLC	high-performance liquid chromatography
MOH	Ministry of Health
CBC	complete blood count

References

1. Kumar, M.; Kargwal, V.; Goel, R.; Debnath, E.; Malhotra, S.; Balyan, K.; Zaidi, M.; Yadav, R. Screening and Diagnosis of Thalassemia and other hemoglobinopathies in North Indian population: Challenges faced. *Pediatr. Hematol. Oncol. J.* **2025**, *10*, 59–65. [CrossRef]
2. Almutairi, G.; Harbi, G.S.A.; Almutairi, L.; Aljarallah, F.S.; Alzaydi, N.M.; Alradaddi, R.; Alofi, A.; Alharbi, M.M.; Alhumaidi, N.H.; Alhomaid, T.A. Knowledge and Attitude toward Hemoglobinopathy Premarital Screening program among students of health colleges at Qassim University. *Cureus* **2025**, *17*, e77081. [CrossRef] [PubMed]
3. Alhowiti, A.; Shaqran, T. Premarital Screening Program Knowledge and Attitude among Saudi University Students in TABUK City 2019. *Int. J. Med. Res. Health Sci.* **2019**, *8*, 75–84.
4. Binshihon, S.M.; Alsulami, M.O.; Alogaibi, W.M.; Mohammedsaleh, A.H.; Mandourah, H.N.; Albaity, B.S.; Qari, M.H. Knowledge and attitude toward hemoglobinopathies premarital screening program among unmarried population in western Saudi Arabia. *Saudi Med. J.* **2018**, *39*, 1226–1231. [CrossRef] [PubMed]
5. Al-Shroby, W.A.; Sulimani, S.M.; Alhurishi, S.A.; Dayel, M.E.B.; Alsanie, N.A.; Alhraiwil, N.J. Awareness of Premarital Screening and Genetic Counseling among Saudis and its Association with Sociodemographic Factors: A National Study. *J. Multidiscip. Healthc.* **2021**, *14*, 389–399. [CrossRef] [PubMed]
6. Gosadi, I.M. National screening programs in Saudi Arabia: Overview, outcomes, and effectiveness. *J. Infect. Public Health* **2019**, *12*, 608–614. [CrossRef] [PubMed]
7. Alsaeed, E.S.; Farhat, G.N.; Assiri, A.M.; Memish, Z.; Ahmed, E.M.; Saeedi, M.Y.; Al-Dossary, M.F.; Bashawri, H. Distribution of hemoglobinopathy disorders in Saudi Arabia based on data from the premarital screening and genetic counseling program, 2011–2015. *J. Epidemiol. Glob. Health* **2017**, *7*, S41. [CrossRef] [PubMed]
8. More, P. A Review of Importance of Premarital Checkup and Counselling among Young Adults. *Psychol. Educ. J.* **2021**, *58*, 6369–6373. [CrossRef]
9. Singh, V.; Biswas, A.K.; Baranwal, A.K.; Asthana, B.; Dahiya, T. Prevalence of hemoglobinopathies using high-performance liquid chromatography as diagnostic tool in anemic patients of tertiary care center of Western India. *Asian J. Transfus. Sci.* **2022**, *18*, 257–263. [CrossRef] [PubMed]
10. Attallah, S.; Alhadad, M.; Alqarni, W.; Filfilan, D.; Zaharani, A.; Alharby, A.; Malki, A.A.; Algabry, N.; Jamil, E.; Hakami, A.; et al. PB2542: Molecular spectrum of alpha thalassemia mutations in the western province of saudi arabia and recommendation for premarital screening. *HemaSphere* **2023**, *7*, e15174c0. [CrossRef]
11. Olwi, D.I.; Merdad, L.A.; Ramadan, E.K. Thalassemia: A prevalent disease yet unknown term among college students in Saudi Arabia. *J. Community Genet.* **2017**, *9*, 277–282. [CrossRef] [PubMed]
12. Alasmari, S.Z. Premarital screening programme in Saudi Arabia: Insights into men's awareness and perceptions. *PubMed* **2024**, *28*, 63–73.
13. Moustafa, A.Z.; Almalki, R.A.; Qhashgry, E.I.; Qari, R.A.; Anwar, Z.S.; Alfahmi, A.M.; Fageeh, S.M.; Hendawy, D.; Balkhair, R. Prevalence of hemoglobin abnormality in the premarital screening Saudi population in Makkah city in a cross-sectional study Abstract. *Deleted J.* **2022**, *2*, 17–25. [CrossRef]

14. Alhuthali, H.M.; Ataya, E.F.; Alsalmi, A.; Elmissbah, T.E.; Alsharif, K.F.; Alzahrani, H.A.; Alsaiari, A.A.; Allahyani, M.; Gharib, A.F.; Qanash, H.; et al. Molecular patterns of alpha-thalassemia in the kingdom of Saudi Arabia: Identification of prevalent genotypes and regions with high incidence. *Thromb. J.* **2023**, *21*, 115. [CrossRef] [PubMed]
15. Al Eissa, M.M.A.; Almsned, F.; Alkharji, R.R.; Aldossary, Y.M.; AlQurashi, R.; Hawsa, E.A.; AlDosari, S.M.; Alqahtani, A.S.; Alotibi, R.S.; Farzan, R.; et al. The perception of genetic diseases and premarital screening tests in the central region of Saudi Arabia. *BMC Public Health* **2024**, *24*, 1556. [CrossRef] [PubMed]
16. AlOtaiby, S.; Alqahtani, A.; Saleh, R.; Mazyad, A.; Albohigan, A.; Kutbi, E. Comprehension of premarital screening and genetic disorders among the population of Riyadh. *J. Taibah Univ. Med. Sci.* **2023**, *18*, 822–830. [CrossRef] [PubMed]
17. Makkawi, M.; Alasmari, S.; Hawan, A.A.; Shahrani, M.M.A.; Dera, A.A. Hemoglobinopathies. *Saudi Med. J.* **2021**, *42*, 784–789. [CrossRef] [PubMed]
18. Aljabry, M.; Sulimani, S.; Alotaibi, G.; Aljabri, H.; Alomary, S.; Aljabri, O.; Sallam, M.; Alsultan, A. Prevalence and Regional Distribution of Beta-Hemoglobin Variants in Saudi Arabia: Insights from the National Premarital Screening Program. *J. Epidemiol. Glob. Health* **2024**, *14*, 1242–1248. [CrossRef] [PubMed]

medicina

MDPI

Article

Using Artificial Neural Network Models (ANNs) to Identify Patients with Idiopathic Normal Pressure Hydrocephalus (INPH) and Alzheimer Dementia (AD): Clinical Psychological Features and Differential Diagnosis

Lara Gitto [1], Carmela Mento [2,*], Giulia Massini [3], Paolo Massimo Buscema [3,4], Giovanni Raffa [2], Antonio Francesco Germanò [2] and Maria Catena Ausilia Quattropani [5]

[1] Department of Economics, University of Messina, 98125 Messina, Italy; lara.gitto@unime.it
[2] Department of Biomedical and Dental Sciences and Morphofunctional Imaging, University of Messina, 98125 Messina, Italy; giovanni.raffa@unime.it (G.R.); antonino.germano@unime.it (A.F.G.)
[3] Semeion Research Center of Sciences of Communication, 00128 Rome, Italy; g.massini@semeion.it (G.M.); m.buscema@semeion.it (P.M.B.)
[4] Department of Mathematical and Statistical Sciences, University of Colorado, 1201 Larimer Street, Denver, CO 80204, USA; paolo.buscema@ucdenver.edu
[5] Department of Educational Sciences, University of Catania, 95124 Catania, Italy; maria.quattropani@unict.it
* Correspondence: cmento@unime.it

Abstract: *Background and Objectives*: Patients with idiopathic normal pressure hydrocephalus (INPH) present similar symptoms as other diseases, such as dementia (AD). However, while dementia is not reversible, INPH dementia can be treated through neurosurgery. This study aims to assess the Rorschach method as a valid tool to identify INPH patients. *Materials and Methods*: The perception characteristics of a small sample of patients (n = 19) were observed through the Rorschach Inblok test. Artificial neural network (ANN) models allowed us to analyze the correlations between patients' cognitive functions and perception characteristics. *Results*: The results obtained revealed significant insights about the independent traits in patients' patterns of response with INPH and AD. In performing the test, patients with INPH and AD concentrated more on the cards displayed and what they perceived, while other patients concentrated on reactions related to the image proposed. *Conclusions*: The Rorschach test is a valid predictor tool to identify INPH patients who could successfully be treated with neurosurgery. Hence, this methodology has potential in differential diagnosis applied to a clinical context.

Keywords: idiopathic normal pressure hydrocephalus (INPH); Alzheimer's dementia (AD); artificial neural network (ANN) models; Rorschach inkblot test

1. Introduction

Idiopathic normal pressure hydrocephalus (INPH) is a brain disorder characterized by the enlargement of the brain's ventricular system and cerebrospinal fluid (CSF) pressure within the normal range. INPH mainly affects men over 65 years of age; it is a progressive, chronic disorder causing cognitive impairment without a specific identifiable cause [1]. The idiopathic form must be distinguished from other chronic forms of hydrocephalus conditions, which can derive from brain surgery, meningitis, or head injury in 50% of cases [2].

INPH is characterized by ventricular enlargement without intracranial hypertension, which causes clinical gait disturbances, urinary incontinence, and dementia (known as the "Adams triad") and accounts for 2–10% of all forms of dementia and 40% of adulthood hydrocephalus.

The classic triad is similar in appearance to other neurological conditions, such as Alzheimer's Dementia (AD) [1]. However, while dementia is not reversible, INPH dementia can be treated through neurosurgical procedures by installing a shunt to drain excess CSF into another part of the body. This treatment may alleviate symptoms and help restore normal cerebrospinal fluid dynamics [3].

In fact, after treatment, clinical improvements have been reported in 30–96% of patients [4]. It was found that 93% of patients experience gait improvements, and more than 50% undergo significant cognitive improvements [5,6].

Despite a large amount of data available, some aspects concerning the differential diagnosis of various forms of dementia and the accuracy of patient selection for ventriculoperitoneal shunts are still controversial [7].

INPH is a significant challenge for the medical community [8]: it is extremely difficult to differentiate between INPH and AD based on neurological deficits and clinical evidence only, such as measuring ventricular size through conventional medical imaging techniques [9]. The distinction is clinically important because INPH is one of the few treatable causes of dementia [10].

Hence, the main costs of INPH derive from its lack of diagnosis. Recently, this issue was analyzed in a conference held at the Italian Ministry of Health (https://www.sanitainformazione.it/idrocefalo-normoteso-attenzione-a-non-confonderlo-con-alzheimer-o-parkinson/, accessed on 7 May 2025). The findings of this conference confirmed the urgent attention this issue requires. Moreover, since there is no formal definition of INPH, discrepancies are encountered when estimating its real incidence, which is thought to range from 2 to 20 per million/people per year. The difficulty of distinguishing INPH from other neurodegenerative disorders is the most likely reason why about 80% of cases remain unrecognized and untreated [11]. Although data report a total of 5/100,000 new cases diagnosed every year, the actual number of people with INPH is predicted to be higher. A percentage ranging from 9 to 14% of the elderly living at home present with INPH symptoms, and a further increase in the number of people suffering from this disease can be assumed considering population aging.

Accurate diagnosis is necessary because conventional hydrocephalus treatments have no benefit in non-hydrocephalus patients: if non-hydrocephalic patients are misdiagnosed as hydrocephalic patients, treatment is not only ineffective but associated with significant morbidity and increased costs [12].

In light of these considerations, since the overall prevalence of dementia rises progressively as the population ages, even if INPH is responsible for only a small proportion of senile dementia, successful treatment could help many patients [13]. They could be treated in a short time and save on resources; costs due to incorrect therapies or inappropriate diagnostic procedures would be lower, and patient's quality of life would be higher.

Regarding the type of treatment and assistance used, the spontaneous course of INPH requires most patients to rely on nursing care [14]. For those patients undergoing surgery, continuous and regular checks are required by a neurosurgeon to ensure that the shunt is working properly [15]; continuous follow-up and assistance can be complemented with physiotherapy treatments, socialization, and psychological support.

A comprehensive estimation of INPH costs has not been performed as of yet. In 2000, more than two decades ago, the cost of treating INPH in the US exceeded USD 1 billion; there were 27,870 patients with treated INPH, while more than 8000 were newly cases diagnosed. However, updated statistics are necessary [16].

Together with considerations of costs, another field of analysis is the implementation of new diagnostic tools. To our knowledge, no clinical or neuroradiological techniques have been validated to clearly identify dementia from INPH, both of which share anatomical and clinical similarities [17]. Magnetic resonance imaging (MRI) depicts ventricle size accurately; however, findings on brain images are not sufficient to establish a diagnosis alone because they provide minimal, if any, evidence of brain damage despite marked deficits in motor skills and cognitive functioning [10,18,19].

In a study describing the advantages and drawbacks of MRI parameters, the importance of finding specific imaging biomarkers likely to distinguish between the two conditions has been emphasized [20]. If a screening tool can identify possible cases, then further workup should be performed to confirm the diagnosis and determine the need for shunting [21–23].

The Rorschach test is usually involved in psychological diagnosis; clinical, personality assessments; and the selection context for the detection of a global personality profile in patterns of response [24–28]. The response process of the inkblot is centered on the identification of mental function, cognitive pattern, and characteristic traits of personality [29,30]. The answers to the questions posed through the perceptual task achieve patterns of cognition alongside visual perception, language processing, or the inhibition of phases of the response process [31–34]. In this study, the Rorschach test is not only a substitute for clinical diagnosis but an exploratory tool to identify potential response patterns that may help generate hypotheses and support the differential diagnosis between iNPH and AD.

Despite the pioneering nature of the present study, its results must be carefully considered since they allow common traits and patterns of response to be identified in patients with INPH and AD.

Hence, this study aims to assess the Rorschach method as a valid tool for identifying INPH patients. The information collected by administering the test is analyzed through the implementation of three different methods: Population, Self-Organizing Maps (SOMs), and artificial neural networks (ANNs). The characteristics of INPH vs. AD patients are outlined and commented on. Some comments on the advantages of adopting the Rorschach test in complex diagnoses will conclude the study. The innovative aspect of this work lies in the proposal of an alternative methodology to support the identification of patients presenting with cognitive decline. Importantly, the findings are intended to generate hypotheses and do not serve a confirmatory diagnostic purpose.

2. Materials and Methods

A small sample of patients ($n = 19$) was observed at the Polyclinic of Messina, Southern Italy, in the year 2015. Eleven patients suffered from INPH, while the remaining 8 presented with AD dementia. The observed patients (or their caregivers) provided written informed consent, and the study was conducted in accordance with the Declaration of Helsinki and approved by the Ethics Committee at the University Hospital of Messina (Prot. 28/219, 26 November 2014).

Two psychological tests were carried out.

The patient's mental status was measured through the Mini-Mental State Examination (MMSE) [35], an 11-item questionnaire testing areas of cognitive function (orientation, registration, attention, calculation, recall, and language). A low score is indicative of cognitive impairment.

Perception characteristics and personality traits were observed through the Personality Rorschach Inkblot test [26,28,36–39]. The test comprises 10 symmetrical inkblots: 5 monochrome, 2 two-tone, and 3 colored inkblots. The images are brought to the attention of the subject, one by one; there is no time limit imposed, and each response comprises an interpretation of the characteristics of each image, i.e., its form, content, and the determinants; codified as form, color, shading, and movement [40–43]. The coding of the responses is based on the time needed to provide or refuse an answer and provide any additional comments [28,30].

The information provided on the general aspects of the inkblot (shape, color, etc.) and the location (such as its details) are often considered more important than the content itself; considering the originality of the response, this is considered positive or negative (+ or −) in relation to good and poor form [37]. Considering the theme of the image, the content (whether it is human, natural, animal, abstract, etc.) is classified into categories according to the frequency of the interpretation [26,28,36]; the emotional life of the subject is centered on the colors and its shading [41,43].

The literature provides an example of the clinical application of the inkblot task in a sample of elderly subjects or suspected dementia patients [30,31] for the differential diagnosis of brain impairment [44,45]. Organic signs were also observed in brain subcortical and cortical involvement and in cognitive deficiency in the performance that occurred in organic lesions [33,44,46,47]. The Inkblot task can detect perceptive and visuo-spatial functions from a neuropsychological perspective in a clinical assessment [48–50].

The information collected from the administration of the Rorschach Inkblot Test was analyzed using computational methods applying different algorithms.

These methods are as follows and in the Appendix A:

- **Populations**: This is a Multi-Dimensional Scaling algorithm that projects the observed individuals on a bi-dimensional plane with coordinates X and Y [51];
- **Self-Organizing Map (SOM)**: This is an example of an unsupervised neural network, clustering the observed individuals and focusing on input variables on a bi-dimensional matrix [52];
- **Auto Contractive Map (AutoCM)**: This is an unsupervised neural network that detects existing relationships between variables based on the values that can be attributed to everyone; the results can be represented through a graph (the *Maximally Regular Graph*, MRG) [53,54].

3. Results

The descriptive statistics of the sample examined can be observed in Table 1.

Table 1. Descriptive statistics.

Variable	Mean	Std. Dev.	Min	Max
Age	76.11	7.32	59	88
Age > 75	0.58	0.51	0	1
Gender (1 = female; 0 = male)	0.58	0.51	0	1
Compulsory education	0.63	0.50	0	1
Married (1 = yes; 0 = no)	0.89	0.32	0	1
Number of answers	10.32	3.83	4	18
MMSE total score	17.89	5.15	8	27
Localization:				
Global (G)	5.42	2.81	1	13
Details (D)	4.58	3.06	0	10
Little details (Dd)	0.11	0.32	0	1
Details → global (DG)	0.21	0.71	0	1

Table 1. *Cont.*

Variable	Mean	Std. Dev.	Min	Max
Determinants:				
F (shape)	8.53	4.14	2	16
F+ (positive shape)	5.63	3.20	1	12
F− (negative shape)	2.89	2.21	0	8
M (Human kinesthetic activity)	0.74	0.73	0	3
FM (Animal kinesthetic activity)	0.74	1.24	0	4
m (inanimate movement)	0.05	0.23	0	1
CF (color and shame)	0.05	0.23	0	1
FCho (diffuse shading)	0.11	0.32	0	1
Cho (pure shading)	0.05	0.23	0	1
Contents:				
A (animals)	5.84	2.59	0	10
Ad (animal details)	0.47	1.02	0	4
H (human)	1.26	1.48	0	5
(h) (fantastic human)	0.11	0.32	0	1
Hd human details	0.37	0.83	0	3
Obj object	0.95	1.31	0	4
Cibo food	0.16	0.37	0	1
Nat nature	0.11	0.32	0	1
Botanic	0.58	0.96	0	3
Anatomical	0.32	0.75	0	3
Smoke	0.05	0.23	0	1
Cartoon	0.11	0.32	0	1
Art	0.11	0.32	0	1
Popular	2.21	1.17	0	4
Original	0.11	0.32	0	1
TRI I (Erleibniss typus I)	1.74	0.99	1	3
TRI II (Erleibniss typus II)	2.16	0.96	1	3
IR (reality index)	3.58	1.80	0	6
Particular phenomena				
Perseveration	0.37	0.50	0	1
Inadequacy	0.21	0.42	0	1
Insecurity	0.26	0.45	0	1
Stereotyped	0.05	0.23	0	1
Refuse	0.63	0.50	0	1
Confabulation	0.21	0.42	0	1
Abstraction	0.05	0.23	0	1
Contamination	0.05	0.23	0	1
Difficulty of naming	0.05	0.23	0	1
Self-reference	0.11	0.32	0	1
Devitalization	0.11	0.32	0	1
Sensation	0.11	0.32	0	1

The mean age of the observed patients was 76 years old (min 59 years; max 88 years old). The sample included 11 males and 8 women; all male patients, apart from one, suffered from INPH. Twelve patients were older than 75 years, and 89% were married. The average number of answers was 10.32 for the ten tables (min 4; max 18).

Despite the small number of subjects in the sample, the methods employed for the analysis allowed the two groups of patients to be clustered.

3.1. Results with Populations

In Table 2, the input data employed in the calculations carried out with *Populations* are shown. On each line, 19 subjects (also called "cases" or "records") are reported; on each column, 45 variables are employed.

The *Populations* method organized the 19 subjects on a two-dimensional plane. Each subject is, therefore, represented by the point with coordinates x and y. The distance between the points is the difference between the values of the 45 variables in the records.

The distribution obtained shows that, except for one subject (which we will refer to as "dementia 1"), the system distinguished between the two populations of patients (Figure 1).

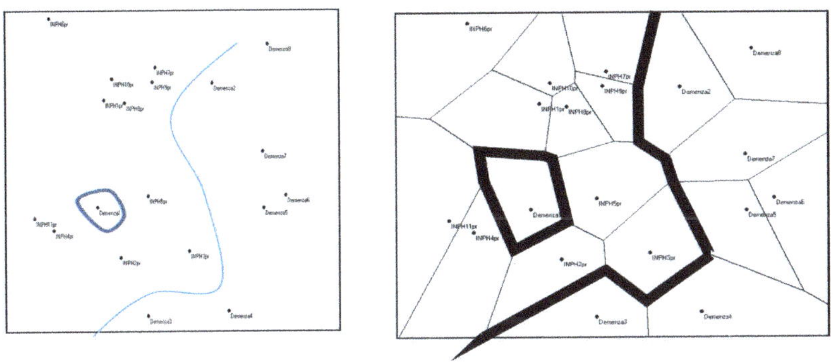

Figure 1. Results with the *Population* algorithm.

Hence, according to this algorithm, the variables included in the analysis are sufficient for the identification of the two types of subjects.

3.2. Results with SOM Algorithm

An SOM was set up with an output matrix measuring 5 × 5; therefore, it was potentially possible to obtain 25 classes.

Given the reduced number of records (19) out of 25 "virtual" classes, SOM located each subject in a class. Only in one case did two subjects share the same class (in the output, this was class 5.2; the subjects were INPH9 and INPH7).

In Figure 2, it can be noted how the two populations were distributed in different areas of the matrix.

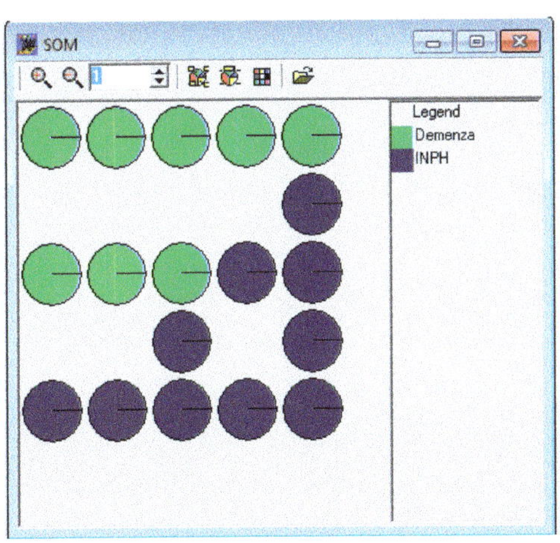

Figure 2. The results with SOM.

Table 2. The data set used in machine learning. There are 19 subjects represented by the lines; 45 variables are represented in the columns.

Caso	Numero Risposte	G	D	Dd	DG	F	F+	F−	M	FM	m	CF	Fcho	CHO	BAN	ORIG	ORIG+	A	Ad	U	(u)	Ud	Obj	Cibo	Nat	Bot	Anat	Fumo	Cartoon	Art	IR	TRI I	TRI II	Perseverazioni	Inadeguatezza	Insicurezza	Stereotipie	Rifiuti	Confabulazione	Astrazione	Contaminazione	Diff. Denominazione	Autoriferimento	Devitalizzazione	Sensazione
Demenza 1	8	8	0	0	0	8	5	3	0	0	0	0	0	0	0	0	0	6	0	0	0	0	2	0	0	0	0	0	1	0	0	3	3	0	0	0	0	1	0	0	0	0	0	0	0
Demenza 2	7	2	5	0	0	5	1	4	1	0	0	0	1	0	2	0	0	5	0	1	0	0	0	0	0	1	0	0	0	0	4	1	3	0	1	0	0	1	1	0	0	0	0	0	0
Demenza 3	10	4	3	0	3	8	3	5	0	0	1	1	0	0	1	0	0	3	0	0	0	2	4	1	0	0	0	0	0	0	2	3	2	1	0	1	0	1	0	0	0	0	0	0	0
Demenza 4	15	7	8	0	0	14	12	2	1	0	0	0	0	0	4	1	1	9	0	3	0	0	2	0	1	0	0	0	0	0	5	1	3	1	0	1	1	1	0	0	0	0	0	0	0
Demenza 5	9	1	7	1	0	9	7	2	0	0	0	0	0	0	1	0	0	5	2	0	0	0	0	0	0	2	0	0	0	0	2	3	3	1	1	1	0	1	1	0	0	0	0	0	0
Demenza 6	13	3	9	0	1	11	8	3	1	0	0	0	1	0	3	1	1	7	1	2	0	0	0	1	0	2	0	0	0	0	4	1	2	0	1	1	0	1	0	0	0	0	1	0	0
Demenza 7	8	2	6	0	0	7	7	0	1	0	0	0	0	0	2	0	0	3	0	2	0	3	0	0	0	0	0	0	0	0	4	1	3	0	1	1	0	0	0	0	0	0	1	0	0
Demenza 8	7	5	2	0	0	4	2	2	3	0	0	0	0	0	1	0	0	0	0	5	0	0	0	0	0	2	0	0	0	0	2	1	3	1	0	0	0	1	1	1	0	1	0	0	1
INPH 1 pr	10	7	3	0	0	6	5	1	0	4	0	0	0	0	1	0	0	9	0	0	0	0	1	0	0	0	0	0	0	0	2	3	1	0	0	0	0	0	0	0	0	0	0	0	0
INPH 2 pr	13	5	8	0	0	13	7	6	0	0	0	0	0	0	4	0	0	7	4	0	0	0	1	0	0	0	1	0	0	0	6	3	3	0	0	0	0	0	1	0	0	0	0	0	0
INPH 3 pr	13	6	7	0	0	13	10	3	0	0	0	0	0	0	4	0	0	10	0	0	0	0	0	0	0	3	0	0	0	0	5	3	3	1	0	0	0	1	0	0	0	0	0	0	0
INPH 4 pr	16	13	3	0	0	15	7	8	1	0	0	0	0	0	4	0	0	6	1	2	0	1	3	1	0	0	1	0	1	0	6	1	3	0	0	0	0	0	0	0	0	0	0	1	0
INPH 5 pr	7	7	0	0	0	7	7	0	0	0	0	0	0	0	2	0	0	7	0	0	0	0	0	0	0	0	0	0	0	0	2	3	3	1	0	0	0	0	0	0	0	0	0	0	0
INPH 6 pr	12	7	5	0	0	7	3	4	1	3	0	0	0	1	3	0	0	6	0	0	1	1	0	0	1	0	3	1	0	0	4	1	1	0	0	0	0	0	0	0	0	0	0	0	1
INPH 7 pr	4	3	1	0	0	2	2	0	1	1	0	0	0	0	3	0	0	3	0	1	0	0	0	0	0	0	0	0	0	0	6	1	1	0	0	0	0	1	0	0	0	0	0	0	0
INPH 8 pr	11	6	5	0	0	8	4	4	1	1	0	0	0	0	1	0	0	6	1	1	0	0	2	0	0	0	0	0	0	1	2	1	1	0	0	0	0	1	0	0	0	0	0	0	0
INPH 9 pr	4	3	1	0	0	2	2	0	1	1	0	0	0	0	3	0	0	3	0	1	0	0	0	0	0	0	0	0	0	0	6	1	1	0	0	0	0	1	0	0	0	0	0	0	0
INPH 10 pr	11	7	4	0	0	7	4	3	1	3	0	0	0	0	2	0	0	7	0	2	0	0	0	0	0	1	1	0	0	0	4	1	1	0	0	0	0	1	0	0	0	0	0	1	0
INPH 11 pr	18	7	10	1	0	16	11	5	1	1	0	0	0	0	1	0	0	9	0	4	1	0	3	0	0	0	0	0	0	1	2	1	1	1	0	0	0	0	0	0	1	0	0	0	0

The results confirm the findings obtained using the *Populations* method; therefore, the 45 variables are good indicators to distinguish between the two pathologies: INPH vs. AD. More specifically, when processing the data, some variables, among which there were, for example, the determining variables "Global", "Detail", "Form", "Good form", etc., did not show a specific distribution. Instead, other variables, such as "Form over diffuse shading", "Original", "Original characterized by good form", and "Inadequacy", showed a high value in some classes only.

3.3. Results with AutoCM

Lastly, the AutoCM model is helpful in understanding the relationship between each variable and the two populations of patients.

The web input was set up using the same 45 variables included in the two previous experiments by adding two variables that discriminated between subjects according to their pathology (see the last column of Table 3); in the graphical representation, the characteristics of the two pathologies are highlighted.

The AutoCM learned the records made by the 19 subjects. Every layer of the web (input, hidden, and output) was composed of 47 units. When the processing was finished, the most relevant connections among the 47 variables were highlighted by the MRG.

Figures 3 and 4 show the graphs obtained with the ANNs, respectively, both with and without the values showing the relationship among variables. Some variables connected to Rorschach's interpretation are more closely linked to the diagnosis of INPH and AD.

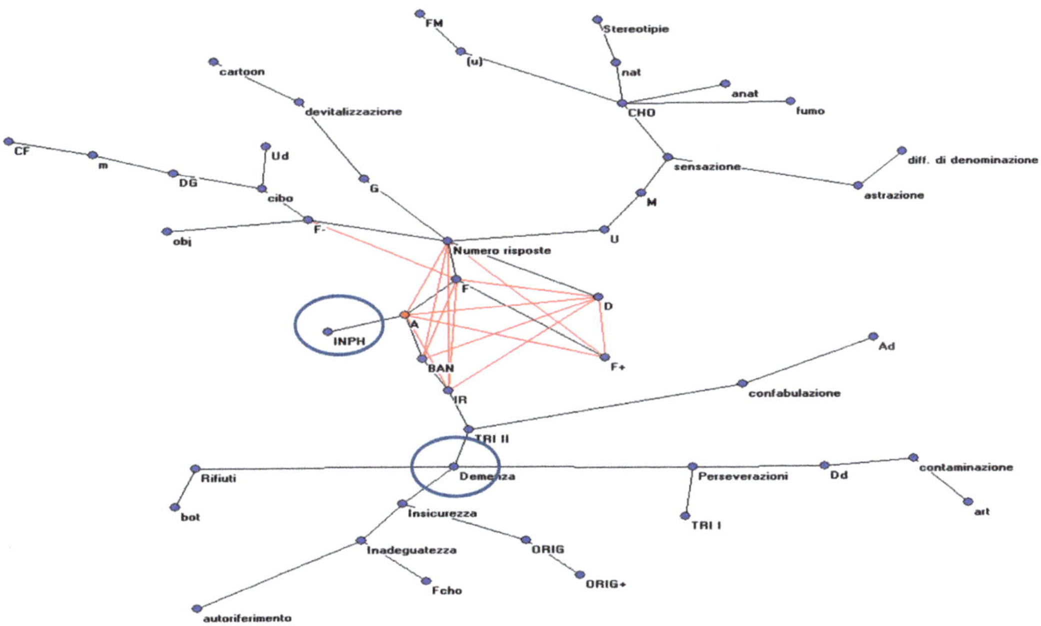

Figure 3. The MRG obtained by analyzing the connections between the hidden and output units of the ANNs.

Table 3. The data set used as the input of the AutoCM network. Nineteen subjects are included in the rows; 47 variables are employed in the columns.

Caso	Numero Risposte	G	D	Dd	DG	F	F+	F−	M	FM	m	CF	Fcho	CHO	BAN	ORIG	ORIG+	A	Ad	U	(u)	Ud	Obj	Cibo	Nat	Bot	Anat	Fumo	Cartoon	Art	IR	TRI I	TRI II	Perseverazioni	Inadeguatezza	Insicurezza	Stereotipie	Rifiuti	Confabulazione	Astrazione	Contaminazione	Diff. Di Denominazione	Autoriferimento	Devitalizzazione	Sensazione
Demenza 1	8	8	0	0	0	8	5	3	0	0	0	0	0	0	0	0	0	6	0	0	0	0	2	0	0	0	0	0	1	0	0	3	3	0	0	0	0	1	0	0	0	0	0	0	0
Demenza 2	7	2	5	0	0	5	1	4	1	0	0	0	1	0	2	0	0	5	0	1	0	0	0	0	0	1	0	0	0	0	4	1	3	0	1	0	0	1	1	0	0	0	0	0	0
Demenza 3	10	4	3	0	3	8	3	5	0	0	1	1	0	0	1	0	0	3	0	0	0	2	4	1	0	0	0	0	0	0	2	3	2	1	0	1	0	1	0	0	0	0	0	0	0
Demenza 4	15	7	8	0	0	14	12	2	1	0	0	0	0	0	4	1	1	9	0	3	0	0	2	0	1	0	0	0	0	0	5	1	3	1	0	1	1	1	0	0	0	0	0	0	0
Demenza 5	9	1	7	1	0	9	7	2	0	0	0	0	0	0	1	0	0	5	2	0	0	0	0	0	0	2	0	0	0	0	2	3	3	1	1	1	0	1	1	0	0	0	0	0	0
Demenza 6	13	3	9	0	1	11	8	3	1	0	0	0	1	0	3	1	1	7	1	2	0	0	0	1	0	2	0	0	0	0	4	1	2	0	1	1	0	1	0	0	0	0	1	0	0
Demenza 7	8	2	6	0	0	7	7	0	1	0	0	0	0	0	2	0	0	3	0	2	0	3	0	0	0	0	0	0	0	0	4	1	3	0	1	1	0	0	0	0	0	0	1	0	0
Demenza 8	7	5	2	0	0	4	2	2	3	0	0	0	0	0	1	0	0	0	0	5	0	0	0	0	0	2	0	0	0	0	2	1	3	1	0	0	0	1	1	1	0	1	0	0	1
INPH 1 pr	10	7	3	0	0	6	5	1	0	4	0	0	0	0	1	0	0	9	0	0	0	0	1	0	0	0	0	0	0	0	2	3	1	0	0	0	0	0	0	0	0	0	0	0	0
INPH 2 pr	13	5	8	0	0	13	7	6	0	0	0	0	0	0	4	0	0	7	4	0	0	0	1	0	0	0	1	0	0	0	6	3	3	0	0	0	0	0	1	0	0	0	0	0	0
INPH 3 pr	13	6	7	0	0	13	10	3	0	0	0	0	0	0	4	0	0	10	0	0	0	0	0	0	0	3	0	0	0	0	5	3	3	1	0	0	0	1	0	0	0	0	0	0	0
INPH 4 pr	16	13	3	0	0	15	7	8	1	0	0	0	0	0	4	0	0	6	1	2	0	1	3	1	0	0	1	0	1	0	6	1	3	0	0	0	0	0	0	0	0	0	0	1	0
INPH 5 pr	7	7	0	0	0	7	7	0	0	0	0	0	0	0	2	0	0	7	0	0	0	0	0	0	0	0	0	0	0	0	2	3	3	1	0	0	0	0	0	0	0	0	0	0	0
INPH 6 pr	12	7	5	0	0	7	3	4	1	3	0	0	0	1	3	0	0	6	0	0	1	1	0	0	1	0	3	1	0	0	4	1	1	0	0	0	0	0	0	0	0	0	0	0	1
INPH 7 pr	4	3	1	0	0	2	2	0	1	1	0	0	0	0	3	0	0	3	0	1	0	0	0	0	0	0	0	0	0	0	6	1	1	0	0	0	0	1	0	0	0	0	0	0	
INPH 8 pr	11	6	5	0	0	8	4	4	1	1	0	0	0	0	1	0	0	6	1	1	0	0	2	0	0	0	0	0	0	1	2	1	1	0	0	0	0	1	0	0	0	0	0	0	0
INPH 9 pr	4	3	1	0	0	2	2	0	1	1	0	0	0	0	3	0	0	3	0	1	0	0	0	0	0	0	0	0	0	0	6	1	1	0	0	0	0	1	0	0	0	0	0	0	0
INPH 10 pr	11	7	4	0	0	7	4	3	1	3	0	0	0	0	2	0	0	7	0	2	0	0	0	0	0	1	1	0	0	0	4	1	1	0	0	0	0	1	0	0	0	0	0	1	0
INPH 11 pr	18	7	10	1	0	16	11	5	1	1	0	0	0	0	1	0	0	9	0	4	1	0	3	0	0	0	0	0	0	1	2	1	1	1	0	0	0	0	0	0	1	0	0	0	0

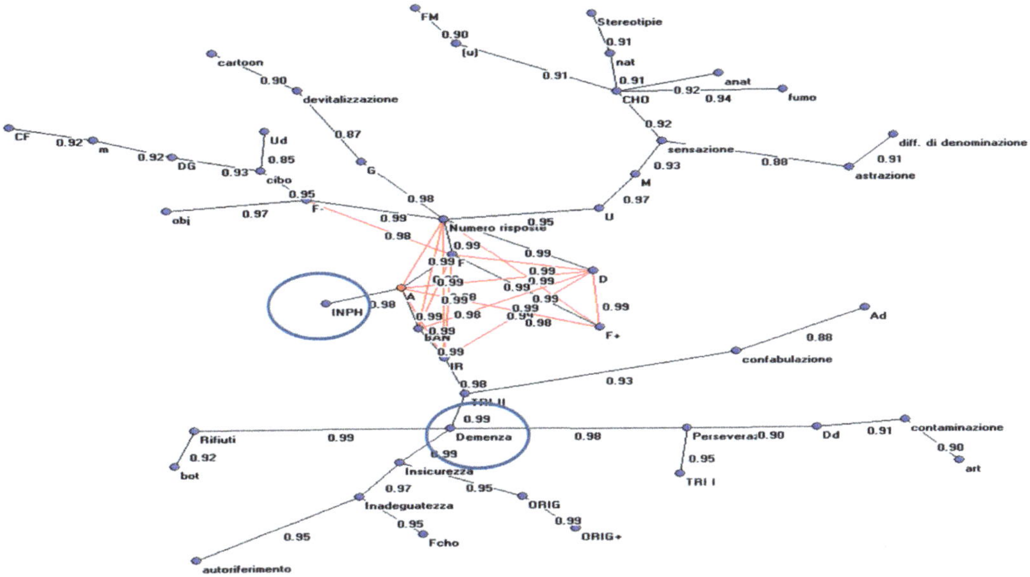

Figure 4. The MRG obtained by analyzing the connections between the hidden and output units of the ANNs (with indications for each value).

We can summarize the evidence obtained by these graphical representations.

For the INPH group, the most relevant variables were animal contents (A); form response (F); details (D); popular response; and adequacy of index of reality (IR).

In AD, the most relevant variables were perseveration phenomena, inadequacy, and particular phenomena, such as card rejection and linguistic errors.

That means that INPH (and, consequently, patients' behavior) is strictly linked (connection value = 0.99) to animal forms, indicating higher emotional inhibition to common responses (popular) and well-formed responses (connection value between popular responses and forms = 0.99). The number of responses, strictly linked to shape, was also connected to the perception of details in the interpretation, well-formed responses, and the reality index.

The data shows how the structure highlighted in this typology of patients has better adaptation to reality with perception levels closer to the average population in comparison to psychopathological phenomena observed in AD cases (i.e., perseveration, card rejection, and linguistic errors).

Instead, patients with AD are more closely linked to phenomena highlighting the behavior of subjects in relation to the stimulus represented on the board (i.e., particular phenomena, for example, waste (0.99); subjects' reactions are uncertainty (0.99) and preserved (0.98). The latter is connected to inadequacy in the response.

4. Discussion

This study highlights the implications of using the Inkblot task in clinical practice and neuropsychological assessments for the differential diagnosis of patients suffering from organic and neurodegenerative diseases, such as Idiopathic Normal Pressure Hydrocephalus (INPH) and Alzheimer's disease (AD).

As specified in the Introduction, INPH is a syndrome characterized by gait impairment, cognitive decline, and urinary incontinence and is associated with ventriculomegaly in the absence of high cerebrospinal fluid (CSF) pressure [55]. It is different from AD, which is a chronic neurodegenerative disease that usually worsens slowly over time.

The Rorschach method can be considered a neuropsychological method to detect alterations in psychic functions [28,37,46,48]. In other contributions, alterations in psychic functions have been studied in relation to memory deficits, poor emotional and impulse control, linguistic errors, and processes of response [31,32,34,44]. In cognitive impairment, elderly patients are unable to synthesize perceptual details or the organization of complex forms, which is centered on the deficit of visual perception, recognition, a lack of awareness, and signs of organicity [32,46]. Unlike patients with AD, those with INPH present an interpretative awareness and do not make linguistic errors. Other authors highlight the potential of this test in neuropsychological assessments related to response processes and psychic functions as well as perceptual processing, attention, memory, and executive functioning [32,45,48–50].

The first analysis technique employed showed how the two subsamples of patients are distinct. Then, we processed data with the SOM. This technique, in line with the literature, was a good indicator to distinguish between the two groups of patients.

In addition, the AutoCM model was useful in understanding the relationship between variables (such as animal contents (A); form response (F); details (D); popular response; and index of reality (IR)) that are strictly connected to INPH diagnosis. Variables connected to AD diagnosis can be identified in perseveration phenomena, inadequacy, particular phenomena, card rejection, and linguistic errors. As far as INPH is concerned, higher emotional inhibition can be found in animal responses along with a higher adaptation rate to reality, which differs from AD patients. These patients have a good adaptation to reality and retain perception levels closer to the average population compared to the psychopathological signs that are observed in patients with AD, i.e., rejection, perseveration processes, and linguistic mistakes. The neuropsychological aspects of patients with cognitive deficits include an inability to grasp the theme regarding the difficulty of reenacting memory and a low control of pulses, usually identified as C, CF, or extra-tensive resonance, codified in the form of subjective Erlebnistypus [26,32,43,45,46].

The results obtained through the implementation of ANNs demonstrate the potential of the Rorschach test to identify patients presenting with INPH, even within a small sample. During the assessment, patients concentrated more on what the table displayed and their perceptions, while AD patients concentrated on personal reactions (such as particular phenomena) in relation to the image used.

The group INPH did not show clear signs of organic dysfunction, as is found specifically in people with AD. The cognitive patterns connected to AD, as stated in the literature, include signs of perplexity in the interpretation process, the perseveration of the content, visuospatial deficit, and language mistakes in the response process [32,44,50].

This evidence shows that the Rorschach method is a cognitive task involving the global brain in the response process and is suitable for detecting perceptual deficits, including visual perception patterns, object recognition, and language production [30,34].

5. Conclusions

A neuropsychological approach to clinical assessments represents a milestone for empirical research in differential diagnosis from a clinical viewpoint.

The neuropsychological approach based on the signs of the Inkblot task has been shown to distinguish between two different diagnoses. Overall, the test detected mental alterations linked to each disease, identifying a pattern of cognitive functions (such as signs of memory impairment, recognition, emotions and control impulses, visual attention, and executive functioning, and language processes).Since it can be used on all individuals without the limitations of education level, this test is a valid predictor task in broader neuropsychological evaluations and is able to identify the cognitive patterns of INPH patients.

The three distinct methods used led to the same conclusions. Even if carried out on a small sample, the present study suggests original and innovative results in the assessment and clinical research of reversible dementia. If correctly and timely diagnosed, INPH can be corrected through neurosurgical treatment, achieving an improvement in patients' wellbeing and quality of life, together with a reduction in the cost of illness.

Author Contributions: Conceptualization, L.G., C.M., A.F.G. and M.C.A.Q.; data curation, C.M. and A.F.G.; formal analysis, G.M. and P.M.B.; methodology, L.G.; supervision, C.M.; writing—original draft, L.G., A.F.G. and M.C.A.Q.; writing—review and editing, G.R., C.M. and M.C.A.Q. All authors have read and agreed to the published version of the manuscript.

Funding: This research received no external funding.

Institutional Review Board Statement: This study was conducted in accordance with the Declaration of Helsinki and approved by the Ethics Committee at the University Hospital of Messina (Prot. 28/219, 6 November 2014).

Informed Consent Statement: All the observed patients (or their caregivers) gave their written informed consent.

Data Availability Statement: The original contributions presented in this study are included in the article. Further inquiries can be directed to the corresponding author.

Acknowledgments: The authors are grateful to Carmen Sindorio and Rosaria Abbritti for their collaboration in collecting the data.

Conflicts of Interest: The authors have no conflicts of interest to declare.

Appendix A. Notes About the Methodology Used

Appendix A.1. Analysis Through Populations

The *Populations* algorithm [51] can be used as a framed framework within Multi-Dimensional Scaling techniques. Reducing the dimensionality of a data set is a frequent problem in the analysis of data and is of leading importance in the field of exploratory analysis.

The *Populations* algorithm can compress N records of M-dimensional space (the "source space") into a subspace of Q dimensions (called the "projected space") where Q << M, maintaining the greatest possible number of existing relationships contained in the original N records. *Populations* is an iterative algorithm based on the calculation of local fitness and the distance between two points and is considered optimal when the differences between the matrix of the distances of the source space and the matrix of the distances of projected space are near zero.

This characteristic of *Populations* is its ability to converge on a solution without calculating the global fitness, which determines the speed with which it finds a solution, minimizing the global error compared to other algorithms of Multi-Dimensional Scaling.

Appendix A.2. Analysis Through the SOM

The SOM [52] classifies the input vectors, creating a prototype of the classes and a projection of the prototypes on a two-dimensional map, which can record the relative proximity between the same classes.

Therefore, the network offers the following important synthetic information on the input:

1. It performs the classification of the input vectors on the basis of their vector similarity and assigns them to a class.
2. It creates a prototypical model of the classes with the same cardinality (number of variables) as the input vector.
3. It provides a measurement, expressed as a numerical value, of the distance/proximity of the various classes.
4. It creates a relational map of the various classes, placing each class on the map itself.
5. It provides a measurement of the distance/proximity that exists between the input vectors from the class they belong to and between the input vectors and other classes.

A typical SOM network is made up of two layers of units: a one-dimensional input and a two-dimensional output layer, also known as "Kohonen's map". A matrix of the weights records the relationship between each unit of the output layer and each unit of the input layer (W matrix). The weight vector connecting each output unit to an input unit is called a "codebook". Within the SOM network, each output unit can be interpreted as a class with a codebook that represents the prototype.

Appendix A.3. Analysis Through AutoCM

The AutoContractive Map neural network AutoCM has an architecture based on three layers of nodes: an input layer that captures the signal from the environment, a hidden layer that modulates the signal within the network, and an output layer that returns a response to the environment based on the processing that occurs [56]. These three layers have the same number (N) of nodes. The connections between the input layer and the hidden layer are mono-dedicated, whereas those between this hidden layer and the output layer are completely connected.

Each connection is assigned a weight: v_i for connections between the ith input node and the corresponding hidden node; $w_{i,j}$ for those between the generic jth node of the hidden layer and the ith node of the output layer.

At the end of the analysis, the results are displayed in a graph. The minimum spanning tree (MST) graph is often used as a filter on the correlations matrix between objects to highlight their most significant relationships. Instead, the Maximally Regular Graph (MRG) reaches the highest value among all the graphs generated by adding the original MST to the most relevant data set connections [56–58].

References

1. Xiao, H.; Hu, F.; Ding, J.; Ye, Z. Cognitive impairment in idiopathic normal pressure hydrocephalus. *Neurosci. Bull.* **2022**, *38*, 1085–1096. [CrossRef] [PubMed]
2. Fife, T.D. Clinical features of normal pressure hydrocephalus. *Barrow Q.* **2003**, *19*, 10–15.
3. Clarfield, A.M. The reversible dementias: Do they reverse? *Ann. Intern. Med.* **1988**, *109*, 476–486. [CrossRef] [PubMed]
4. Klinge, P.; Marmarou, A.; Bergsneider, M.; Relkin, N.; Black, P.M. Outcome of shunting in idiopathic normal-pressure hydrocephalus and the value of outcome assessment in shunted patients. *Neurosurgery* **2005**, *57*, 40–52. [CrossRef] [PubMed]
5. Duinkerke, A.; Williams, M.A.; Rigamonti, D.; Hillis, A.E. Cognitive recovery in idiopathic normal pressure hydrocephalus after shunt. *Cogn. Behav. Neurol.* **2004**, *17*, 179–184. [CrossRef] [PubMed]
6. Thomas, G.; McGirt, M.J.; Woodworth, G.; Heidler, J.; Rigamonti, D.; Hillis, A.E.; Williams, M.A. Baseline neuropsychological profile and cognitive response to cerebrospinal fluid shunting for idiopathic normal pressure hydrocephalus. *Dement. Geriatr. Cogn. Disord.* **2005**, *20*, 163–168. [CrossRef] [PubMed]
7. Sindorio, C.; Abbritti, R.V.; Raffa, G.; Priola, S.M.; Germanò, A.; Visocchi, M.; Quattropani, M.C. Neuropsychological Assessment in the Differential Diagnosis of Idiopathic Normal Pressure Hydrocephalus. An Important Tool for the Maintenance and Restoration of Neuronal and Neuropsychological Functions. *Acta. Neurochir. Suppl.* **2017**, *124*, 283–288. [CrossRef] [PubMed]
8. Holodny, A.I.; Waxman, R.; George, A.E.; Rusinek, H.; Kalnin, A.J.; Leon, M.d. MR differential diagnosis of normal-pressure hydrocephalus and Alzheimer disease: Significance of perihippocampal fissures. *Am. J. Neuroradiol.* **1998**, *19*, 813–819. [PubMed] [PubMed Central]

9. Laurent, M.S. Normal pressure hydrocephalus in geriatric medicine: A challenge. *J. Geriatr. Psychiatry Neurol.* **1988**, *1*, 163–168. [CrossRef] [PubMed]
10. Gallia, G.L.; Rigamonti, D.; Williams, M.A. The diagnosis and treatment of idiopathic normal pressure hydrocephalus. *Nat. Clin. Pr. Neurol.* **2006**, *2*, 375–381. [CrossRef] [PubMed]
11. Siraj, S. An overview of normal pressure hydrocephalus and its importance: How much do we really know? *J. Am. Med. Dir. Assoc.* **2011**, *12*, 19–21. [CrossRef] [PubMed]
12. Shprecher, D.; Schwalb, J.; Kurlan, R. Normal Pressure Hydrocephalus: Diagnosis and Treatment. *Curr. Neurol. Neurosci. Rep.* **2008**, *8*, 371–376. [CrossRef] [PubMed]
13. Grossman, H.; Bergmann, C.; Parker, S. Dementia: A brief review. *Mt. Sinai. J. Med.* **2006**, *73*, 985–992. [PubMed]
14. Kiefer, M.; Unterberg, A. The differential diagnosis and treatment of normal-pressure hydrocephalus. *Dtsch. Arztebl. Int.* **2012**, *109*, 15–25. [CrossRef] [PubMed]
15. Patwardhan, R.V.; Nanda, A. Implanted ventricular shunts in the United States: The billion-dollar-a-year cost of hydrocephalus treatment. *Neurosurgery* **2005**, *56*, 139–145. [CrossRef] [PubMed]
16. Vacca, V. Diagnosis and Treatment of Idiopathic Normal Pressure Hydrocephalus. *J. Neurosci. Nurs.* **2007**, *39*, 107–111. [CrossRef] [PubMed]
17. Factora, R.; Luciano, M. Normal pressure hydrocephalus: Diagnosis and new approaches to treatment. *Clin. Geriatr. Med.* **2006**, *22*, 645–657. [CrossRef] [PubMed]
18. Marmarou, A.; Bergsneider, M.; Klinge, P.; Relkin, N.; Black, P.M. The value of supplemental prognostic tests for the preoperative assessment of idiopathic normal-pressure hydrocephalus. *Neurosurgery* **2005**, *57*, 17–28. [CrossRef] [PubMed]
19. Krauss, J.K.; Halve, B. Normal pressure hydrocephalus: Survey on contemporary diagnostic algorithms and therapeutic decision-making in clinical practice. *Acta. Neurochir.* **2004**, *146*, 379–388. [CrossRef] [PubMed]
20. Di Ieva, A.; Valli, M.; Cusimano, M.D. Distinguishing Alzheimer's disease from normal pressure hydrocephalus: A search for MRI biomarkers. *J. Alzheimers. Dis.* **2014**, *38*, 331–335. [CrossRef] [PubMed]
21. Pickard, J.D.; Spiegelhalter, D.; Czosnyka, M. Health economics and the search for shunt-responsive symptomatic hydrocephalus in the elderly. *J. Neurosurg.* **2006**, *105*, 811–813. [CrossRef] [PubMed]
22. Williams, M.A.; Sharkey, P.; van Doren, D.; Thomas, G.; Rigamonti, D. Influence of shunt surgery on healthcare expenditures of elderly fee-for-service Medicare beneficiaries with hydrocephalus. *J. Neurosurg.* **2007**, *107*, 21–28. [CrossRef] [PubMed]
23. Kazui, H.; Mori, E.; Hashimoto, M.; Ishikawa, M.; Hirono, N.; Takeda, M. Effect of Shunt Operation on Idiopathic Normal Pressure Hydrocephalus Patients in Reducing Caregiver Burden: Evidence from Sinphoni. *Dement. Geriatr. Cogn. Disord* **2011**, *31*, 363–370. [CrossRef] [PubMed]
24. Barison, F.; Tognazzo, D.P. *Il Rorschach Fenomenologico*; Franco Angeli: Milano, Italy, 1982.
25. Mihura, J.L.; Jowers, C.E.; Dumitrascu, N.; van den Hurk, A.W.V.; Keddy, P.J. The specific uses of the Rorschach in clinical practice. *Rorschachiana* **2022**, *43*, 14–35. [CrossRef]
26. Tognazzo, D.P. *Il Metodo Rorschach*; Giunti: Firenze, Italy, 1994.
27. Acklin, M.W. Some contributions of cognitive science to the Rorschach test. *Rorschachiana* **1994**, *19*, 129–145. [CrossRef]
28. Weiner, I.B. Using the Rorschach properly in practice and research. *J. Clin. Psychol.* **2000**, *56*, 435–438, discussion 441–448. [CrossRef]
29. Smith, S.R.; Bistis, K.; Zahka, N.E.; Blais, M.A. Perceptual-organizational characteristics of the Rorschach task. *Clin. Neuropsychol.* **2007**, *21*, 789–799. [CrossRef] [PubMed]
30. Schott, G.D. Revisiting the Rorschach inkblots: From iconography and psychology to neuroscience. *J. Neurol. Neurosurg. Psychiatry* **2014**, *85*, 699–706. [CrossRef] [PubMed]
31. Insùa, A.M.; Loza, S.M. Psychometric patterns of the Rorschach of healthy elderly persons and patients with suspected dementia. *Percept. Mot. Ski.* **1986**, *63*, 931–936. [CrossRef] [PubMed]
32. Perry, W.; Potterat, E.; Auslander, L.; Kaplan, E.; Jeste, D. A Neuropsychological approach to the Rorschach in patients with Dementia of the Alzheimer Type. *Assessment* **1996**, *3*, 351–363. [CrossRef]
33. Makoto, S.; Nishio, Y.; Kanno, S.; Uchiyama, M.; Hayashi, A.; Takagi, M.; Kikuchi, H.; Yamasaki, H.; Shimomura, T.; Iizuka, O.; et al. Cognitive profile of Idiopathic Normal pressure Hydrocephalus. *Extra Dement. Geriatr. Cogn. Disord.* **2011**, *1*, 202–211. [CrossRef]
34. Sànchez, H.S. Rorschach y la psicobiología de la personalidad. *Univ. Psychol.* **2016**, *15*, 15–39. [CrossRef]
35. Cockrell, J.R.; Folstein, M.F. Mini-mental state examination. In *Principles and Practice of Geriatric Psychiatry*, 2nd ed.; Sadavoy, J., Lazarus, L.W., Jarvik, L.F., Eds.; John Wiley & Sons: Chichester, UK, 2002; pp. 140–141. [CrossRef]
36. Rorschach, H. *Psychodiagnostics: A Diagnostic Test Based on Perception*; Reading Read Books: Virginia Beach, VA, USA, 2011.
37. Schachtel, E.G. *Experiential Foundations of Rorschach's Test*; Analytic Press: Hillsdale, NJ, USA, 2001.
38. Groth-Marnat, G. *Handbook of Psychological Assessment*; John Wiley & Sons: New York, NY, USA, 2003.
39. Pelto, J.; Pelto, G.H. *Anthropological Research: The Structure of Inquiry*; Cambridge University Press: Cambridge, UK, 1996.

40. Malmgren, H. Rorschach's idea of a "movement" response in the light of recent philosophy and psychology of perception. *Rorschachiana* **2000**, *24*, 1–27. [CrossRef]
41. Kron, A.; Cohen, A.; Benziman, H.; Ben-Shakha, G. What is it that color determinants determine? The relation between the Rorschach inkblot method and cognitive object-recognition processes. *J. Pers. Assess.* **2009**, *91*, 137–142. [CrossRef] [PubMed]
42. Giromini, L.; Porcelli, P.; Viglione, D.J.; Parolin, L.; Pineda, J.A. The feeling of movement: EEG evidence for mirroring activity during the observations of static, ambiguous stimuli in the Rorschach cards. *Biol. Psychol.* **2010**, *85*, 233–241. [CrossRef] [PubMed]
43. Malone, J.C.; Stein, M.B.; Slavin-Mulford, J.; Bello, I.; Sinclair, S.J.; Blais, M.A. Seeing red: Affect modulation and chromatic color responses on the Rorschach. *Bull. Menninger. Clin.* **2013**, *77*, 70–93. [CrossRef] [PubMed]
44. Insùa, A.M.; Loza, S.M. Evaluation of Piotrowsky's organic signs in the Rorschach test of patients with an early stage of dementia. *Acta. Psiquiatr. Psicol. Am. Lat.* **1988**, *34*, 243–250. [PubMed]
45. Zillmer, E.A.; Perry, W. Cognitive-neuropsychological abilities and related psychological disturbance: A factor model of Neuropsychological, Rorschach and MMPI indices. *Psychol. Assess* **1996**, *3*, 209–224. [CrossRef]
46. Piotrowski, C. The Rorschach in research on neurocognitive dysfunction: An historical overview, 1936–2016. *SIS J. Proj. Psychol. Ment. Health.* **2018**, *25*, 44–53.
47. Acklin, M.W.; Decato, C.M. Piotrowski's enduring contributions to the Rorschach: A review of Perceptanalysis. *J. Personal. Assess Dec.* **1993**, *61*, 584–595. [CrossRef] [PubMed]
48. Acklin, M.W.; Wu-Holt, P. Contributions of cognitive science to the Rorschach Technique: Cognitive and neuropsychological correlates of the response process. *J. Pers. Assess.* **1996**, *67*, 169–178. [CrossRef] [PubMed]
49. Kimoto, A.; Iseki, E.; Ota, K.; Murayama, N.; Sato, K.; Ogura, N.; Arai, H. Differences in responses to the Rorschach test between patients with dementia with Lewy bodies and Alzheimer's disease from the perspective of visuoperceptual impairment. *Psychiatry Res.* **2017**, *257*, 456–461. [CrossRef] [PubMed]
50. Massini, G.; Terzi, S.; Buscema, P.M. Population Algorithm: A New Method of Multi-Dimensional Scaling. In *Data Mining Applications Using Artificial Adaptive Systems*; Tastle, W.J., Ed.; Springer Science+Business Media: New York, NY, USA, 2013; Chapter 3, pp. 63–74. [CrossRef]
51. Kohonen, T. *Self-Organizing Maps. Series in Information Sciences*; Springer: Heidelberg, Germany, 1995; Volume 30.
52. Buscema, P.M. A general presentation of Artificial Neural Networks in Substance Use & Misuse. *Int. J. Addict.* **1997**, *32*, 97–112.
53. Buscema, P.M.; Massini, G.; Breda, M.; Lodwick, W.A.; Newman, F.; Asadi-Zeydabadi, M. *Artificial Adaptive Systems Using Auto Contractive Maps: Theory, Applications and Extensions*; Springer: Cham, Switzerland, 2018. [CrossRef]
54. Buscema, P.M.; Lodwick, W.A.; Massini, G.; Sacco, P.L.; Asadi-Zeydabadi, M.; Newman, F.; Petritoli, R.; Marco Breda, M. *AI: A Broad and a Different Perspective*; Springer Briefs in Applied Sciences and Technology. Computational Intelligence; Springer: Cham, Switzerland, 2025. [CrossRef]
55. Ogata, Y.; Ozaki, A.; Ota, M.; Oka, Y.; Nishida, N.; Tabu, H.; Sato, N.; Hanakawa, T. Interhemispheric resting-state functional connectivity predicts severity of idiopathic normal pressure hydrocephalus. *Front. Neurosci.* **2017**, *11*, 470. [CrossRef] [PubMed]
56. Singh, A. An artificial bee colony algorithm for the leaf-constrained minimum spanning tree problem. *Appl. Soft Comput.* **2009**, *9*, 625–631. [CrossRef]
57. Graham, R.L.; Hell, P. On the history of the minimum spanning tree problem. *Ann. Hist. Comput.* **1985**, *7*, 43–57. [CrossRef]
58. Grygorash, O.; Zhou, Y.; Jorgensen, Z. Minimum spanning tree based clustering algorithms. In Proceedings of the 2006 18th IEEE International Conference on Tools with Artificial Intelligence (ICTAI'06), Arlington, VA, USA, 13–15 November 2006; IEEE: New York, NY, USA, 2006; pp. 73–81. [CrossRef]

medicina

MDPI

Article

Age-Related Trends in Dual-Energy X-Ray Absorptiometry–Measured Adiposity and Their Clinical Relevance: A Multicenter Cross-Sectional Study of Korean Peri- and Postmenopausal Women

Jung Yoon Park [1], Hyoung Moo Park [2], Youn-Jee Chung [1], Mee-Ran Kim [1], Kyung Jin Hwang [2] and Jae-Yen Song [1,*]

[1] Department of Obstetrics and Gynecology, Seoul St. Mary's Hospital, College of Medicine, The Catholic University of Korea, Seoul 06591, Republic of Korea; aurorix86@naver.com (J.Y.P.); porshe80@catholic.ac.kr (Y.-J.C.); drmrkim@gmail.com (M.-R.K.)

[2] Department of Obstetrics and Gynecology, Menopause Clinic Grace Women's Hospital, Goyang 10444, Republic of Korea; hmpark52@hanmail.net (H.M.P.); drhkj@naver.com (K.J.H.)

* Correspondence: jaeyen77@catholic.ac.kr; Tel.: +82-2-2258-6166

Abstract: *Background and Objectives:* Body composition changes with aging and menopause, often leading to increased adiposity and a shift in fat distribution. While BMI is commonly used in clinical practice, it does not accurately reflect fat mass or distribution. This study aims to evaluate age-related changes in both total and regional adiposity using DXA-derived indices in Korean women aged ≥ 40 years and to assess the limitations of BMI-based obesity classification. *Materials and Methods:* This retrospective multicenter study analyzed the DXA scans and clinical records of 914 Korean women aged 40–80 years who attended menopause clinics across multiple institutions between 2018 and 2021. We analyzed five adiposity indices: body mass index (BMI), total body fat percentage (TB%F), fat mass index (FMI), visceral adipose tissue (VAT) area, and android-to-gynoid (A/G) fat ratio. Excess adiposity was defined as BMI ≥ 23 kg/m^2, TB%F ≥ 40%, FMI ≥ 9 kg/m^2, VAT > 100 cm^2, or A/G ratio > 1.0. Age group comparisons were made using ANOVA, and misclassification was assessed by comparing BMI with other indices. *Results*: Mean BMI increased with age, peaking in the 60s before declining in the 70s. TB%F and FMI peaked in the 50s, while VAT and A/G ratio increased continuously with age. Excess adiposity was found in 41.9% of women by TB%F, 40.5% by FMI, and 59.4% by VAT in the 70s. Notably, 22% of women with normal BMI (<23 kg/m^2) had VAT > 100 cm^2, and 35.7% had A/G > 1.0, indicating central obesity. *Conclusions*: DXA-based indices provide a more accurate assessment of adiposity and associated cardiometabolic risks in aging women than BMI alone. Clinical screening strategies should consider incorporating regional fat distribution markers, particularly in midlife and postmenopausal populations, to better identify individuals at risk.

Keywords: body composition; adiposity; menopause; abdominal fat; absorptiometry

1. Introduction

Obesity is a multifactorial health issue with rising global prevalence, especially in aging populations [1,2]. In women, the menopausal transition accelerates changes in body composition, including an increase in fat mass and a redistribution toward central fat accumulation. These alterations are driven by hormonal shifts, reduced energy expenditure, and lifestyle factors [3,4].

1.1. Biological and Hormonal Mechanisms of Aging in Women

Midlife represents a critical period during which biological aging and hormonal changes converge to influence body composition and metabolic health. As part of the physiological aging process, adults typically experience a gradual decline in organ and tissue function, with estimates suggesting a reduction of up to 2% annually. This decline contributes to a progressive loss of skeletal muscle mass and a concomitant increase in adipose tissue, even in the absence of overt disease [5]. In young adults, skeletal muscle turnover—comprising both protein synthesis and degradation—is tightly regulated to preserve lean body mass [6,7]. However, aging disrupts this balance. Muscle mass, which accounts for approximately 30% of total body protein turnover in youth, may decline to below 20% in older adults. Beginning around the age of 50, skeletal muscle mass decreases by an estimated 1–2% per year, a trajectory that may accelerate with sedentary behavior or chronic disease [8,9].

Longitudinal analyses indicate that between ages 30 and 60, adults may gain roughly 0.45 kg of fat and lose 0.23 kg of lean mass per year. Over several decades, this pattern can culminate in a net increase of over 14 kg in fat and a loss exceeding 6 kg in muscle, contributing to a body composition profile increasingly characterized by sarcopenic adiposity [10]. In women, these age-related changes are compounded by the hormonal alterations of menopause. The sharp decline in estrogen during the menopausal transition facilitates a shift in fat storage patterns—from predominantly subcutaneous depots to increased visceral adipose tissue (VAT) accumulation [11]. This redistribution has important clinical implications, as the proportion of VAT typically rises from 5–8% of total fat mass in premenopausal women to 15–20% following menopause [12].

These physiological alterations have important clinical consequences, as women in midlife are particularly vulnerable to cardiometabolic complications associated with obesity. Epidemiological data suggest that the burden of obesity is disproportionately higher in women than in men; for example, findings from the National Health and Nutrition Examination Survey (NHANES) report a higher prevalence of obesity among women (40.4%) compared to men (35.0%) in the United States [13]. While midlife weight gain has traditionally been regarded as a natural consequence of chronological aging, evidence from the longitudinal Study of Women's Health Across the Nation (SWAN), which followed more than 3300 women, indicates that hormonal shifts—particularly the decline in circulating estrogen—play a pivotal role in driving fat redistribution and adverse changes in body composition during the menopausal transition [14].

1.2. Limitations of BMI and the Clinical Value of DXA in Midlife Women

Menopause is now recognized as a pivotal period in women's metabolic health, during which the decline in estrogen contributes to profound changes in adipose tissue biology [15]. Postmenopausal women experience a shift from subcutaneous to visceral fat deposition, along with adipocyte hypertrophy, chronic low-grade inflammation, and impaired insulin signaling [16,17]. This adipose tissue remodeling, characterized by increased macrophage infiltration and pro-inflammatory cytokine release, promotes systemic metabolic dysfunction [18]. These alterations not only increase total fat mass but also disproportionately affect the quality and distribution of fat, thereby increasing the risk of cardiometabolic diseases such as type 2 diabetes, hypertension, and atherosclerosis—even in women with normal BMI [19].

Central obesity, particularly the accumulation of visceral adipose tissue (VAT), is strongly associated with adverse cardiometabolic outcomes [20]. Traditionally, obesity has been assessed using body mass index (BMI), a simple and widely used metric derived from weight and height [21,22]. However, BMI does not differentiate between fat and lean mass, nor does it capture regional fat distribution—especially VAT—which has a closer relationship with metabolic risk [23].

Dual-energy X-ray absorptiometry (DXA) is a validated method for assessing body composition that offers accurate and reproducible measurements of total and regional adiposity. DXA-derived indices, including total body fat percentage (TB%F), fat mass index (FMI), VAT area, and android-to-gynoid (A/G) fat ratio, provide a more nuanced view of adiposity and its health implications [24,25].

Notably, there is a lack of population-based data examining how DXA-derived adiposity indices change with age in Asian women, particularly in the Korean population [26,27]. Understanding these age-related trends is critical for identifying women at elevated cardiometabolic risk who may be misclassified by BMI-based criteria alone [28].

Therefore, the primary aim of this study was to investigate age-related trends in body fat distribution using DXA-derived adiposity indices—including VAT, A/G ratio, TB%F, and FMI—in Korean women aged 40 years and older. The secondary aim was to examine the discordance between BMI-based obesity classification and DXA-derived adiposity patterns, with particular emphasis on identifying women with metabolically unfavorable fat distribution despite normal BMI. These objectives aim to inform more accurate risk stratification strategies and support the integration of advanced adiposity indices into routine clinical assessment for aging women.

2. Methods

This multicenter retrospective cross-sectional study analyzed 914 women aged 40–80 years who underwent DXA scans between June 2018 and June 2021 at a university hospital and a regional medical hospital in Korea. All women had visited the menopause clinic for routine evaluation or health screening. Exclusion criteria included a history of malignancy, autoimmune disease, or any chronic illness known to affect body composition.

This study adhered to the STROBE (Strengthening the Reporting of Observational Studies in Epidemiology) guidelines for cross-sectional studies. The STROBE checklist has been submitted as a supplementary file [29].

Height and weight were measured using standardized protocols, and BMI was calculated as weight (kg) divided by height (m^2) [30]. Whole-body DXA scans were performed using a Hologic DXA system (Hologic Inc., Marlborough, MA, USA) with Horizon software for analysis. All participating institutions used the same model of DXA device and identical software versions to ensure methodological consistency. All DXA scans were conducted by trained radiologic technologists following a standardized protocol across both sites to ensure consistency. Centralized calibration and quality assurance procedures were performed regularly to minimize inter-institutional variability. The following indices were derived:

The adiposity indices assessed in this study included total body fat percentage (TB%F), fat mass index (FMI), visceral adipose tissue (VAT) area, and the android-to-gynoid (A/G) fat ratio. Total body fat percentage reflects the proportion of an individual's weight composed of fat mass. The fat mass index (FMI) is calculated by dividing the total fat mass in kilograms by the square of the individual's height in meters (kg/m^2), offering a height-adjusted measure of adiposity [25]. The VAT area, measured in square centimeters, quantifies the amount of visceral fat—fat stored within the abdominal cavity, surrounding internal organs [24]. The A/G fat ratio represents the distribution of body fat between the android (abdominal) and gynoid (hip and thigh) regions, with higher values indicating a greater degree of central (abdominal) fat accumulation [31].

Excess adiposity was defined based on established clinical thresholds. Overweight and obesity were defined as a BMI of $\geq$23 kg/m^2 and $\geq$25 kg/m^2, respectively, according to the

WHO Asia-Pacific and Korean Society for the Study of Obesity (KSSO) guidelines [32]. A TB%F of ≥40% was considered indicative of excess fat, as suggested by Dufour et al. [33–35]. An FMI of ≥9 kg/m^2, as proposed by Kelly et al., was used to define elevated fat mass [25]. Central obesity was defined as a VAT area greater than 100 cm^2 [24], and an A/G fat ratio exceeding 1.0 was considered indicative of an android or abdominal fat distribution pattern [36,37].

Statistical analysis was performed using SPSS version 23.0 (IBM, Armonk, NY, USA). Between-group comparisons used ANOVA with Bonferroni correction; chi-square tests compared prevalence across age groups. Statistical significance was defined as $p < 0.05$.

3. Results

A total of 917 Korean women aged 40 years and older were included in the analysis. Participants were categorized into four age groups: 40–49 years (n = 128), 50–59 years (n = 545), 60–69 years (n = 209), and ≥70 years (n = 35). The mean age was 56.2 years. The overall mean height was 157.7 cm, the mean body weight was 56.2 kg, and the mean body mass index (BMI) was 22.8 kg/m^2 (Table 1).

Table 1. General Characteristics of Study Participants by Age Group.

Age Group (Years)	n	Mean Age (Years)	Mean Weight (kg)	Mean Height (cm)	Mean BMI (kg/m^2)
40–49	128	46.9	55.5	159.8	21.7
50–59	545	54.7	56.5	158.4	22.8
60–69	209	63.1	56.2	156.3	23.6
≥70	35	72.7	54.2	154.2	22.8
Total	917	56.2	56.2	157.7	22.8

BMI, body mass index.

DXA-derived adiposity indices showed distinct patterns according to age. Mean BMI increased with age and peaked in the 60s (23.6 kg/m^2), followed by a slight decrease in the 70s (22.8 kg/m^2). TB%F was highest in the 50s (39.0%), with a mild decline thereafter. Fat mass index (FMI) demonstrated a similar peak in the 50s (8.85 kg/m^2). In contrast, visceral adipose tissue (VAT) and android-to-gynoid fat ratio (A/G ratio) increased consistently with age, peaking in the 70s at 107.6 cm^2 and 1.06, respectively (Table 2).

Table 2. DXA-Derived Adiposity Indices by Age Group.

Age Group (Years)	BMI (kg/m^2)	TB%F (%)	FMI (kg/m^2)	A/G Ratio	VAT (cm^2)
40–49	21.7	38.2	8.34	0.93	87.7
50–59	22.8	39.0	8.85	1.09	99.6
60–69	23.6	38.6	8.72	1.01	102.2
≥70	22.8	38.4	8.64	1.06	107.6
Total (Mean ± SD)	22.8 ± 7.2	38.8 ± 4.8	8.74 ± 2.38	1.05 ± 1.82	98.8 ± 40.4

BMI, body mass index; TB%F, total body fat percentage; FMI, fat mass index; A/G ratio, android-to-gynoid fat ratio; VAT, visceral adipose tissue area.

Excess adiposity was prevalent across all age groups. The proportion of overweight and obese individuals (BMI ≥ 23 kg/m^2) was 38.8%, with the highest prevalence in the 60–69 age group (44.5%). A TB%F ≥ 40% was observed in 41.9% of participants, most commonly in women in their 50s (44.6%). FMI ≥ 9 kg/m^2 was found in 37.6% of the cohort, with the highest prevalence in the 60s (43.5%). The proportion of participants with VAT > 100 cm^2 increased steadily with age, from 22.6% in the 40s to 48.5% in the 70s. An

A/G ratio > 1.0, indicative of central adiposity, was observed in 49.2% of participants and showed a progressive increase across age groups, from 31.3% in the 40s to 60.0% in the 70s.

A more detailed breakdown of high-risk adiposity indices by age group is presented in Table 3. The highest proportion of women with TB%F ≥ 40% was observed in the 50s (44.6%), whereas FMI ≥ 9 kg/m^2 peaked in the 60s (43.5%). VAT >100 cm^2 increased consistently with age, suggesting age-related accumulation of visceral fat. The detailed adiposity outcomes for each individual by age in the total cohort are provided in Supplementary Data S1.

Table 3. Prevalence of Excess Adiposity According to DXA-Based Indices by Age Group.

Age Group (Years)	BMI ≥ 23 (%)	TB%F ≥ 40% (%)	FMI ≥ 9 kg/m^2 (%)	A/G Ratio > 1.0 (%)
40–49	28.9	33.6	28.9	31.3
50–59	38.7	44.6	37.4	50.1
60–69	44.5	39.7	43.5	55.9
≥70	42.8	42.9	37.4	60.0
Total	38.8	41.9	37.6	49.2

BMI represents the combined proportion of individuals classified as overweight (BMI 23.0–24.9 kg/m^2) and obese (BMI ≥ 25.0 kg/m^2), based on WHO Asia-Pacific and KSSO criteria. BMI, body mass index; TB%F, total body fat percentage; FMI, fat mass index; A/G ratio, android-to-gynoid fat ratio; VAT, visceral adipose tissue area.

3.1. *Adiposity Characteristics According to BMI Categories in Women over Age 40*

In this study, we analyzed adiposity indices including total body fat percentage (TB%F), fat mass index (FMI), visceral adipose tissue (VAT), and android-to-gynoid (A/G) fat ratio according to BMI categories in Korean women aged 40 years and older (Table 4).

Table 4. Adiposity Distribution by BMI Category.

BMI Category	TB%F (Mean ± SD)	FMI (Mean ± SD)	VAT			Apple Shape (%)	Pear Shape (%)
			Normal >100 (%)	Borderline 100–160 (%)	High Risk ≤160 (%)		
Underweight	32.2 ± 3.7	5.6 ± 0.8	100	0	0	8.3	91.7
Normal	37.3 ± 3.9	7.9 ± 2.2	78.0	21.6	0.4	35.7	64.3
Overweight	40.5 ± 3.7	9.5 ± 1.0	31.2	62.8	6.0	67.3	32.7
Obese ≥ 25	43.0 ± 3.5	11.3 ± 1.3	7.6	55.4	36.9	82.8	17.2
Severe Obese ≥ 30	47.9 ± 10.1	13.6 ± 2.8					

BMI, body mass index; TB%F, total body fat percentage; FMI, fat mass index; VAT, visceral adipose tissue area.

3.1.1. General Trends in Body Fat Accumulation (TB%F, FMI)

Both TB%F and FMI demonstrated a progressive increase across BMI categories. Underweight women had a mean TB%F of 32.2% and an FMI of 5.6 kg/m^2, while those with obesity (BMI ≥ 25 kg/m^2) had markedly elevated values (TB%F 43.0%, FMI 11.3 kg/m^2). The severely obese group (BMI ≥ 30 kg/m^2) showed the highest TB%F (47.9%) and FMI (13.6 kg/m^2), with standard deviations indicating greater variability within this group. These findings suggest that while total adiposity increases with BMI, the variance in fat composition becomes more prominent in the highest BMI category.

3.1.2. Visceral Fat Accumulation (VAT Stratification)

VAT distribution varied significantly across BMI categories. Notably, 100% of underweight women and 78.0% of those with normal BMI had VAT < 100 cm^2 (classified as "normal"). However, among overweight women, only 31.2% remained in this normal range, while 62.8% had VAT between 100 and 160 cm^2 (borderline), and 6.0% exceeded 160 cm^2 (high risk). In the obese group, the prevalence of VAT > 160 cm^2 rose dramatically to 36.9%. These findings highlight that even within the overweight category, visceral adiposity becomes prominent and potentially harmful.

3.1.3. Central Fat Distribution Pattern (A/G Ratio and Body Shape)

An age-related and BMI-dependent shift from gynoid (pear-shaped) to android (apple-shaped) fat distribution was clearly observed. Among women with normal BMI, 35.7% had an android body shape. This proportion increased to 67.3% in overweight women and further to 82.8% in those classified as obese. In contrast, pear-shaped distribution was dominant in the underweight (91.7%) and normal BMI groups (64.3%) but diminished with increasing BMI.

In summary, while BMI, TB%F, and FMI peaked during midlife and plateaued or declined thereafter, VAT and A/G ratio continued to increase into older age. These findings highlight the progressive nature of central fat accumulation with aging and the need for comprehensive adiposity assessment beyond BMI in postmenopausal women.

4. Discussion

This study investigated age-related changes in adiposity patterns among Korean women aged 40 years and older using DXA-derived body composition indices. The findings demonstrate that while general adiposity indices such as BMI, TB%F, and FMI tend to peak during midlife (50s–60s), regional adiposity markers, particularly VAT and A/G ratio, show a continuous upward trend into older age. This progressive increase in central adiposity with age has significant implications for cardiometabolic health in postmenopausal women [19].

The results are consistent with previous studies suggesting that the menopausal transition accelerates the redistribution of fat from peripheral to central compartments, driven by estrogen deficiency, changes in energy balance, and age-related metabolic decline [3,15]. Notably, our study revealed that nearly half of all participants had an A/G ratio > 1.0 and that VAT > 100 cm^2 was observed in over 40% of the cohort. These proportions increased markedly with age, underscoring the need to evaluate regional fat accumulation as women age [24].

An important observation was the discrepancy between BMI and DXA-derived adiposity indices. A substantial proportion of women classified as having normal BMI (<23 kg/m^2) demonstrated excess VAT and elevated A/G ratios, suggesting the presence of metabolically unfavorable fat distribution that may not be detected through BMI alone. These findings reinforce concerns that reliance on BMI may lead to the underestimation of central obesity and associated health risks, particularly in aging Asian women who may exhibit normal-weight obesity (NWO) phenotypes [19,24].

Furthermore, the strong correlation between general obesity (BMI $\geq$ 25 kg/m^2) and A/G ratio > 1.0 in over 80% of participants in this category highlights that central adiposity commonly accompanies overt obesity. However, its presence in normal-weight individuals warrants targeted screening using DXA or other imaging modalities, especially for preventive cardiometabolic risk stratification [38].

The continuous rise in VAT and A/G ratio into the 70s contrasts with the plateau observed in BMI and TB%F, suggesting that age-related metabolic risk increases may be more closely associated with fat distribution than with absolute fat mass [39,40]. These findings support the incorporation of regional adiposity indices in routine assessment, particularly for older women who may be misclassified by conventional BMI-based criteria [41].

4.1. Clinical Implications and Integration with Updated Obesity Guidelines

The observed age-related increase in central adiposity—particularly in VAT and the android-to-gynoid (A/G) fat ratio—has critical implications for clinical screening and intervention strategies in midlife and older women. These regional fat indices revealed substantial proportions of women with metabolically adverse fat profiles despite normal BMI classifications. Notably, 22% of women with BMI < 23 kg/m^2 had VAT > 100 cm^2, and 35.7% had A/G ratio > 1.0, highlighting the presence of hidden central adiposity. These findings suggest that traditional reliance on BMI alone may overlook women at high cardiometabolic risk due to normal-weight obesity (NWO), especially prevalent in Asian populations [42,43].

To address this diagnostic gap, our study aligns with the 2025 definition of obesity recently proposed by The Lancet Diabetes & Endocrinology Commission, which introduces a paradigm shift from BMI-centric classification to a function- and organ-impairment-based approach [44]. This framework distinguishes between preclinical obesity—characterized by excess adiposity without overt metabolic dysfunction—and clinical obesity, where functional limitations or organ impairment are present [44]. Importantly, the Commission recommends direct body fat measurement tools such as DXA as core diagnostic components. Our use of DXA-derived VAT and A/G ratio thus offers practical validation of this model and supports its application in real-world settings, particularly in resource-equipped clinical environments [44].

In line with this emerging perspective, we propose that clinicians incorporate regional adiposity markers into routine evaluation protocols, particularly for peri- and postmenopausal women. Targeted DXA screening may be especially warranted for women over 50 years of age, even when BMI is within the normal range. In low-resource settings where DXA is unavailable, bioelectrical impedance analysis (BIA)—as a low-cost and widely accessible method—may offer a viable alternative for estimating visceral fat and body composition with greater precision than traditional anthropometric indices [45,46]. Waist circumference also remains a useful surrogate marker for central fat accumulation [47–49].

Furthermore, these findings support the need to develop population-specific guidelines that consider cultural and ethnic variations in body composition. For example, the Korean Society for the Study of Obesity (KSSO) defines overweight as BMI $\geq$ 23 kg/m^2 and obesity as BMI $\geq$ 25 kg/m^2, thresholds that better reflect the elevated cardiometabolic risk in Asian populations compared to Western criteria [32]. Additionally, these findings highlight the need for further epidemiological research to define population-specific thresholds for regional adiposity indices—such as VAT area and A/G ratio—and to clarify their associations with cardiovascular and metabolic outcomes across different ethnic and geographic populations.

Together, our findings advocate for a more nuanced, function-oriented framework for obesity diagnosis and risk stratification in women across midlife and aging, consistent with both international and national recommendations.

4.2. Study Limitations: Methodological, Demographic, and Measurement Considerations

This study has several limitations that must be acknowledged. First, the retrospective cross-sectional design precludes causal inference regarding the relationship between age and adiposity changes. Second, the sample size was unevenly distributed across age groups, with a markedly smaller number of participants aged $\geq$ 70 years. This imbalance may have limited statistical power and increased variability in estimates for the oldest group. Although our primary aim was to assess overall trends across midlife and aging, the interpretation of findings in the $\geq$70 group should be made with caution. Third, menopausal status was not directly measured and was instead inferred based on age, which may have led to misclassification. Fourth, while participants were recruited from both a university hospital and a regional medical center, the cohort may not be fully representative of the general Korean female population. Cultural, behavioral, and environmental factors unique to this population—such as dietary patterns, physical activity, and healthcare access—may limit generalizability to other populations. Moreover, as the entire cohort consisted exclusively of Korean women, our findings may not be generalizable to non-Asian populations. Prior studies have demonstrated significant ethnic differences in fat distribution patterns and in the relationship between BMI and body fatness, particularly between Asian and Western populations. Therefore, caution is warranted when extrapolating these results to ethnically diverse or global populations. Fifth, although DXA is a validated method for body composition analysis, its estimation of visceral fat remains indirect compared to gold-standard imaging modalities such as CT or MRI. Lastly, several potential confounders—including socioeconomic status, dietary intake, physical activity, and hormone therapy use—were not assessed and could have influenced the observed adiposity patterns. Future prospective studies with larger and more balanced sample sizes across age groups, as well as the direct assessment of menopausal status and inclusion of diverse populations, are warranted to validate and extend these findings.

4.3. Study Strengths: Comprehensive DXA-Based Assessment and Clinical Relevance

This study has several notable strengths. It included a relatively large and age-diverse sample of 917 Korean women aged 40 years and older, allowing for robust comparisons across age groups. Second, we utilized standardized whole-body DXA measurements to assess not only general adiposity indices such as BMI and total body fat percentage (TB%F), but also regional fat distribution markers including fat mass index (FMI), visceral adipose tissue (VAT), and the android-to-gynoid fat ratio (A/G ratio). This comprehensive approach enhances the precision of body composition assessment and highlights the limitations of BMI-based obesity classification. This study provides valuable population-specific data on Asian women, particularly on Korean women, a group underrepresented in existing DXA research. Lastly, our findings emphasize the presence of metabolically unfavorable fat distribution—such as excess VAT and elevated A/G ratio—even in women with normal BMI, thereby underscoring the need for improved risk stratification methods beyond BMI.

Importantly, to the best of our knowledge, this is the first study to focus specifically on adiposity changes from the perimenopausal to postmenopausal period in Korean women using DXA-derived indices. By identifying progressive central fat accumulation during this transitional stage, our findings offer clinically relevant insights for the early detection of cardiometabolic risk in aging women.

5. Conclusions

This study highlights distinct age-related trends in body fat distribution among Korean women aged 40 years and older. While general adiposity measures plateau in later life, central adiposity—as reflected by increasing VAT and A/G ratio—continues to rise with age. A significant proportion of women with normal BMI exhibited excess visceral fat and unfavorable fat distribution, indicating the limitations of BMI in detecting metabolically relevant adiposity. These results underscore the clinical value of incorporating DXA-derived indices into obesity assessment to more accurately identify women at elevated cardiometabolic risk. Comprehensive body composition evaluation may contribute to earlier identification and intervention in aging women, ultimately improving long-term health outcomes. Our findings support the integration of regional fat distribution indices into clinical screening protocols, particularly for midlife and older women who may be misclassified by BMI alone.

Supplementary Materials: The following supporting information can be downloaded at: https://www.mdpi.com/article/10.3390/medicina61071301/s1, Table S1: The STROBE checklist

Author Contributions: Conceptualization, J.Y.P., M.-R.K., and J.-Y.S.; data analysis, J.Y.P., H.M.P., and K.J.H.; methodology, J.Y.P., Y.-J.C., and J.-Y.S.; writing—original draft, J.Y.P.; writing—review and editing, J.Y.P., H.M.P., M.-R.K., and J.-Y.S. All authors have read and agreed to the published version of the manuscript.

Funding: This study was supported by a grant from Korea Research Foundation for Gynecologic Cancer (2024-1).

Institutional Review Board Statement: This study was conducted in accordance with the ethical standards of the Declaration of Helsinki and was approved by the Institutional Review Board of Seoul St. Mary's Hospital (approval number: KC25RASI0416, approval date: 27 June 2025).

Informed Consent Statement: This study was granted exemption by the Institutional Review Board (IRB) of The Catholic University of Korea, Seoul, St, Mary's Hospital.

Data Availability Statement: The datasets generated during and/or analyzed during the current study are available from the corresponding author on reasonable request.

Conflicts of Interest: The authors have no conflicts of interest to declare.

References

1. GBD 2021 Risk Factor Collaborators. Global burden of 88 risk factors in 204 countries and territories, 1990–2021: A systematic analysis for the Global Burden of Disease study 2021. *Lancet* **2024**, *403*, 2162–2203. [CrossRef]
2. Okunogbe, O.; Nugent, R.; Spencer, G.; Powis, J.; Ralston, J.; Wilding, J.E. *Economic Impacts of Overweight and Obesity: 2nd Edition with Estimates for 161 Countries*; World Obesity Federation: London, UK, 2022.
3. Marlatt, K.L.; Pitynski-Miller, D.R.; Gavin, K.M.; Moreau, K.L.; Melanson, E.L.; Santoro, N.; Kohrt, W.M. Body composition and cardiometabolic health across the menopause transition. *Obes. Silver Spring* **2022**, *30*, 14–27. [CrossRef]
4. Moccia, P.; Belda-Montesinos, R.; Monllor-Tormos, A.; Chedraui, P.; Cano, A. Body weight and fat mass across the menopausal transition: Hormonal modulators. *Gynecol. Endocrinol.* **2022**, *38*, 99–104. [CrossRef]
5. Sehl, M.E.; Yates, F.E. Kinetics of human aging: I. Rates of senescence between ages 30 and 70 years in healthy people. *J. Gerontol. A Biol. Sci. Med. Sci.* **2001**, *56*, B198–B208. [CrossRef] [PubMed]
6. Balagopal, P.; Rooyackers, O.E.; Adey, D.B.; Nair, K.S. Effects of aging on in vivo synthesis of skeletal muscle myosin heavy-chain and sarcoplasmic protein in humans. *Am. J. Physiol.* **1997**, *273*, E790–E800. [CrossRef] [PubMed]
7. Volpi, E.; Sheffield-Moore, M.; Rasmussen, B.B.; Wolfe, R.R. Basal muscle amino acid kinetics and protein synthesis in healthy young and older men. *J. Am. Med. Assoc.* **2001**, *286*, 1206–1212. [CrossRef]
8. Young, V.R. Amino acids and proteins in relation to the nutrition of elderly people. *Age Ageing* **1990**, *19* (Suppl. 1), S10–S24. [CrossRef]
9. Baumgartner, R.N.; Stauber, P.M.; McHugh, D.; Koehler, K.M.; Garry, P.J. Cross-sectional age differences in body composition in persons 60+ years of age. *J. Gerontol. A Biol. Sci. Med. Sci.* **1995**, *50*, M307–M316. [CrossRef]
10. Forbes, G.B. Longitudinal changes in adult fat-free mass: Influence of body weight. *Am. J. Clin. Nutr.* **1999**, *70*, 1025–1031. [CrossRef]
11. Lizcano, F.; Guzmán, G. Estrogen deficiency and the origin of obesity during menopause. *Biomed. Res. Int.* **2014**, *2014*, 757461. [CrossRef]
12. Karvonen-Gutierrez, C.; Kim, C. Association of mid-life changes in body size, body composition and obesity status with the menopausal transition. *Healthcare* **2016**, *4*, 42. [CrossRef]
13. Flegal, K.M.; Kruszon-Moran, D.; Carroll, M.D.; Fryar, C.D.; Ogden, C.L. Trends in obesity among adults in the United States, 2005 to 2014. *J. Am. Med. Assoc.* **2016**, *315*, 2284–2291. [CrossRef]
14. El Khoudary, S.R.; Greendale, G.; Crawford, S.L.; Avis, N.E.; Brooks, M.M.; Thurston, R.C.; Karvonen-Gutierrez, C.; Waetjen, L.E.; Matthews, K. The menopause transition and women's health at midlife: A progress report from the Study of Women's Health Across the Nation (SWAN). *Menopause* **2019**, *26*, 1213–1227. [CrossRef]
15. Marsh, M.L.; Oliveira, M.N.; Vieira-Potter, V.J. Adipocyte metabolism and health after the menopause: The role of exercise. *Nutrients* **2023**, *15*, 444. [CrossRef] [PubMed]
16. Steiner, B.M.; Berry, D.C. The regulation of adipose tissue health by estrogens. *Front. Endocrinol.* **2022**, *13*, 889923. [CrossRef] [PubMed]

17. Abildgaard, J.; Ploug, T.; Al-Saoudi, E.; Wagner, T.; Thomsen, C.; Ewertsen, C.; Bzorek, M.; Pedersen, B.K.; Pedersen, A.T.; Lindegaard, B. Changes in abdominal subcutaneous adipose tissue phenotype following menopause is associated with increased visceral fat mass. *Sci. Rep.* **2021**, *11*, 14750. [CrossRef] [PubMed]
18. Li, X.; Ren, Y.; Chang, K.; Wu, W.; Griffiths, H.R.; Lu, S.; Gao, D. Adipose tissue macrophages as potential targets for obesity and metabolic diseases. *Front. Immunol.* **2023**, *14*, 1153915. [CrossRef]
19. Wu, J.; Lin, X.; Yin, X.; Xu, Z.; Wu, N.; Zhang, Z.; Zhou, J.; Li, H. Comparison of incidence of metabolic syndrome and five obesity- and lipid-linked indicators for predicting metabolic syndrome among normal-weight and overweight adults. *Diabetes Metab. Syndr. Obes.* **2024**, *17*, 3509–3520. [CrossRef]
20. Cesaro, A.; De Michele, G.; Fimiani, F.; Acerbo, V.; Scherillo, G.; Signore, G.; Rotolo, F.P.; Scialla, F.; Raucci, G.; Panico, D.; et al. Visceral adipose tissue and residual cardiovascular risk: A pathological link and new therapeutic options. *Front. Cardiovasc. Med.* **2023**, *10*, 1187735. [CrossRef]
21. World Health Organization. *Physical Status: The Use and Interpretation of Anthropometry*; WHO: Geneva, Switzerland, 1995.
22. Sweatt, K.; Garvey, W.T.; Martins, C. Strengths and limitations of BMI in the diagnosis of obesity: What is the path forward? *Curr. Obes. Rep.* **2024**, *13*, 584–595. [CrossRef]
23. Weber, D.R.; Leonard, M.B.; Shults, J.; Zemel, B.S. A comparison of fat and lean body mass index to BMI for the identification of metabolic syndrome in children and adolescents. *J. Clin. Endocrinol. Metab.* **2014**, *99*, 3208–3216. [CrossRef] [PubMed]
24. Messina, C.; Albano, D.; Gitto, S.; Tofanelli, L.; Bazzocchi, A.; Ulivieri, F.M.; Guglielmi, G.; Sconfienza, L.M. Body composition with dual energy X-ray absorptiometry: From basics to new tools. *Quant. Imaging Med. Surg.* **2020**, *10*, 1687–1698. [CrossRef] [PubMed]
25. Hinton, B.J.; Fan, B.; Ng, B.K.; Shepherd, J.A.; Thomas, D.M. Dual energy X-ray absorptiometry body composition reference values of limbs and trunk from NHANES 1999–2004 with additional visualization methods. *PLoS ONE* **2017**, *12*, e0174180. [CrossRef] [PubMed]
26. Jeong, S.M.; Lee, D.H.; Rezende, L.F.M.; Giovannucc, E.L. Different correlation of body mass index with body fatness and obesity-related biomarker according to age, sex and race-ethnicity. *Sci. Rep.* **2023**, *13*, 3472. [CrossRef]
27. Lim, U.; Ernst, T.; Buchthal, S.D.; Latch, M.; Albright, C.L.; Wilkens, L.R.; Kolonel, L.N.; Murphy, S.P.; Chang, L.; Novotny, R.; et al. Asian women have greater abdominal and visceral adiposity than Caucasian women with similar body mass index. *Nutr. Diabetes* **2011**, *1*, e6. [CrossRef]
28. Hyman, M.H.; Peled, T.J.; Hyman, N.M.; Tan, J.; Guo, X.; Rotter, J.I. Differences in BMI obesity measures in a workers compensation population: A cross-sectional study. *Ann. Med. Surg. Lond* **2023**, *85*, 1607–1613. [CrossRef]
29. von Elm, E.; Altman, D.G.; Egger, M.; Pocock, S.J.; Gøtzsche, P.C.; Vandenbroucke, J.P. The Strengthening the Reporting of Observational Studies in Epidemiology (STROBE) statement: Guidelines for reporting observational studies. *Ann. Intern. Med.* **2007**, *147*, 573–577. [CrossRef]
30. WHO Expert Consultation. Appropriate body-mass index for Asian populations and its implications for policy and intervention strategies. *Lancet* **2004**, *363*, 157–163. [CrossRef]
31. Ma, W.; Zhu, H.; Yu, X.; Zhai, X.; Li, S.; Huang, N.; Liu, K.; Shirai, K.; Sheerah, H.A.; Cao, J. Association between android fat mass, gynoid fat mass and cardiovascular and all-cause mortality in adults: NHANES 2003–2007. *Front. Cardiovasc. Med.* **2023**, *10*, 1055223. [CrossRef]
32. Korean Society for the Study of Obesity (KSSO). Obesity Fact Sheet 2023. Available online: https://www.kosso.or.kr/ (accessed on 8 June 2025).
33. Dufour, A.B.; Hannan, M.T.; Murabito, J.M.; Kiel, D.P.; McLean, R.R. Sarcopenia definitions considering body size and fat mass are associated with mobility limitations: The Framingham Study. *J. Gerontol. A Biol. Sci. Med. Sci.* **2013**, *68*, 168–174. [CrossRef]
34. Davison, K.K.; Ford, E.S.; Cogswell, M.E.; Dietz, W.H. Percentage of body fat and body mass index are associated with mobility limitations in people aged 70 and older from NHANES III. *J. Am. Geriatr. Soc.* **2002**, *50*, 1802–1809. [CrossRef]
35. Macek, P.; Biskup, M.; Terek-Derszniak, M.; Krol, H.; Smok-Kalwat, J.; Gozdz, S.; Zak, M. Optimal cut-off values for anthropometric measures of obesity in screening for cardiometabolic disorders in adults. *Sci. Rep.* **2020**, *10*, 11253. [CrossRef] [PubMed]
36. Nistor, I.M.; Fica, S.; Martin, S.C.; Mustata, T.; Oprea, T.E.; Sirbu, A.E.; Barbu, C.G. DXA android-to-gynoid ratio and cardiovascular risk assessment in age and BMI propensity-matched early postmenopausal women. *Medicina* **2024**, *60*, 1096. [CrossRef] [PubMed]
37. Yang, L.; Huang, H.; Liu, Z.; Ruan, J.; Xu, C. Association of the android to gynoid fat ratio with nonalcoholic fatty liver disease: A cross-sectional study. *Front. Nutr.* **2023**, *10*, 1162079. [CrossRef] [PubMed]
38. Tchernof, A.; Després, J.P. Pathophysiology of human visceral obesity: An update. *Physiol. Rev.* **2013**, *93*, 359–404. [CrossRef]
39. Moreira, V.C.; Silva, C.M.S.; Welker, A.F.; da Silva, I.C.R.; Balistreri, C.R. Visceral adipose tissue influence on health problem development and its relationship with serum biochemical parameters in middle-aged and older adults: A literature review. *J. Aging Res.* **2022**, *2022*, 8350527. [CrossRef]

40. van der Leeuw, J.; Wassink, A.M.; van der Graaf, Y.; Westerveld, H.E.; Visseren, F.L.J. Age-related differences in abdominal fat distribution in premenopausal and postmenopausal women with cardiovascular disease. *Menopause* **2013**, *20*, 409–417. [CrossRef]
41. Riaz, M.; Lodhi, S. Beyond BMI: Exploring obesity trends in the South Asian region. *Obes. Pillars* **2024**, *13*, 100156. [CrossRef]
42. Franco, L.P.; Morais, C.C.; Cominetti, C. Normal-weight obesity syndrome: Diagnosis, prevalence, and clinical implications. *Nutr. Rev.* **2016**, *74*, 558–570. [CrossRef]
43. Kim, J.; Kang, S.; Kang, H. Normal-weight obesity and metabolic syndrome in Korean adults: A population-based cross-sectional study. *Healthcare* **2023**, *11*, 2303. [CrossRef]
44. Rubino, F.; Cummings, D.E.; Eckel, R.H.; Cohen, R.V.; Wilding, J.P.H.; A Brown, W.; Stanford, F.C.; Batterham, R.L.; Farooqi, I.S.; Farpour-Lambert, N.J.; et al. Definition and diagnostic criteria of clinical obesity. *Lancet Diabetes Endocrinol.* **2025**, *13*, 221–262. [CrossRef] [PubMed]
45. Ogawa, H.; Fujitani, K.; Tsujinaka, T.; Imanishi, K.; Shirakata, H.; Kantani, A.; Hirao, M.; Kurokawa, Y.; Utsumi, S. InBody 720 as a new method of evaluating visceral obesity. *Hepato Gastroenterol.* **2011**, *58*, 42–44.
46. Brunani, A.; Perna, S.; Soranna, D.; Rondanelli, M.; Zambon, A.; Bertoli, S.; Vinci, C.; Capodaglio, P.; Lukaski, H.; Cancello, R. Body composition assessment using bioelectrical impedance analysis (BIA) in a wide cohort of patients affected with mild to severe obesity. *Clin. Nutr.* **2021**, *40*, 3973–3981. [CrossRef] [PubMed]
47. Browning, L.M.; Hsieh, S.D.; Ashwell, M. A systematic review of waist-to-height ratio as a screening tool for the prediction of cardiovascular disease and diabetes: 0.5 could be a suitable global boundary value. *Nutr. Res. Rev.* **2010**, *23*, 247–269. [CrossRef]
48. Bosomworth, N.J. Normal-weight central obesity: Unique hazard of the toxic waist. *Can. Fam. Physician* **2019**, *65*, 399–408.
49. Nahorna, A.; Baur, H. Evaluating abdominal obesity by waist circumference, anthropometric indices and bioelectrical impedance analysis: A comparative pilot study. *Obes. Sci. Pract.* **2025**, *11*, e70078. [CrossRef]

medicina

MDPI

Article

Five-Year Sales Trends of Osteoporosis Medications in Korea: A Market Analysis Based on IMS Health Sales Audit Data (2018–2023)

Jung Yoon Park, Youn-Jee Chung, Mee-Ran Kim and Jae-Yen Song *

Division of Reproductive Endocrinology, Department of Obstetrics and Gynecology, Seoul St. Mary's Hospital, College of Medicine, The Catholic University of Korea, 222 Banpo-daero, Seocho-gu, Seoul 06591, Republic of Korea; aurorix86@naver.com (J.Y.P.); porshe80@catholic.ac.kr (Y.-J.C.); drmrkim@gmail.com (M.-R.K.)

* Correspondence: jaeyen77@nate.com; Tel.: +82-2-2258-6166

Abstract: *Background and Objectives*: Osteoporosis is a common chronic condition after menopause that increases the risk of fractures. In South Korea, the prevalence of osteoporosis among adults aged 50 and older is 22.4%, with 94.4% of treated patients being women, highlighting its significant impact on postmenopausal health. In this study, we examine the sales trends of osteoporosis medications in Korea from 2018 to 2023 to understand current usage patterns and market dynamics. *Materials and Methods*: This study is a retrospective analysis based on pre-recorded sales data from Intercontinental Marketing Services (IMS). Data covering a five-year period (2018–2023) were analyzed to examine the sales trends of osteoporosis medications, including bisphosphonates, selective estrogen receptor modulators (SERMs), parathyroid hormone analogs, denosumab, romosozumab, and others. Romosozumab, approved in November 2019, was included in the analysis. Given the nature of this study, no direct patient data or clinical interventions were involved. *Results*: The total market size for osteoporosis medications in South Korea reached USD 285.42 million in 2023, reflecting a 15.3% increase from 2022. Bisphosphonates, previously the dominant therapy, experienced an 11% decline in market share over five years. Meanwhile, denosumab, a receptor activator of the nuclear factor-κB ligand inhibitor, showed a remarkable growth rate of 957.6% from 2018 to 2023, surpassing bisphosphonates in their market share. Romosozumab, a newly introduced anabolic agent, accounted for 7.4% of the market, with sales increasing by 59% in 2023. *Conclusions*: This analysis revealed major shifts in treatment preferences, with newer drugs like denosumab and romosozumab gaining prominence over traditional bisphosphonates. These trends highlight the increasing clinical adoption of anabolic agents for high-risk patients and the impact of expanded reimbursement policies on osteoporosis management. Given the increasing use of advanced therapies, it is essential to monitor treatment access, patient adherence, and long-term clinical outcomes. Understanding these sales trends can aid healthcare professionals and policymakers in optimizing osteoporosis treatment strategies and ensuring better patient care.

Keywords: osteoporosis; romosozumab; denosumab; hormone replacement therapy; menopause; marketing; retrospective studies

1. Introduction

The World Health Organization (WHO) defines osteoporosis as "a systemic skeletal disease characterized by low bone mass, deterioration of bone tissue, and disruption of bone microarchitecture, leading to compromised bone strength and an increase in the risk of fractures [1]." The US National Institutes of Health simply defines it as "a skeletal disease in which the risk of fracture increases due to weakening of bone strength [2]." The WHO estimates that over 200 million people worldwide suffer from osteoporosis, contributing to 8.9 million fractures annually, or approximately one fracture every three seconds [3,4]. Osteoporosis is a major global health issue, particularly among postmenopausal women, due to the associated risk of fractures and increased healthcare burden.

National Health Insurance data indicate that the prevalence of osteoporosis in South Korean adults aged 50 or older is 22.4%, while that of osteopenia is 48%. More than 5000 out of 100,000 people are counted as suffering from osteoporosis in South Korea [5].

From 2018 to 2023, the number of patients treated for osteoporosis steadily increased at an average annual rate of 4.8%, from 9.8 million in 2018 to 11.8 million in 2022. As of 2022, female patients accounted for 94.4% of the total, indicating that the frequency of osteoporosis in women is about 17 times greater than that in men [6]. Along with this trend, the total medical expenses for osteoporosis increased by 51% from 2015 to 2019 (from USD 155 million to USD 234 million), while the medical expenses per patient increased by 3.7% annually, reaching USD 216 [7].

Osteoporosis treatment can be broadly divided into general lifestyle recommendations, which can benefit most postmenopausal women, and specific pharmaceutical treatments [8]. General recommendations include using non-pharmacological strategies such as calcium and vitamin D supplementation, performing appropriate weight-bearing and muscle-strengthening exercises, avoiding smoking and excessive alcohol consumption, and preventing falls [9]. Antiresorptive and osteoanabolic drugs are used as pharmaceutical treatments in patients with osteoporotic fractures and in those with increased fracture risk due to osteoporosis [10].

Since the WHO declared the coronavirus disease (COVID-19) a pandemic in 2020, prolonged restrictions on healthcare accessibility, reduced outdoor activity, and increased indoor living have heightened the risk of vitamin D deficiency in patients with osteoporosis [11,12]. Vitamin D is an essential nutrient that facilitates calcium absorption and regulates bone formation, playing a crucial role in the prevention and treatment of osteoporosis [13]. Notably, during the COVID-19 pandemic, the use of vitamin D supplements increased, and some studies have suggested that vitamin D may exert immunomodulatory effects, potentially offering protective benefits against viral infections [14]. These findings underscore how the importance and consumption of specific treatments can be significantly influenced by changing global circumstances.

Bisphosphonates represent a class of antiresorptive drugs that currently dominate pharmaceutical treatment worldwide, but their use is limited because they only inhibit bone resorption and have been associated with various side effects such as atypical femoral fractures, osteonecrosis of the jaw, and gastrointestinal irritation [15,16]. However, the recent development of denosumab, the most powerful antiresorptive agent, and the osteoanabolic drug romosozumab have increased treatment options for patients with osteoporosis. With the continuous introduction of new medications and changes in usage standards, the trend of use is also changing.

Our primary objective in this study was to analyze the market dynamics of osteoporosis medications in South Korea from 2018 to 2023 using data from Intercontinental Marketing Services (IMS). Specifically, we aimed to assess sales trends, shifts in market share among drug classes, and the impact of newer treatments, such as denosumab and romosozumab, on prescribing patterns. The secondary objectives were to evaluate factors influencing these market trends, including changes in osteoporosis treatment guidelines, reimbursement policies, and the potential impact of external factors such as the COVID-19 pandemic on drug utilization.

2. Methods

The list of drugs approved for the treatment of osteoporosis in South Korea in 2023 is provided in Supplementary Table S1 [17]. Among them, the costs of items and drugs sold for osteoporosis prevention and treatment between 2018 and 2023 were calculated based on IMS data (in USD).

Osteoporosis drugs were divided into general treatments (calcium and vitamin D supplementation) and pharmaceutical agents (hormone and non-hormonal therapies). In accordance with IMS recommendations, the analysis of hormone therapy included female hormones (estrogen only or an estrogen–progesterone combination), tibolone, and a tissue-selective estrogen complex (TSEC). Non-hormonal therapies included bisphosphonates; selective estrogen receptor modulators (SERMs); raloxifene and bazedoxifene; calcitonin; parathyroid hormones (PTHs); denosumab, the recently approved receptor activator of nuclear factor-κB ligand (RANKL); and romosozumab, the monoclonal anti-sclerostin antibody. This study was granted an exemption by the Institutional Review Board (IRB) of The Catholic University of Korea, Seoul, St, Mary's Hospital (IRB No KC21ZASI1011). This study followed the Reporting of Studies Conducted Using Observational Routinely Collected Data (RECORD) guidelines to ensure transparency and reproducibility in reporting pharmaceutical sales data. RECORD provides a structured framework for studies using administrative and healthcare databases. Additionally, the Consolidated Health Economic Evaluation Reporting Standards (CHEERS) checklist was applied to enhance the clarity of the economic analysis. CHEERS ensures the standardized reporting of key elements in health economic evaluations. By adhering to these guidelines, we aimed to improve the methodological rigor and clarity of our findings [18,19].

Statistical Analysis

To evaluate temporal trends in the annual sales volumes of osteoporosis medications between 2018 and 2023, we conducted a linear trend analysis using simple linear regression. For each medication, the year was treated as a continuous independent variable, and the annual sales volume was treated as the dependent variable. The slope and p-value of each regression model were examined to determine the presence of a statistically significant increasing or decreasing trend over time. A p-value of less than 0.05 was considered indicative of a significant trend. The coefficient of determination (R^2) was also reported to evaluate the goodness-of-fit for each model. All statistical analyses were performed using SPSS version 23.0 (IBM Corp., Armonk, NY, USA).

3. Results

3.1. Market Size for Osteoporosis Medications in Korea in 2023

The total market size of osteoporosis medications in 2023 was USD 285.42 million, which is a 15.3% increase from USD 257.38 million in 2022. Denosumab accounted for 39.2%, followed by bisphosphonates at 30.0% of the total market size (USD 85.69 million), menopausal hormone therapy at 10.2%, SERMs at 7.1%, and anabolic agents at 13.5% (Figure 1). Among pharmaceutical treatments, hormonal and non-hormonal drugs for osteoporosis accounted for 10.2% (USD 30.38 million) and 89.8% (USD 266.31 million) of the total market, respectively.

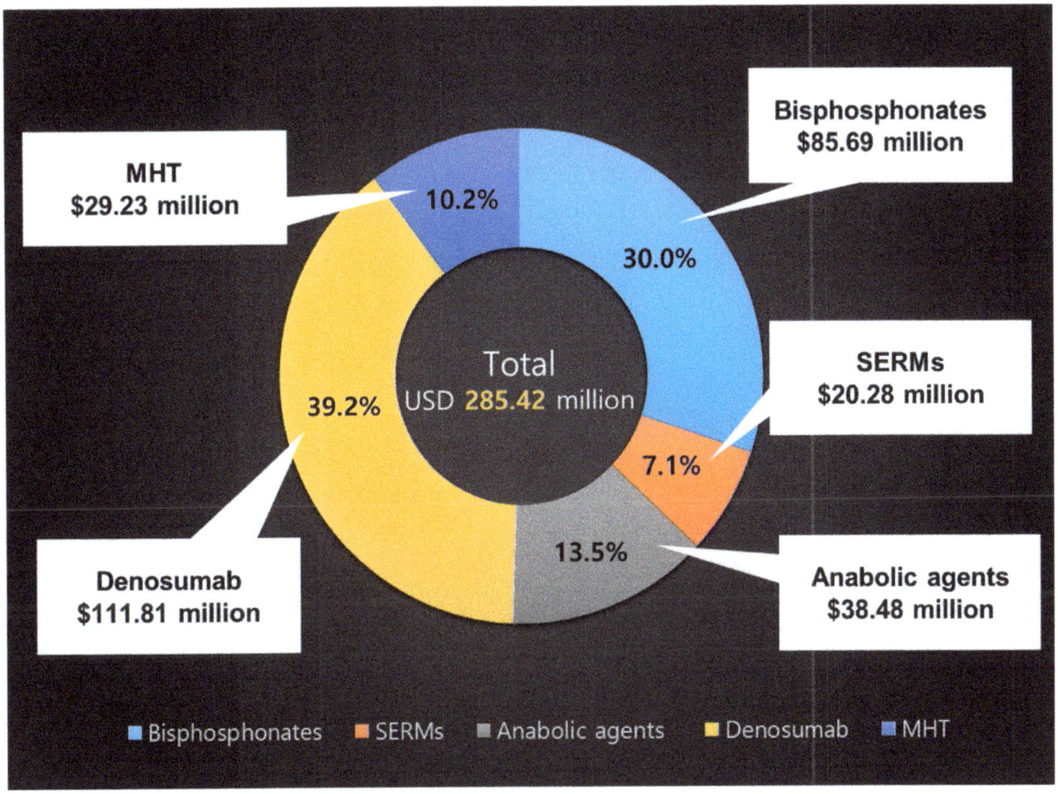

Figure 1. Market size for osteoporosis treatment in Korea in 2023. SERMs, selective estrogen receptor modulators; MHT, menopausal hormone therapy; USD, US dollar.

3.2. Hormonal Treatments

Postmenopausal female hormone therapy includes estrogen-only (ET) treatment, estrogen–progestogen therapy (EPT), tibolone, and TSEC. The total cost of hormonal agents used in 2023 was USD 30.38 million, showing no significant change compared to USD 30.31 million in 2018. In 2023, ET and EPT treatments represented 51.4% of the total market share, followed by tibolone at 46.1% and TSEC at approximately 2.5%. A linear trend analysis was conducted to assess annual changes in the sales volumes of four osteoporosis medications from 2018 to 2023. Among the four agents, TSEC showed a statistically significant decreasing trend over the 6-year period (slope = −1.028, p = 0.033, R^2 = 0.718), whereas tibolone exhibited a significant increasing trend (slope = +0.877, p = 0.023, R^2 = 0.764). No statistically significant trend was observed for EPT (slope = −0.039, p = 0.833, R^2 = 0.013) or ET (slope = +0.172, p = 0.278, R^2 = 0.282), although ET demonstrated a slight upward trend over time. (Figure 2).

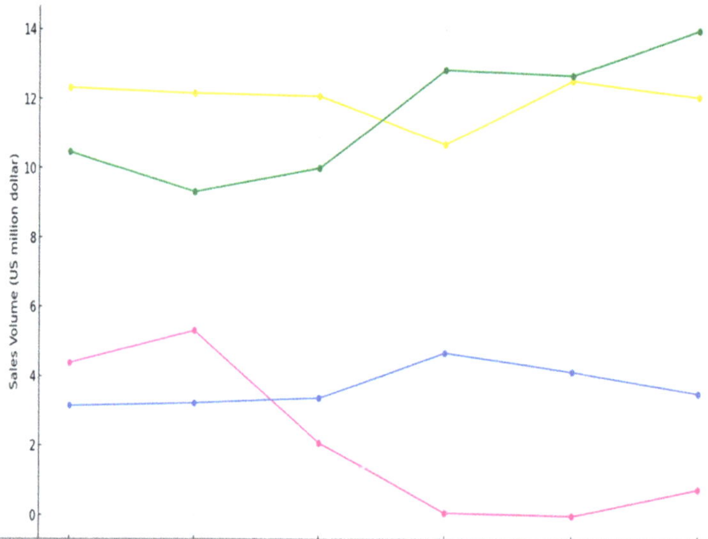

(US million dollar)

Drug	2018	2019	2020	2021	2022	2023	Slope	*p*_value	R^2
EPT	12.31	12.15	12.08	10.69	12.54	12.08	-0.04	0.83	0.01
TSEC	4.38	5.31	2.08	0.08	0	0.77	-1.03	0.03	0.72
ET	3.15	3.23	3.38	4.69	4.15	3.54	0.17	0.28	0.28
Tibolone	10.46	9.31	10	12.85	12.69	14	0.88	0.02	0.76

Figure 2. Trends in hormonal treatments for osteoporosis (2018–2023). EPT, estrogen–progestogen therapy; TSEC, tissue-selective estrogen complex; ET, estrogen-only therapy.

3.3. Non-Hormonal Treatments

Excluding hormonal treatments, the total sales of osteoporosis drugs in 2023 was USD 266.31 million, with bisphosphonates accounting for approximately one-third of the market share (33.4%, USD 89.08 million). Denosumab, a RANKL inhibitor, accounted for the largest share of the market at 43.6% (USD 116.23 million). Sales rose from USD 11 million in 2018 to USD 36.38 million in 2019 and further to USD 116.23 million in 2023, representing a 957.6% increase. In 2023, denosumab experienced a 31.6% increase compared to the previous year and ranked first in sales among single-agent components. SERMs (including bazedoxifene and raloxifene) accounted for 7.1% of the market share (USD 20.28 million), while anabolic agents such as teriparatide and romosozumab accounted for another 13.5% (USD 38.48 million). Romosozumab has been available in the South Korean market since 2020, accounting for 7.4% (USD 21.31 million) of the market share in 2023. (Figure 3).

A linear trend analysis was conducted to evaluate changes in the annual sales volumes of five major osteoporosis medications from 2018 to 2023. Bisphosphonates showed a statistically significant decreasing trend over this period (slope = −2.83, $p = 0.0262$, $R^2 = 0.748$), while RANKL inhibitors demonstrated the most substantial increase (slope = +19.92, $p < 0.0001$, $R^2 = 0.990$). Sales of sclerostin inhibitors also increased significantly (slope = +4.38, $p = 0.0021$, $R^2 = 0.927$), reflecting the emerging role of anabolic agents in osteoporosis treatment. In contrast, there were no statistically significant trends observed for SERMs (slope = +0.11, $p = 0.6611$, $R^2 = 0.053$) or PTH analogs (slope = −0.49, $p = 0.4835$, $R^2 = 0.130$), suggesting a relatively stable market trend for these agents during the study period.

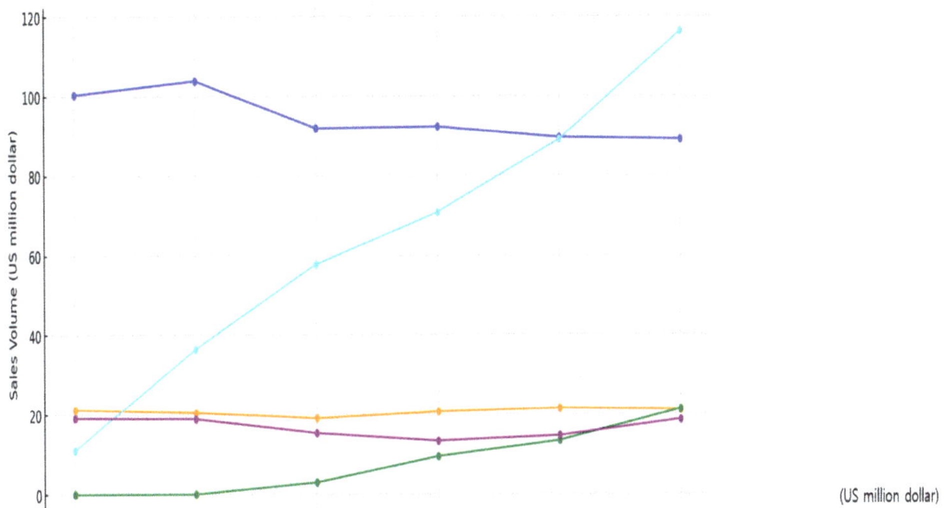

(US million dollar)

Drug	2018	2019	2020	2021	2022	2023	Slope	*p*-value	R^2
Bisphosphonates	100.38	103.85	91.92	92.31	89.54	89.08	-2.83	0.03	0.75
SERM	21.23	20.47	19	20.62	21.47	21.07	0.11	0.66	0.05
Sclerostin inhibitor	0	0	2.92	9.46	13.38	21.31	4.38	0.00	0.93
RANKL inhibitor	11	36.38	57.77	70.85	89	116.23	19.92	0.00	0.99
PTH	19.15	18.92	15.31	13.31	14.62	18.69	-0.49	0.48	0.13

Figure 3. Trends in non-hormonal treatments for osteoporosis (2018–2023). SERM, selective estrogen receptor modulator; RANKL, receptor activator of nuclear factor kappa-B ligand inhibitor; PTH, parathyroid hormone.

3.4. Changes in Prescription Patterns for Bisphosphonates

The analysis of bisphosphonate usage trends from 2018 to 2023 revealed a decline in the overall market volume, with a 5-year reduction of 11% (100.38 in 2018 to 89.08 in 2023). While oral bisphosphonates, such as alendronate and ibandronate, have shown consistent decreases in their usage over the years (−19% and −25%, respectively), risedronate demonstrated a modest recovery with a 2% increase in 2023 compared to 2022. Intravenous bisphosphonates present a contrasting trend; while zoledronate usage decreased significantly by 36% over five years, intravenous ibandronate stood out with a 20% increase during the same period, and its upward trend was sustained in the most recent year (Table 1).

Table 1. Evolving prescription trends for oral and intravenous bisphosphonates.

Category	Therapy	2018	2022	2023	1-Year Growth Rate (2022 vs. 2023)	5-Year Growth Rate (2018 vs. 2023)
Oral BP agent	Alendronate	25.15	20.92	20.46	−2%	−19%
	Risedronate	26.08	19.85	20.31	2%	−22%
	Ibandronate	11.77	9.08	8.85	−3%	−25%
IV BP agent	Zoledronate	9.69	6.92	6.23	−10%	−36%
	Ibandronate	27.69	32.77	33.23	1%	20%
Total Bisphosphonates		100.38	89.54	89.08	−1%	−11%

(US million dollar). BP, bisphosphonates; IV, intravenous.

3.5. Global Trends in Osteoporosis Drug Sales

Three Year Sales Trends in the United States, Japan, and South Korea (2021–2023)

From 2021 to 2023, the total sales of osteoporosis drugs increased significantly in the United States by 37.45%, highlighting its robust market expansion. This is primarily attributed to the significant growth in RANKL and sclerostin inhibitors. South Korea also experienced a substantial growth rate of 28.97%, reflecting its emerging market potential. In contrast, Japan recorded a modest growth of only 1.16%, indicating a stagnant or mature market with limited expansion during this period. This appears to have been impacted by the decreased use of bisphosphonates and PTH (Figure 4).

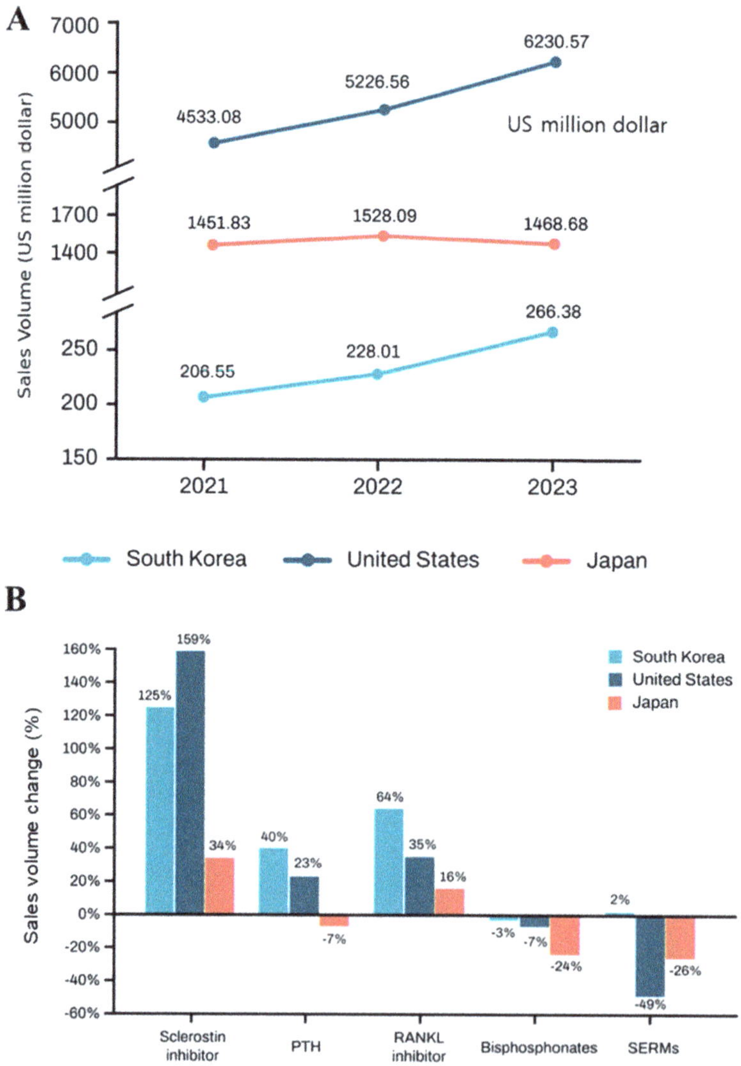

Figure 4. Three-year sales trends in the United States, Japan, and South Korea (2021–2023). (**A**). Total sales of osteoporosis medications over three years in the United States, Japan, and South Korea. (**B**). The growth rate of each osteoporosis medication by country. SERMs, selective estrogen receptor modulator; RANKL, receptor activator of nuclear factor kappa-B ligand inhibitor; PTH, parathyroid hormone.

4. Discussion

Currently, 200 million people worldwide have osteoporosis, with estimates indicating that even more are living with osteopenia [20]. More than 8.9 million fractures are caused by osteoporosis every year, occurring approximately once every 3 s [21]. The number of patients with osteoporotic compression fractures in South Korea increased from 117,361 in 2012 to 139,889 in 2016, and 54.3% of these patients received hospital treatment [22]. Along with the increase in the number of fractures, treatment costs have also increased rapidly [22]. In 2003, the estimated total socio-economic loss associated with osteoporosis in South Korea was USD 871.7 million, with annual medical expenses and loss of productivity costs reaching USD 364.6 million and USD 566.4 million, respectively [22]. Similarly, the osteoporosis drug market also continues to expand, and the seven major markets for osteoporosis treatment in the United States, Japan, and Europe are expected to grow from approximately USD 6.1 billion in 2014 to USD 9.34 billion in 2024 [23]

This study aimed to analyze the size and trends of the osteoporosis drug market in South Korea from 2018 to 2023. According to a previous study that evaluated markets for hormonal and osteoporosis treatments in South Korea from 2016 to 2019, the osteoporosis drug market has expanded from approximately USD 133.4 million in 2016 to USD 210 million in 2019, with bisphosphonates accounting for the largest share and exhibiting a steady increase [24]. In the analysis of hormonal therapies for the prevention and treatment of postmenopausal osteoporosis, the authors noted that sales of TSEC increased annually while EPT sales gradually decreased [24]. However, in the case of TSEC, the product was withdrawn from the market in 2019 due to a defect in the aluminum laminate packaging, which allowed oxygen ingress and subsequently reduced the dissolution rate of the active pharmaceutical ingredient. After quality improvements were made, its supply was resumed in 2023 [25]. From 2019 to 2023, the sharp decline in TSEC sales, accompanied by a gradual increase in tibolone use, resulted in a stagnation in the overall market share of postmenopausal hormonal agents in 2023 compared to 2018.

Denosumab received approval for reimbursement as a second-line treatment for osteoporosis in October 2017 in Korea [26]. Initially, the criteria for the reimbursement of Prolia as a second-line treatment were restrictive, requiring patients to have experienced new fractures or a decrease in their T-score on bone density tests after using bisphosphonates for more than one year [26]. However, in April 2019, the approval was expanded to include denosumab as a first-line treatment, leading to a significant increase in sales [26]. Denosumab is a human monoclonal antibody against RANKL that inhibits differentiation and bone resorption in osteoclasts [27]. Previous clinical studies have highlighted the excellent efficacy and safety of denosumab treatment in reducing fracture incidence in various patient groups [27]. The most important study that demonstrated the efficacy of denosumab in postmenopausal women with osteoporosis was the Fracture Reduction Evaluation of Denosumab in Osteoporosis Every Six Months (FREEDOM) study [28]. Subsequently, the FREEDOM Extension study, which evaluated the efficacy and safety of the drug over 10 years by extending the study period by 7 years, revealed that the incidence of new vertebral fractures was 0.90–1.86%, while the incidence of non-vertebral fractures was 0.84–2.55% [29]. The Determining Efficacy: Comparison of Initiating Denosumab versus Alendronate (DECIDE) study compared the effects of bisphosphonates and denosumab [30]. The denosumab administration group exhibited significantly higher bone densities in the lumbar spine, femoral neck, and femur than the alendronate administration group (with increases of 1.1%, 0.6%, and 1.0%, respectively), indicating that its effects were superior to those of existing drugs [30]. Furthermore, the FREEDOM Extension study reported that the incidence of adverse reactions such as severe infections, cellulitis, eczema, and malignant tumors was low in patients treated with denosumab [29]. In addition, osteonecrosis of the jaw occurred in only 5.2 cases per 10,000 patient years, indicating that denosumab administration does not require an off period during long-term use in contrast to bisphosphonates [29]. Based on the current analysis, the use of denosumab is predicted to increase due to its demonstrated efficacy, low risk of side effects, and the expansion of insurance standards in 2019.

Romosozumab is the latest osteoporosis treatment to be approved by the U.S. FDA (April 2019) [31]. PTH agents, which represent the only anabolic agents approved for osteoporosis prior to April 2019, increase both bone formation and resorption [32]. In contrast, despite being a single drug, romosozumab inhibits bone resorption while promoting bone formation [33]. In the FRActure study in postmenopausal woMen with osteoporosis (FRAME), a phase 3 clinical trial of romosozumab showed vertebral and femoral bone densities to increase by 13.3% and 6.8%, respectively, after one year of treatment with romosozumab when compared to those observed in the placebo group [34].

The STRUCTURE trial compared outcomes for romosozumab treatment with those for treatment with teriparatide, which is the same type of anabolic agent, reporting better results in the romosozumab group, showing a more positive effect on hip bone mineral density in particular [35].

In the Active-Controlled Fracture Study in Postmenopausal Women With Osteoporosis at High Risk (ARCH) study comparing the outcomes of romosozumab and alendronate treatment after 1 year, there was a 2.5% incidence of cardiovascular adverse events in the romosozumab group compared to 1.9% in the alendronate group, even though the incidence of fractures was significantly reduced in the romosozumab group [36]. Hence, the FDA approved the use of romosozumab with the stipulation that it cannot be used in patients who have recently experienced a myocardial infarction or stroke [37]. Recently, osteoporosis treatment groups have been classified according to fracture risk, and the use of anabolic agents is primarily recommended in groups with a very high risk of fracture (e.g., patients with severe osteoporosis accompanied by fractures or multiple vertebral fractures) [38].

In the United States, following FDA approval in April 2019, romosozumab was included in Medicare Part B, the public health insurance system operated by the federal government. Additionally, many major private insurers began covering this medication as a reimbursable treatment starting in 2020 [39]. Through this process, initial reimbursement coverage targeted patients with severe osteoporosis, allowing treatment without prior authorization or step therapy requirements. This increased the acceptance of the new drug among physicians and patients, driving significant growth in the osteoporosis market.

Similarly, in Japan, following its approval in May 2019, the Osteoporosis Fracture Score system was developed to identify high-risk groups for hip fractures and emphasize the importance of proactive early treatment with anabolic agents. Patients diagnosed with osteoporosis continued to receive medical insurance coverage without interruption, as there were no criteria for discontinuing reimbursement, leading to a high proportion of romosozumab usage in treatment [40–42].

Romosozumab was approved by the Ministry of Food and Drug Safety in South Korea in June 2020, allowing its use in the country [43,44]. In South Korea, the current insurance coverage criteria limit its use to patients for whom previous anti-osteoporosis therapies have been ineffective or to patients aged 65 and older with a T-score of −2.5 or below and two or more osteoporotic fractures [45]. Although these restrictions have resulted in a relatively low market share of 7.4% for romosozumab, its high therapeutic efficacy has led to a growing trend in usage, with a notable 59% increase in sales in 2023 compared to 2022. In addition, the recently published guidelines from the American Association of Clinical Endocrinologists (AACE) and the American College of Endocrinology (ACE) recommend romosozumab as a first-line treatment for patients at very high risk of fractures, and its use is expected to increase further [38].

In addition to the shift toward newer agents such as denosumab and romosozumab, notable trends have been observed within the bisphosphonate class. Between 2018 and 2023, the overall market volume of bisphosphonates declined by 11%, reflecting a gradual reduction in the use of oral formulations. Specifically, the use of alendronate and oral ibandronate decreased by 19% and 25%, respectively. In contrast, risedronate showed a modest rebound with a 2% increase in 2023 compared to the previous year. Interestingly, intravenous bisphosphonates exhibited divergent trends; while the usage of zoledronate declined sharply by 36% over five years, intravenous ibandronate experienced a 20% increase during the same period, and this upward trend has been sustained in the most recent year. These findings suggest a growing preference for intravenous agents—particularly ibandronate—likely due to its quarterly dosing regimen and lower gastrointestinal side effects, which may enhance patient adherence [46]. This underscores the increasing importance of treatment convenience and tolerability in the evolving landscape of osteoporosis management.

These findings should also be considered in the context of broader social and healthcare system changes. With the onset of the coronavirus infection in China at the end of 2019, COVID-19 in 2020 was classified as a pandemic by the WHO on 11 March 2020. In response, many countries have implemented unprecedented measures to contain the spread of the virus, including nationwide lockdowns, massive social quarantines, restrictions on public gatherings, and travel bans. These social distancing strategies created difficulties in the management of many chronic diseases. It cannot be ruled out that this social and medical environment may have caused changes in drug treatment.

In osteoporosis medication treatment, a critical focus lies in the treat-to-target strategy for reducing fracture risk and implementing national treatment strategies that ensure the continuity of care through changes in the reimbursement criteria. In South Korea, significant changes in medication usage frequency have been noted following modifications to the reimbursement criteria. For medications with restrictive reimbursement criteria, their usage frequency has been observed to be relatively low despite their clinical efficacy.

However, as of May 2024, reimbursement criteria were revised. Previously, osteoporosis medications were reimbursed only for patients with a T-score of −2.5 or lower [47]. The updated criteria now extend reimbursement eligibility to patients with T-scores exceeding −2.5 but not exceeding −2.0, allowing continuous treatment for up to two years. This revision applies to raloxifene, bazedoxifene, bisphosphonates, and denosumab injections, with flexibility for switching between these treatments based on dosage and administration requirements. This expansion ensures the continuity of treatment.

4.1. *Perspectives for Clinical Practice*

The findings of this study provide valuable insights into the evolving landscape of osteoporosis treatment in South Korea and have significant implications for clinical practice. The increasing use of romosozumab and denosumab indicates a shift toward anabolic and potent antiresorptive agents for high-risk patients with osteoporosis. The 2024 reimbursement revision expanded coverage to T-scores between −2.5 and −2.0 and is expected to improve treatment access and long-term outcomes. The decline in oral bisphosphonate use and the preference for injectables highlight the need for treatment adherence and patient-centered care. Clinicians should consider shared decision-making to optimize therapy selection.

The monitoring of real-world effectiveness and long-term outcomes is essential for refining osteoporosis management and healthcare policies.

4.2. Limitations

First, although hormonal replacement therapy has been indicated to prevent and treat osteoporosis, it is also used to treat other menopausal symptoms. However, our ability to subdivide and understand these different indications was limited. Second, since the market size was determined based only on the total sales, there may be a difference between the actual numbers of prescriptions or agents used. Nonetheless, most drugs, including hormonal replacement therapy, have been analyzed, making it easy to evaluate the overall drug market. Third, the sales trends do not directly capture patient adherence, treatment persistence, or clinical outcomes. Fourth, this study does not quantitatively assess the long-term impact of the COVID-19 pandemic on osteoporosis management. Future research incorporating real-world evidence studies, long-term treatment outcomes, and international comparisons are necessary to refine osteoporosis treatment strategies and improve patient care. Despite these limitations, this study provides critical insights into the evolving osteoporosis drug market and serves as a foundation for future research.

5. Conclusions

This study highlights key trends in the osteoporosis drug market in South Korea from 2018 to 2023, including the increasing use of anabolic agents, such as romosozumab and denosumab, and the impact of the 2024 reimbursement revision, which expands treatment access for patients with T-scores between −2.5 and −2.0.

The shift from oral bisphosphonates to injectable therapies emphasizes the need for patient-centered treatment approaches that improve adherence and convenience. While this study provides valuable market insights, it does not capture patient adherence, treatment persistence, or long-term clinical outcomes.

Future research should incorporate real-world evidence and long-term effectiveness studies to further refine osteoporosis treatment strategies and healthcare policies.

Supplementary Materials: The following supporting information can be downloaded at: https://www.mdpi.com/article/10.3390/medicina61050805/s1, Table S1: Types of osteoporosis treatment.

Author Contributions: Conceptualization: J.Y.P., J.-Y.S., Y.-J.C. and M.-R.K. Data analysis: J.Y.P. Methodology: J.Y.P. and J.-Y.S. Writing—Original draft: J.Y.P. Writing—Review and Editing: J.Y.P., J.-Y.S., Y.-J.C. and M.-R.K. All authors have read and agreed to the published version of the manuscript.

Funding: This study was not supported by any external funding.

Institutional Review Board Statement: This study was granted exemption by the Institutional Review Board (IRB) of The Catholic University of Korea, Seoul, St, Mary's Hospital (IRB No. KC25ZISI0151, approval date 14 March 2025).

Informed Consent Statement: The requirement for informed consent was waived because of this dataset does not include any personally identifiable patient information, obtaining informed consent from individual participants was neither required nor possible.

Data Availability Statement: The datasets generated during and/or analyzed in the current study are available from the corresponding author upon reasonable request.

Conflicts of Interest: The authors have no conflicts of interest to declare for this study.

References

1. World Health Organization. Assessment of fracture risk and its application to screening for postmenopausal osteoporosis: Report of a WHO study group [meeting held in Rome from 22 to 25 June 1992]. In Proceedings of the Assessment of Fracture Risk and Its Application to Screening for Postmenopausal Osteoporosis: Report of a WHO Study Group, Rome, Italy, 22–25 June 1992.
2. NIH CNcs. Osteoporosis prevention, diagnosis, and therapy. *NIH Consens. Statement* **2000**, *17*, 1–45.

3. Johnell, O.; Kanis, J.A. An estimate of the worldwide prevalence and disability associated with osteoporotic fractures. *Osteoporos. Int.* **2006**, *17*, 1726–1733. [CrossRef]
4. Reginster, J.-Y.; Burlet, N.J.B. Osteoporosis: A still increasing prevalence. *Bone* **2006**, *38*, 4–9. [CrossRef] [PubMed]
5. Ahn, S.H.; Park, S.-M.; Park, S.Y.; Yoo, J.-I.; Jung, H.-S.; Nho, J.-H.; Kim, S.H.; Lee, Y.-K.; Ha, Y.-C.; Jang, S. Osteoporosis and osteoporotic fracture fact sheet in Korea. *J. Bone Metab.* **2020**, *27*, 281–290. [CrossRef] [PubMed]
6. Health Insurance Review & Assessment Service (HIRA). *Stc Illness Information View*; Health Insurance Review & AssessmentService (HIRA): Wonju, Republic of Korea, 2023.
7. National Health Insurance Service. *2015–2019 Statistical Reports on Osteoporosis*; National Health Insurance Service: Seoul, Republic of Korea, 2020.
8. Bhatnagar, A.; Kekatpure, A.L. Postmenopausal osteoporosis: A literature review. *Cureus* **2022**, *14*, e29367. [CrossRef]
9. Zaheer, S.; LeBoff, M.S. Osteoporosis: Prevention and treatment. *Endotext* **2022**. Available online: https://www.ncbi.nlm.nih.gov/books/NBK279073/ (accessed on 20 December 2024).
10. Cosman, F.; Lewiecki, E.M.; Eastell, R.; Ebeling, P.R.; Jan De Beur, S.; Langdahl, B.; Rhee, Y.; Fuleihan, G.E.-H.; Kiel, D.P.; Schousboe, J.T. Goal-directed osteoporosis treatment: ASBMR/BHOF task force position statement 2024. *J. Bone Miner. Res.* **2024**, *39*, 1393–1405. [CrossRef]
11. World Health Organization. *Coronavirus Disease 2019 (COVID-19) Situation Report–46*; World Health Organization: Geneva, Switzerland, 2020; Volume 6.
12. Rosenbaum, L. The untold toll—The pandemic's effects on patients without Covid-19. *N. Engl. J. Med.* **2020**, *382*, 2368–2371. [CrossRef]
13. Voulgaridou, G.; Papadopoulou, S.K.; Detopoulou, P.; Tsoumana, D.; Giaginis, C.; Kondyli, F.S.; Lymperaki, E.; Pritsa, A.J.D. Vitamin D and calcium in osteoporosis, and the role of bone turnover markers: A narrative review of recent data from RCTs. *Diseases* **2023**, *11*, 29. [CrossRef]
14. Lordan, R.J.N. Notable developments for vitamin D amid the COVID-19 pandemic, but caution warranted overall: A narrative review. *Nutrients* **2021**, *13*, 740. [CrossRef]
15. Ruggiero, S.L. Bisphosphonate-related osteonecrosis of the jaw: An overview. *Ann. N. Y. Acad. Sci.* **2011**, *1218*, 38–46. [CrossRef] [PubMed]
16. Nguyen, H.H.; van de Laarschot, D.M.; Verkerk, A.J.; Milat, F.; Zillikens, M.C.; Ebeling, P.R. Genetic risk factors for atypical femoral fractures (AFFs): A systematic review. *J. Bone Miner. Res. Plus* **2018**, *2*, 1–11. [CrossRef] [PubMed]
17. Korean Society for Bone and Mineral Research. *2020 Physician's Guide for Osteoporosis*; Korean Society for Bone and Mineral Research: Seoul, Republic of Korea, 2020.
18. Benchimol, E.I.; Smeeth, L.; Guttmann, A.; Harron, K.; Moher, D.; Petersen, I.; Sørensen, H.T.; von Elm, E.; Langan, S.M. The REporting of studies Conducted using Observational Routinely-collected health Data (RECORD) statement. *PLoS Med.* **2015**, *12*, e1001885. [CrossRef]
19. Husereau, D.; Drummond, M.; Petrou, S.; Carswell, C.; Moher, D.; Greenberg, D.; Augustovski, F.; Briggs, A.H.; Mauskopf, J.; Loder, E. Consolidated health economic evaluation reporting standards (CHEERS) statement. *Int. J. Technol. Assess. Health Care* **2013**, *29*, 117–122. [CrossRef]
20. Sözen, T.; Özışık, L.; Başaran, N.Ç. An overview and management of osteoporosis. *Eur. J. Rheumatol.* **2016**, *4*, 46–56. [CrossRef] [PubMed]
21. Johnston, C.B.; Dagar, M. Osteoporosis in older adults. *Med. Clin.* **2020**, *104*, 873–884. [CrossRef]
22. National Health Insurance Service Ilsan Hospital Institute of Health Insurance and Clinical Research. *A Study on the Osteoporotic Compression Fracture Occurrence Frequency According to the Trend of Osteoporosis Treatment and Treatment of Osteoporotic Patients in Korea*; National Health Insurance Service Ilsan Hospital Institute of Health Insurance and Clinical Research: Goyang, Republic of Korea, 2020.
23. Korea Health Industry Development Institute (KHIDI). Global market analysis of osteoporosis treatment. *KHIDI Brief* **2018**, *253*.
24. Lee, E.S.; Kwon, S.; Park, H.M. The Trend in the Sales of Menopausal Hormone and Other Osteoporosis Medications in South Korea from 2016 to 2019. *J. Bone Metab.* **2021**, *28*, 201–206. [CrossRef]
25. Pfizer Korea. Announcement Regarding the Voluntary Recall of Duavive Tablets (0.45/20mg, Lot Numbers: T34122, T42330, W78858, W78860, X34636, AG6437, AG6438, CG3243, CW7990, DC5278). 2020. Available online: https://www.pfizer.co.kr/media/%ED%99%94%EC%9D%B4%EC%9E%90-%EC%86%8C%EC%8B%9D/%EB%93%80%EC%95%84%EB%B9%84%EB%B8%8C%EC%A0%95-04520mg-%EC%A0%9C%EC%A1%B0%EB%B2%88%ED%98%B8-t34122-t42330-w78858-w78860-x34636-ag6437-ag6438-cg3243-cw7990-dc5278-%EC%9E%90%EC%A7%84%ED%9A%8C%EC%88%98%EC%9D%98-%EA%B1%B4 (accessed on 23 April 2025).
26. Health Insurance Review & Assessment Service (HIRA). *Criteria for Reimbursement of Denosumab*; Health Insurance Review & Assessment Service (HIRA)): Wonju, Republic of Korea, 2019.

27. Raggatt, L.J.; Partridge, N.C. Cellular and molecular mechanisms of bone remodeling. *J. Biol. Chem.* **2010**, *285*, 25103–25108. [CrossRef]
28. Cummings, S.R.; Martin, J.S.; McClung, M.R.; Siris, E.S.; Eastell, R.; Reid, I.R.; Delmas, P.; Zoog, H.B.; Austin, M.; Wang, A. Denosumab for prevention of fractures in postmenopausal women with osteoporosis. *N. Engl. J. Med.* **2009**, *361*, 756–765. [CrossRef]
29. Bone, H.G.; Wagman, R.B.; Brandi, M.L.; Brown, J.P.; Chapurlat, R.; Cummings, S.R.; Czerwiński, E.; Fahrleitner-Pammer, A.; Kendler, D.L.; Lippuner, K.; et al. 10 years of denosumab treatment in postmenopausal women with osteoporosis: Results from the phase 3 randomised FREEDOM trial and open-label extension. *Lancet Diabetes Endocrinol.* **2017**, *5*, 513–523. [CrossRef]
30. Brown, J.P.; Prince, R.L.; Deal, C.; Recker, R.R.; Kiel, D.P.; De Gregorio, L.H.; Hadji, P.; Hofbauer, L.C.; Álvaro-Gracia, J.M.; Wang, H.; et al. Comparison of the effect of denosumab and alendronate on BMD and biochemical markers of bone turnover in postmenopausal women with low bone mass: A randomized, blinded, phase 3 trial. *J. Bone Miner. Res.* **2009**, *24*, 153–161. [CrossRef] [PubMed]
31. Mullard, A. FDA approves first-in-class osteoporosis drug. *Nat. Rev. Drug Discov.* **2019**, *18*, 411. [CrossRef]
32. Silva, B.C.; Bilezikian, J.P. Parathyroid hormone: Anabolic and catabolic actions on the skeleton. *Curr. Opin. Pharmacol.* **2015**, *22*, 41–50. [CrossRef] [PubMed]
33. Sølling, A.S.K.; Harsløf, T.; Langdahl, B. The clinical potential of romosozumab for the prevention of fractures in postmenopausal women with osteoporosis. *Ther. Adv. Musculoskelet. Dis.* **2018**, *10*, 105–115. [CrossRef]
34. Cosman, F.; Crittenden, D.B.; Ferrari, S.; Lewiecki, E.M.; Jaller-Raad, J.; Zerbini, C.; Milmont, C.E.; Meisner, P.D.; Libanati, C.; Grauer, A. Romosozumab FRAME study: A post hoc analysis of the role of regional background fracture risk on nonvertebral fracture outcome. *J. Bone Miner. Res.* **2018**, *33*, 1407–1416. [CrossRef] [PubMed]
35. Langdahl, B.L.; Libanati, C.; Crittenden, D.B.; Bolognese, M.A.; Brown, J.P.; Daizadeh, N.S.; Dokoupilova, E.; Engelke, K.; Finkelstein, J.S.; Genant, H.K. Romosozumab (sclerostin monoclonal antibody) versus teriparatide in postmenopausal women with osteoporosis transitioning from oral bisphosphonate therapy: A randomised, open-label, phase 3 trial. *Lancet* **2017**, *390*, 1585–1594. [CrossRef]
36. Saag, K.G.; Petersen, J.; Brandi, M.L.; Karaplis, A.C.; Lorentzon, M.; Thomas, T.; Maddox, J.; Fan, M.; Meisner, P.D.; Grauer, A. Romosozumab or alendronate for fracture prevention in women with osteoporosis. *N. Engl. J. Med.* **2017**, *377*, 1417–1427. [CrossRef]
37. Camacho, P.M.; Petak, S.M.; Binkley, N.; Diab, D.L.; Eldeiry, L.S.; Farooki, A.; Harris, S.T.; Hurley, D.L.; Kelly, J.; Lewiecki, E.M. American Association of Clinical Endocrinologists/American College of Endocrinology Clinical Practice Guidelines for the Diagnosis and Treatment of Postmenopausal Osteoporosis—2020 Update. *Endocr. Pract.* **2020**, *26*, 1–46. [CrossRef]
38. Chandran, M. AACE/ACE clinical practice guidelines for the diagnosis and treatment of postmenopausal osteoporosis—2020 update: Risk stratification and intervention thresholds. *Endocr. Pract.* **2021**, *27*, 378. [CrossRef]
39. Centers for Medicare & Medicaid Services (CMS). *Medicare Part B coverage for Romosozumab Following FDA Approval*; Centers for Medicare & Medicaid Services (CMS): Baltimore, MD, USA, 2019. Available online: https://www.cms.gov (accessed on 20 December 2024).
40. Amgen. *Evenity (Romosozumab) Receives Approval in Japan for the Treatment of Osteoporosis in Patients at High Risk of Fracture*; Amgen: Thousand Oaks, CA, USA, 2019; Available online: https://www.amgen.com/newsroom/press-releases/2019/01/evenity-romosozumab-receives-approval-in-japan-for-the-treatment-of-osteoporosis-in-patients-at-high-risk-of-fracture (accessed on 20 December 2024).
41. Japanese Society for Bone and Mineral Research (JSBMR). Development of the Fracture Risk Assessment Tool (FRAX) in Japan. *Endocr. J.* **2017**, *65*, 109–117. Available online: https://www.jstage.jst.go.jp/article/endocrj/65/2/65_EJ17-0331/_article/-char/ja (accessed on 20 December 2024).
42. Nojiri, S.; Burge, R.T.; Flynn, J.A.; Foster, S.A.; Sowa, H. Osteoporosis and treatments in Japan: Management for preventing subsequent fractures. *J. Bone Miner. Metab.* **2013**, *31*, 367–380. [CrossRef] [PubMed]
43. U.S. Food and Drug Administration. *FDA Approves New Treatment for Osteoporosis in Postmenopausal Women at High Risk for Fracture*; U.S. Food and Drug Administration: Silver Spring, MD, USA, 2019. Available online: https://www.fda.gov/news-events/press-announcements/fda-approves-new-treatment-osteoporosis-postmenopausal-women-high-risk-fracture (accessed on 20 December 2024).
44. Ministry of Food and Drug Safety (MFDS). *Approval of Romosozumab (Evenity) for Osteoporosis Treatment*; Ministry of Food and Drug Safety (MFDS): Sejong, Republic of Korea, 2020. Available online: https://www.mfds.go.kr (accessed on 23 January 2025).
45. Health Insurance Review & Assessment Service (HIRA). *(n.d.) Reimbursement Criteria for Romosozumab [로모소주맙 급여 기준]*; Health Insurance Review & Assessment Service (HIRA): Wonju, Republic of Korea, 2024; Available online: https://www.hira.or.kr/rc/insu/insuadtcrtr/InsuAdtCrtrList.do (accessed on 24 December 2024).

46. Lewiecki, E.M.; Babbitt, A.M.; Piziak, V.K.; Ozturk, Z.E.; Bone, H.G. Adherence to and gastrointestinal tolerability of monthly oral or quarterly intravenous ibandronate therapy in women with previous intolerance to oral bisphosphonates: A 12-month, open-label, prospective evaluation. *Clin. Ther.* **2008**, *30*, 605–621. [CrossRef] [PubMed]
47. Ministry of Health and Welfare (MOHW). *Revision of Reimbursement Criteria for Osteoporosis Medications;* Ministry of Health and Welfare (MOHW): Sejong, Republic of Korea, 2024. Available online: https://www.mohw.go.kr/boardDownload.es?bid=0026&list_no=1482116&seq=7 (accessed on 23 January 2025).

medicina

MDPI

Article

The Impact of Standard Care Versus Intrinsic Relaxation at Home on Physiological Parameters in Patients with Fibromyalgia: A Comparative Cohort Study from Romania

Theodora Florica Borze (Ursu) [1,2], Annamaria Pallag [1,3,*], Emilian Tarcău [2], Doriana Ioana Ciobanu [2], Felicia Liana Andronie-Cioară [4], Carmen Delia Nistor-Cseppento [4], Gabriela Ciavoi [1,5] and Mariana Mureșan [1,6]

1 Doctoral School of Biomedical Sciences, Faculty of Medicine and Pharmacy, University of Oradea, 410073 Oradea, Romania; borze.theodoraflorica@student.uoradea.ro (T.F.B.); gciavoi@uoradea.ro (G.C.); mmuresan@uoradea.ro (M.M.)
2 Department of Physical Education, Sport and Physical Therapy, Faculty of Geography, Tourism and Sports, University of Oradea, 410087 Oradea, Romania; emilian.tarcau@didactic.uoradea.ro (E.T.); dciobanu@uoradea.ro (D.I.C.)
3 Department of Pharmacy, Faculty of Medicine and Pharmacy University of Oradea, 410073 Oradea, Romania
4 Department of Psycho-Neuroscience and Recovery, Faculty of Medicine and Pharmacy University of Oradea, 410073 Oradea, Romania; fcioara@uoradea.ro (F.L.A.-C.); dcseppento@uoradea.ro (C.D.N.-C.)
5 Department of Dental Medicine, Faculty of Medicine and Pharmacy University of Oradea, 410073 Oradea, Romania
6 Department of Preclinical Disciplines, Faculty of Medicine and Pharmacy University of Oradea, 410073 Oradea, Romania
* Correspondence: apallag@uoradea.ro; Tel.: +40-770-904-739

Abstract: *Background and Objectives*: Fibromyalgia (FM), through the presence of widespread chronic pain, stiffens the musculoskeletal system and causes sleep disturbances and fatigue. Through this study, we aimed to compare the effectiveness of two different recovery interventions for improving sleep quality: a standard, multidisciplinary intervention in a recovery hospital versus a therapy focused on intrinsic relaxation at home. *Materials and Methods*: This study included 60 adult patients who participated voluntarily and were diagnosed with FM by a rheumatologist, randomly divided into two groups. During this study, 30 patients out of the 60 were randomly assigned to experimental group 1 and underwent treatment at the Recovery Clinical Hospital in Băile Felix. The other 30 patients were assigned to experimental group 2 and underwent treatment at home. They were assessed on the first and last day of the recovery program using the Fatigue Severity Scale (FSS) and the Pittsburgh Sleep Quality Index (PSQI). *Results*: In experimental group 1, where by patients underwent hospital recovery (EG1), the results show that the severity of fatigue (FSS) was significantly reduced, with $p = 0.00$ and an effect size of 0.77, which suggests a general improvement in the state of fatigue, as well as in the quality of sleep evaluated with the PSQI ($p = 0.00$, effect size = 0.55). In experimental group 2 (EG2), no change was observed between assessments in terms of the FSS, but in terms of the quality of sleep, there was a small decrease in the PSQI score ($p = 0.083$), with a small effect size of 0.09. *Conclusions*: The results show that, from a clinical point of view, a complex treatment carried out daily improves sleep quality and reduces fatigue.

Keywords: fibromyalgia; sleep quality; fatigue; chronic pain

1. Introduction

Fibromyalgia is a complex syndrome characterized by chronic pain, joint stiffness, fatigue, sleep disturbances, brain dysfunction, and depression [1,2]. The history of fibromyalgia is complex and has evolved gradually as doctors and researchers have tried to better understand the condition. However, the terms and explanations varied a lot [3]. In 1970, FM was associated with a central nervous system condition [4]; then, in 1976, the link between sleep disorders and chronic pain was first described [5]. In 1981, the Yunus criteria included in FM diagnosis comprised fatigue, sleep problems, sensitivity to weather, and chronic pain, all of which are aggravated by the presence of stress and anxiety [6]. Patients with fibromyalgia have been observed to have an increased sensitivity to stimuli that would not normally cause pain, a phenomenon known as allodynia [7]. In addition, research has shown that the neurotransmitters responsible for pain, such as substance P and serotonin, are involved in the exacerbation of symptoms [8]. Reflex phenomena are considered among the most important factors triggering FM, and they are associated with deep chronic pain produced by the activation of a pain–spasm cycle through the presence of repeated trauma or postural stress [9]. The exact causes and pathogenic mechanisms of fibromyalgia are unknown. Biological, psychological, and socio-cultural factors have been suggested as possible contributors, including abnormal pain signaling, abnormal activity of the neuroendocrine and autonomic systems, genetic predisposition, certain environmental triggers, and sleep disturbances [10]. These factors hypersensitize patients to pain [11]. Since the pathogenesis of this disease is not well known, the diagnosis is only made clinically at this time. Oxidative stress, mitochondrial dysfunction, mineral and vitamin deficiencies, and disproportions in other components are interesting and attractive topics from a clinical point of view, which require further studies to clarify the status and development of FM [12]. It is necessary to find the most appropriate solutions to reduce the permanent fatigue faced by these patients.

The European League against Rheumatism states that, for the management of FM, physical exercises represent the only effective recommendation over time, being adapted according to the needs of patients, with some patients not being able to tolerate strength and flexibility exercises even though they seem to be the most beneficial [13]. Regarding the management of FM [14], treatment requires a comprehensive approach that combines non-pharmacological interventions, such as exercise, and pharmacological management with duloxetine, pregabalin, milnacipran, and amitriptyline, which have remarkable benefits for fibromyalgia symptoms. Pure mu-opioid agonists such as NSAIDs and acetaminophen do not have effective results, and methylphenidate, despite improving mental status and fatigue, requires further studies [15]. However, pharmacological therapy is only useful for individual symptoms [16], with non-pharmacological interventions being more effective according to systematic reviews, because combining aerobic exercise with resistance and stretching reduces FM symptoms and the stress response [17]. Some authors believe that accepting pain without daily attempts to reduce it has positive effects on improving daily functioning [18].

Psychological factors should be considered alongside the management of FM, as they contribute significantly to both symptomatology and the functioning of the treatment. Relaxation therapy is an autonomous process, representing a main goal in the prophylaxis and recovery of a patient, because it brings a state of rest to the muscles and inhibits nervous tension. Intrinsic relaxation rebalances the well-being inside the body. Studies on mind–body recovery are limited, and further research is needed. Published studies have limited effects due to low-quality evidence or lack of recent studies [19]. At the same time, mind–body therapies are favorable in pathologies that have affected psychological function [20], aiming to induce the body's relaxation response [21]. The author Liraz Cohen-Biton concludes that holistic therapies focusing on body, mind, and soul provide an appropriate response that promotes the health status of patients with FM [22]. A study of this therapy was conducted with 28 women with FM via the Zoom platform.

This study showed that performing eight sessions of conscious breathing and listening to one's own body for 8 weeks reduced physical and mental suffering, fatigue, fear, and disabilities, $p < 0.001$ [23]. During home therapy, FM patients were assessed on several dimensions such as the presence of stress in their daily environment, program resilience, and coping to check the effectiveness of treatments and to understand the weaknesses they face [24]. Also, according to Theadom [25], mind–body therapies could be good therapeutic strategies for physical and psychological improvement because mind, body, and behaviors are interconnected. Another purpose of using relaxation through online consultations is the permanent adherence of patients to recovery, something that would be impossible during pandemics such as SARS-CoV-2, which negatively affected the management of chronic health conditions by imposing isolation restrictions [26–28].

Regarding sleep, it is known that there are two types of sleep, i.e., REM and non-REM. The non-REM period has four stages with waves that have certain electroencephalographic characteristics [29,30]. In fibromyalgia, there are disturbances in the fourth phase of non-REM sleep, which are translated by the appearance of alpha waves that overlap the normal delta waves. The results from specialized literature show that sleep disorders are one of the most important aspects of FM [31] poor sleep quality being a fundamental index in the pathophysiology of FM, together with fatigue and pain. The prevalence of sleep quality shows that only 11% of FM patients reported good sleep quality, while up to 99% of patients report having problems with the amount, initiation, and maintenance of sleep during the night, with long refresh times or waking up too early in the morning, which makes it difficult to start their daily activities [32]. Kline et al. [33] mentioned that the definition of sleep quality should be related to the personal experience of each person, depending on the stage that affects them. Poor sleep quality has a negative impact because it lowers the pain threshold and increases the level of its catastrophizing. At the same time, this cycle of sleep impairment causes a high level of fatigue; studies show that poor sleep quality leads to the appearance of cognitive, social, and integration problems [34], having a tendency to become chronic [35]. Patients with fibromyalgia complain of sleep disturbances and the intensification of pain, stiffness, and fatigue after waking up [36]. Often, when patients are asked if they wake up rested, the answer is negative, with sleep being impaired in over 80% of FM patients [37]. Often sleepless nights are followed by worsening pains [38]. Some studies suggest that fatigue is a cause of FM and not a symptom [39]. In the anamnesis, there are frequent associations with diseases that recognize a stress etiology, such as ulcerative hemorrhagic colitis, irritable colon, migraine, hypertension, and so on [40].

We created this study by observing the negative impact of FM on patients' lives and the lack of evidence for the introduction of programs focused on relaxation. The aim of this study is to compare the effects of applying two different types of intervention on sleep quality and fatigue in fibromyalgia patients, respectively, a therapy without additional costs, focused only on intrinsic relaxation carried out at home in relation to a multidisciplinary therapy.

2. Materials and Methods

Following visits to the rheumatologist, 67 patients with fibromyalgia were invited, by the physical therapist, to participate in the present study. Seven of them withdrew before the start of the initial assessments at the time of the study presentation. A total of 60 patients participated in this study. Patients were chosen following the inclusion and exclusion criteria. The main inclusion criteria were the age of at least 18 years, the presence of a diagnosis of fibromyalgia, voluntary and independent participation in this study, and the absence of contraindications for the intervention. At the same time, pregnant women and those who were absent from the evaluation were excluded from this study.

The allocation of patients was carried out by the method of simple randomization, without knowing the severity of the symptoms, so that at the end of this study, the chance of specific recovery would be given to the group with more effective intervention. Furthermore, 30 patients out of 60 were randomly assigned to experimental group 1 and underwent treatment at the Recovery Clinical Hospital in Băile Felix. The other 30 patients were assigned to experimental group 2 and performed the treatment at home. The period of this study is January–November 2024. All 60 patients also administered the pharmacological treatment received during the study period upon learning the diagnosis.

The two groups received treatment for 2 weeks. EG1 performed 10 standard recovery sessions in the presence of a physical therapist. They had a complex recovery program consisting of 30 min of individual physical therapy that included warm-up exercises and mobilization exercises for all joints, followed by muscle-strengthening exercises and stretching at the end for increased flexibility [41–47]. Each exercise was performed in 4 sets of 10 repetitions. The exercises were performed from dorsal decubitus, ventral decubitus, standing, and quadrupedal positions and were performed in breathing rhythm. Patients also had electrotherapy sessions at the BTL 5000 machine with low frequency (80–130 Hz) transcutaneous electrical nerve stimulation (TENS) for 15 min to reduce chronic pain and classic Swedish massage for 10 min. They also had group hydrokinetotherapy for 20 min from orthostatism at a water temperature of 36–37 degrees Celsius, which facilitates movement and reduces gravitational forces [48], the benefits of thermal water being known since ancient times [49]. Exercise is part of managing fibromyalgia as it reduces pain and improves sleep and overall functioning [45]. Physiotherapy is the most important basis because it is based on movement, which is essential for life. Mobilizations, tractions, active exercises, active exercises with resistance, isometrics, and stretching are performed because people with FM have low endurance and muscle strength [46]. Massage brings a general and local state of well-being, reduces pain, and improves circulation and is useful when the patient's mobility is reduced, helping to rebalance the posture, improve muscle relaxation, and eliminate acute pain [47]. Electrotherapy reduces pain and can be used for medical purposes because the human body works mostly electrically [50]. Hydrokinetic therapy is one of the main forms of restoring diminished functions because water can support 90% of the body's weight, reducing the muscle effort required to perform movements and increasing the amplitude of movements [48].

Experimental group 2 (EG2) performed at home for 2 weeks without the physical supervision of a physiotherapist, 20 min of intrinsic relaxation specific to the author Parow, every evening before going to bed. Parow's relaxation technique is based on intrinsic relaxation, which helps to actively induce relaxation and ensures mutual inhibition between muscles and psyche. It is performed without other auxiliary tools and can be performed at home. The author recommends maintaining the supine position in bed for 20 min, breathing freely. During this time, it is recommended to inhale through the nose and exhale with a long "sh" to automatically induce general muscle relaxation. All patients in this group were helped before the start of the 10 recovery sessions to perform the breathing technique correctly and communicated daily, online, with the physiotherapist to record the session performed and to offer them help if they needed it. This intervention, focused only on intrinsic relaxation, is based on the need to integrate a recuperative program as simplified as possible and accessible to anyone, the specialists in the field claiming that notable improvements in the clinical profile occur in people who have a high adherence to the treatment.

Each group was analyzed after signing consent for the processing of personal data to ensure voluntary participation. After signing the documents, the first assessment was carried out one day before the start of the treatment, and the final assessment was carried out at the end of the recovery sessions, after the two weeks of treatment.

The data collected were used for this study only, and patients could withdraw from this study at any time. In the studies, only patients' initials were used, and no pictures were taken during this period. To respect their right to privacy, the recovery was carried out only in the presence of the physical therapist.

2.1. *Instruments*

To find out information about the subjects, an assessment form was drawn up that included questions about independent variables such as age, height, sex, weight, duration of the condition, associated diagnoses, symptoms, triggers, background, occupation, and medication. The following two questionnaires were assigned to the dependent variables: the Fatigue Severity Scale (FSS) questionnaire to assess fatigue and the Pittsburgh Sleep Quality Index (PSQI) for sleep quality.

2.1.1. Assessment of Fatigability and Fatigue

Fatigue severity was assessed using the Fatigue Severity Scale (FSS) [51]. The Fatigue Scale is used to measure the severity, frequency, and impact of fatigue, typically in patients with chronic conditions such as cancer, multiple sclerosis (MS), or other long-term illnesses such as fibromyalgia. Fatigue is a common symptom that affects a person's physical, emotional, and mental well-being, and these scales help clinicians and researchers provide better diagnosis, monitoring, and treatment. The scale is self-reported, requiring only paper and pen. Subjects responded to the 9 items using a 7-point Likert scale (1 = strongly disagree, 7 = strongly agree). The minimum score is 9 and the maximum is 63, which indicates a severe state of fatigue.

2.1.2. Assessment of Overall Sleep Quality

Sleep quality has a clinically relevant influence on a person's daytime functioning. The degree of sleep disturbance has been studied most with the help of the Pittsburgh Sleep Quality Index (PSQI) questionnaire [52], which comprises 19 items related to 7 subcategories: subjective sleep quality, latency period, sleep duration, usual sleep efficiency, sleep disorders, sleep medication use, and daytime dysfunction. Five additional roommate-rated questions are included for clinical purposes but are not scored. The questionnaire is validated for patients with major depressive disorders, sleep initiation and maintenance disorders, excessive sleepiness disorders, insomnia, depression, chronic pain, and other health conditions, cancer, and fibromyalgia. It is also used in research studies to investigate how sleep quality is related to various health outcomes. The questionnaire consists of a combination of Likert-type and open-ended questions that will later be converted to scaled scores using guidelines provided by the authors. Patients are asked to indicate how often they have experienced certain sleep difficulties in the last month. Scores for each question range from 0 to 3, with higher scores indicating more disturbed sleep [53]. The component scores are then summed to give a global PSQI score, ranging from 0 to 21, where scores ≤ 5 indicate good sleep quality, scores > 5 indicate poor sleep quality, and scores > 10 suggest a potential sleep disorder.

2.2. *Statistical Analysis*

The results were interpreted, and the statistical analysis aimed at improving the variables after treatment for each group. The IBM SPSS Statistics for Windows software, Version 29.0, was used for the statistical processing of the study data (30-day trial version; Armonk, NY, USA: IBM Corp). Nominal data were described as frequency and percentage and continuous variables as mean, median, standard deviation, frequency ranges, minimum, and maximum. Differences between groups and time points were assessed using Student's *t*-test and Chi-square test, with a significance threshold of $p < 0.05$ and high significance defined as $p < 0.01$. The independent samples *t*-test was used to compare the means with respect to the dichotomous variables in this study. To compare two dependent or paired datasets, we used the *t*-test for dependent (paired) samples. The *t*-test for dependent samples (pairs) is used in research protocols that involve repeated measurements on the same individuals or on individuals with similar characteristics (even twins). The data are considered paired because for each value there is a matched value. The test evaluates the difference score within each pair so that subjects are compared only with themselves or their pair. The *t*-test of the difference between the means of two dependent samples allows the evaluation of the significance of the variation of a certain characteristic in the same individuals in two different situations (for example, "before" and "after" the action of a certain condition, or in two different contexts, regardless of the time of their manifestation). The major advantage of this statistical model is that it captures the so-called "intrasubject" variation by the fact that the basis of calculation is the difference between the two values of each individual subject.

2.3. Sample Size

The general formula for calculating the size of the patient sample used in this study was is expressed as follows:

$$n = (Z\alpha/2 + Z\beta)2 \cdot (2\sigma 2)/d2,$$

where

- n is the sample size.
- $Z\alpha/2 = 1.96$ is the critical value of the standard normal distribution (Z) corresponding to the significance level α (0.05).
- $Z\beta = 0.80$ is the critical value of the standard normal distribution corresponding to the power of the test $(1 - \beta)$.
- σ is the population standard deviation.
- d is the minimum effect size we want to detect.

Thus, $n = (1.96 + 0.84)2 \cdot (2 \cdot 102)/52 = 62.7$.

In this study, 67 patients were recruited.

3. Results

The results include the evaluation of the two analyzed groups.

3.1. Patient Data

In Table 1, the average age difference between EG1 (46.97 years) and EG2 (44.73 years) is 2.233 years, and the *p*-value is 0.484. This is a relatively small difference, suggesting that, in terms of age, the two groups are comparable.

Table 1. Distribution by age of patients.

Group	N	Mean	SD
EG1	30	46.97	13.163
EG2	30	44.73	11.317

SD = standard deviation.

The gender distribution, observed in Table 2, shows a female prevalence of FM in both EG1 and EG2. In other words, there is no significant association between gender and the group to which the participants are assigned.

Table 2. Distribution according to patient gender.

Group		Gender		Total
		Male	Female	
EG 1	Count	2	28	30
	%	6.7%	93.3%	100.0%
EG 2	Count	3	27	30
	%	10.0%	90.0%	100.0%
Total	Count	5	55	60
	%	8.33%	91.6%	100.0%

Below, in Table 3, it can be seen that all patients followed a pharmacological treatment based on non-steroidal anti-inflammatory drugs, which shows the homogeneity of the study groups.

Table 3. Distribution according to pharmacological treatment.

Pharmacological Treatment	EG1 (Count/%)	EG2 (Count/%)	Total EG1 + EG2 (Count/%)
Ibuprofen	16 (52)	14 (48)	30 (50)
Acetaminophen	14 (48)	16 (52)	30 (50)

The distribution by body mass index (BMI) shows, in Table 4, that the *p*-value (0.426) is much higher than the usual significance threshold of 0.05, indicating that the difference between the groups is not statistically significant. Thus, there is insufficient evidence to state that the BMI between experimental groups 1 and 2 is significantly different.

Table 4. Distribution of patients according to BMI.

Group	N	SD	Mean	t	df	*p*	Mean Difference
EG1	30	24.4207	4.41671	0.801	58	0.426	0.78600
EG2	30	23.6347	3.05794				

N = the number of patients; SD = standard deviation; t = the *t*-test of the difference in means; df = the difference between the two values; *p* = statistical significance coefficient.

Table 5 shows the distribution of symptoms reported by participants in the two groups. Both groups experience a significant number of symptoms, with a similar prevalence for many of them. However, EG1 reports a higher prevalence for certain symptoms, such as migraines, paresthesias, and anxiety, and EG2 reports a higher prevalence for chronic fatigue. In general, symptoms such as chronic pain, fatigue, and sleep disturbances are common in both groups.

Table 5. Distribution of symptoms reported by EG1 and EG2 participants.

Symptom [a]	U.M.	Group		Total
		EG1	EG2	
Chronic diffuse pain	Count	29	29	58
	%	96.7%	96.7%	
Fatigability	Count	19	15	34
	%	63.3%	50.0%	
Headache	Count	15	13	28
	%	50.0%	43.3%	
Migraines	Count	12	7	19
	%	40.0%	23.3%	
Paresthesia	Count	14	11	25
	%	46.7%	36.7%	
Myalgia	Count	18	17	35
	%	60.0%	56.7%	
Irritable bowel syndrome	Count	7	6	13
	%	23.3%	20.0%	
Restless legs syndrome	Count	9	4	13
	%	30.0%	13.3%	
Cognitive disorders	Count	2	2	4
	%	6.7%	6.7%	
Sleep disorders	Count	14	15	29
	%	46.7%	50.0%	
Depression	Count	9	6	15
	%	30.0%	20.0%	
Anxiety	Count	17	12	29
	%	56.7%	40.0%	
Chronic fatigue	Count	19	23	42
	%	63.3%	76.7%	
Other	Count	2	0	2
		6.7%	0.0%	
Total	Count	30	30	60

[a] Percentages and totals are based on respondents; U.M. = unit of measure.

Table 6 shows the distribution of frequencies for the triggering factors according to the type of lot. The contingency table shows how many participants in each group reported each trigger. There is a diversity of triggers reported in the two groups, with psychological stress being the main common factor and the most frequently mentioned. Factors such as infections and physical trauma are less relevant in this analysis, and the experimental group tends to have a higher prevalence of psychological stress and hormonal changes.

Table 6. The distribution of patients according to the triggering factors.

The Triggering Factor		EG1	EG2	Total
I do not know	Count	7	9	16
	%	23.3%	30.0%	
Infections (parvovirus or Lyme)	Count	3	0	3
	%	10.0%	0.0%	
Physical trauma	Count	2	0	2
	%	6.7%	0.0%	
Psychological stress	Count	19	14	33
	%	63.3%	46.7%	
Hormonal changes	Count	8	5	13
	%	26.7%	16.7%	
Medicines and vaccines	Count	1	0	1
	%	3.3%	0.0%	
Catastrophic events (war, etc.)	Count	1	1	2
	%	3.3%	3.3%	
Other	Count	1	3	4
	%	3.3%	10.0%	

3.2. The Results of the Evaluation of the State of Fatigue Evaluated with the FSS, Respectively of the Quality of Sleep Evaluated with the PSQI

In Table 7 and Figure 1, the intervention applied to EG1 shows that sleep duration increased, with patients able to fall asleep faster and maintain sleep for a longer period. Diurnal dysfunction caused by lack of sleep was reduced, with patients reporting better overall sleep quality with a moderate effect size of 0.55 points. Fatigue Severity (FSS) was significantly reduced, $p = 0.00$, with a moderate effect size of 0.77 points, suggesting an overall improvement in fatigue status. Overall, the intervention had a significant positive effect on various aspects of sleep and daytime functioning.

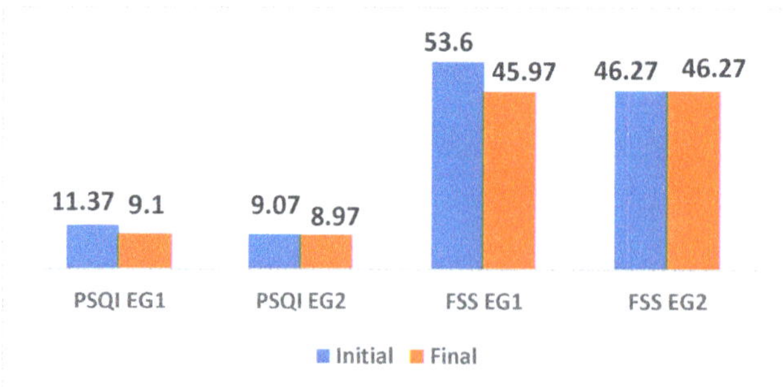

Figure 1. The results of FSS and PSQI scores from the two groups, EG1 and EG2.

In EG2, the intervention had limited effects. No significant changes were observed between baseline and final values in most sleep components, such as sleep quality, sleep duration, sleep efficiency, sleep medication use, and Fatigue Severity Scale. The global sleep quality score (PSQI) decreased slightly, with a low effect size of 0.09 points, and the fatigue state remained at the same value.

Table 7. Comparison of the parameters between the initial and final moment within EG1 and EG2, respectively.

Component	Paired-Sample Statistics						Paired-Sample Test		
			Mean		SD				
	Group	N	Initial	Final	Initial	Final	t	df	*p*
Sleep Quality	EG1	30	2.07	1.53	0.740	0.571	5.757	29	0.000
	EG2	30	1.83 [a]	1.83 [a]	0.834	0.834			
Sleep latency	EG1	30	1.67	1.37	1.155	0.928	3.525	29	0.001
	EG2	30	0.80	0.77	0.925	0.898	1.000	29	0.326
Sleeping duration	EG1	30	1.63	1.20	1.098	0.961	4.709	29	0.000
	EG2	30	1.20 [a]	1.20 [a]	0.761	0.761			
Sleep efficiency	EG1	30	1.73	1.10	1.143	0.995	4.289	29	0.000
	EG2	30	1.03 [a]	1.03 [a]	1.066	1.066			
Sleep disturbance	EG1	30	1.67	1.57	0.547	0.568	1.795	29	0.083
	EG2	30	1.57	1.53	0.504	0.507	1.000	29	0.326
Use of sleeping medication	EG1	30	0.63	0.47	0.890	0.776	2.408	29	0.023
	EG2	30	0.50 [a]	0.50 [a]	0.731	0.731			
Daytime dysfunction	EG1	30	1.97	1.53	0.765	0.571	4.709	29	0.000
	EG2	30	1.93	1.90	0.828	0.803	1.000	29	0.326

[a] The correlation and t cannot be computed because the standard error of the difference is 0; N = the number of patients; SD = standard deviation; t = the *t*-test of the difference in means; df = the difference between the two values; *p* = statistical significance coefficient.

In Table 8, regarding the comparison of the two groups at baseline, significant differences can be observed between EG1 and EG2 for sleep latency, sleep efficiency, PSQI global score, and FSS score. EG1 shows poorer sleep quality and more sleep-related problems compared to EG2. However, no significant differences were observed for sleep quality, sleep disturbances, sleep medication use, and daytime dysfunction. The results of the final evaluation show significant differences between the EG1 and EG2 regarding sleep latency and daytime dysfunction. EG1 had higher latency and lower diurnal dysfunction compared to EG2. Regarding sleep quality, sleep duration, sleep efficiency, sleep disturbances, use of sleep medication, PSQI total score, or FSS total score, no significant differences were observed between the two groups ($p > 0.05$). During the sleep analysis, it can be seen that the patients in EG2 with more negative symptoms have significant improvements regarding latency and daytime dysfunctions compared to the less symptomatic patients in group 2.

Table 8. Comparison of parameters between the two groups at baseline and endpoint (independent samples test).

Component	*p*	
	Initial	Final
Sleep Quality	0.256	0.109
Sleep latency	0.002	0.014
Sleeping duration	0.081	1.000
Sleep efficiency	0.017	0.803

Table 8. *Cont.*

Component	p	
	Initial	Final
Sleep disturbance	0.464	0.811
Use of Sleeping Medication	0.529	0.865
Daytime dysfunction	0.872	0.046
PSQI total	0.048	0.899
FSS total	0.020	0.916

p = statistical significance coefficient.

4. Discussion

The specialized literature confirms the need for more in-depth studies regarding the management of fibromyalgia, especially regarding beneficial therapeutic measures to improve the inner state. Although this study has some limitations, especially the short period of the intervention, significant results can be observed in the case of the multidisciplinary intervention, as the sessions were conducted daily. This study has clinical importance due to the novelty of comparing these two types of intervention.

In terms of age and gender correlation with treatment efficacy, there is no clinical connection, with improvement occurring on average equally across all ages.

The homogeneity of the groups in terms of age, gender, muscle mass index, pharmacological treatment, and felt symptoms demonstrates that the changes occurring during the treatment are due only to the recovery intervention.

In terms of symptoms, FM patients show symptoms of fatigue, headaches, paresthesias, myalgias, irritable bowel syndrome, micturition disorders, cognitive and sleep disorders including depression and anxiety that lead to the inability to perform daily activities [54]. These symptoms are also present in the study carried out, in different percentages, each having a role in maintaining chronic pain that leads to a state of general fatigue and disturbed sleep quality.

The use of massage as a decontracting means applied externally to the body helps to reduce the state of muscle tension and stops the stagnation of non-oxygenated blood; patients have a more efficient sleep, managing to fall asleep faster and maintain sleep for a longer period. Electrotherapy applied by means of low-frequency currents has effects on the production of endorphins, reducing pain, the results of the intervention indicating a significant reduction in the use of sleep medications. Exercises for resistance, muscle strengthening, and flexibility help to stimulate circulation and better oxygenation, which reduces fatigue and diminishes the diurnal dysfunctions that most patients face when performing daily activities. Thus, by using these techniques alongside hydrokinetotherapy, which through the action of water reduces physical stress, the fatigue–restless sleep cycle is inhibited. The quality of sleep being improved, the accumulated fatigue is also reduced. Overall, the intervention in the case of EG1 had beneficial effects on the studied variables.

The induction of relaxation through the internal rebalancing of the body based on breathing and muscle rest has limited effects ($p > 0.05$) in the short term on the quality of sleep, slightly improving by eliminating the state of tension during the period of maintaining sleep and helping to reduce diurnal dysfunctions and disorders that occur during sleep, but the difference compared to the first group is visible at the level of fatigue, the patients not having improvements in this chapter.

Regarding within-group variations, at EG1, the decrease in mean score indicates an improvement in patient-reported fatigue between the two assessments, with a general trend observed and improvement in fatigue symptoms for most participants, not just those with score extremes. The standard deviation decreased from 10.811 to 8.763, suggesting a leveling of fatigue severity across participants. At the beginning, the variability of the scores was greater, but at the end, the differences between the participants became smaller, which may indicate a generalized and more even improvement. The decrease in values for each component and the total PSQI suggests an overall improvement in sleep quality and a reduction in sleep-related problems following the intervention.

Intra-group variations within EG2 show that there is no change in the mean score between the initial and final assessment, suggesting that the intervention did not influence the participants' perceived level of fatigue. Both the mean and median constants indicate that the fatigue felt by the group remained uniform before and after. The standard deviation of 12.820 indicates moderate variability between participants, both at baseline and at follow-up.

Referring to the purpose of this study, we can conclude that a multidisciplinary therapy has meaningful effects on FM patients, while the recovery based only on relaxation does not focus on all the weak points of the patients; in this case, the hypothesis is not confirmed. The results of this study have clinical relevance and help specialists in the field to improve management.

Contextualizing the obtained results, the influence of different recovery procedures on fatigue and sleep quality can be seen below. Fibromyalgia has a low incidence; most studies in the specialized literature are conducted on a small sample. The author Andrade C. [55] et al. looked at the effects of water training in women with fibromyalgia. After the 16 weeks of intervention, the amount of VO2 increased in the experimental group ($p = 0.04$), the pressure pain threshold increased ($p = 0.02$), but the effects on sleep quality were insignificant. In this study, it was concluded that aquatic exercises improve cardiovascular function but have no significant effects on the other variables. However, aquatic exercise combined with individual physical therapy, manual therapy, and electrotherapy by EG1 produced a significant difference ($p = 0.00$) between ratings, suggesting a significant decrease in sleep severity. In another article by Hauser et al. [56], it was concluded that aerobic exercises combined with flexibility and muscle-strengthening exercises do not have significant effects on sleep quality (SMD = 0.01), while Steffens et al. [57] showed that aerobic exercise combined with hydrokinetotherapy has a moderate effect on improving sleep quality. Also, Kundakci et al. [58] found that strength training has significant effects of improving sleep quality with a moderate clinical effect (SMD = −0.74), and Busch et al. [59] reached the same conclusion about aerobic exercises. The author Cuenca-Martinez F. et al. [60] explained that relaxation exercises combined with aerobic and strength exercises bring about a real improvement in the quality of sleep that will lead to an improvement in the quality of life, compared to recovery programs isolated.

The author Nadal et al. [61], following the effects of manual therapy, concluded that there are no significant improvements regarding FSS and PSQI, the p-value being greater than 0.05, but this form of therapy decreases the perception of pain, thus concluding that interventions based on relaxation, both intrinsic and extrinsic through massage, do not change the state of fatigue.

Strengths and Limitations of This Study

As, to our knowledge, this is the first study in Romania comparing two types of intervention on patients diagnosed with FM, this is also the strength of our study.

This study has limitations regarding the short duration and the small number of patients due to the incidence of FM because the diagnosis is very difficult to make, and patients find out the exact cause over several years. Short intervention periods are due to country legislation because Romanian legislation only offers 10 free recovery sessions for 2 weeks, once every 6 months. To carry out this study over a longer period, it would have been necessary to change the location, which involved giving up hydrokinetotherapy. EG2 had the same limitation in terms of recovery time because it was desired to follow the effectiveness of two different programs in the same number of sessions. Conducting recovery sessions at home has both positive effects in terms of the psychological state and stress being eliminated, as well as negative effects caused by the lack of permanent supervision. These limitations, together with the performance of a single procedure alone, attracted lower clinical improvements compared to group 1.

To observe the long-term results, the patients in experimental group 1 will be re-evaluated 6 months after the intervention, and the patients in experimental group 2 received the recommendation to continue the relaxation technique at home for 6 months, monitored online by a physiotherapist to avoid biases. The purpose of continuing the program is to observe if a treatment based on a single form of relaxation can improve the state of fatigue by acting on sleep, following this period to begin multidisciplinary treatment if no beneficial results appear on the variables evaluated.

5. Conclusions

Due to the unclear pathogenesis of fibromyalgia, the multidisciplinary approach focused on improving flexibility, extrinsic relaxation, and muscle tone has better effectiveness on sleep quality than therapy focused only on intrinsic relaxation. Although the intervention was of a short duration, the daily sessions made an increased contribution to the recovery. This study offers a new perspective on the integration of simple recovery programs in chronic pathologies. The clinical relevance of our findings helps specialists have better management of FM, since better quality of sleep ultimately improves the quality of life.

Author Contributions: Conceptualization, T.F.B., A.P. and M.M.; methodology, T.F.B. and C.D.N.-C.; software, T.F.B.; validation, A.P., F.L.A.-C., D.I.C. and E.T.; formal analysis, E.T. and M.M.; investigation, T.F.B.; writing—original draft preparation, T.F.B., A.P., G.C. and M.M.; writing—review and editing, E.T., D.I.C., F.L.A.-C. and C.D.N.-C. All authors have read and agreed to the published version of the manuscript.

Funding: The APC was founded by the University of Oradea, Oradea, Romania.

Institutional Review Board Statement: The research was carried out in accordance with the ethical principles of the Nuremberg Code, the Declaration of Helsinki with its amendments, and the approval of the Ethics Commission of the Faculty of Medicine and Pharmacy, Oradea, number 22 of 26 February 2021.

Informed Consent Statement: The documentation of the entire research activity was carried out in compliance with the principles and norms of ethics, the documents prepared for carrying out the activity being kept and archived.

Data Availability Statement: Data is contained within the article.

Acknowledgments: The authors wish to thank the University of Oradea for supporting the payment of the invoice through an internal project.

Conflicts of Interest: The authors declare no conflicts of interest.

References

1. Teodoro, T.; Edwards, M.J.; Isaacs, J.D. A unifying theory for cognitive abnormalities in functional neurological disorders, fibromyalgia and chronic fatigue syndrome: Systematic review. *J. Neurol. Neurosurg. Psychiatry* **2018**, *89*, 1308–1319. [CrossRef] [PubMed]

2. Metyas, C.; Aung, T.T.; Cheun, J.; Joseph, M.; Ballester, A.M.; Metyas, S. Diet and Lifestyle Modifications for Fibromyalgia. *Curr. Rheumatol. Rev.* **2024**, *20*, 405–413. [CrossRef] [PubMed]
3. Wolfe, F.; Rasker, J.J. The Evolution of Fibromyalgia, Its Concepts, and Criteria. *Cureus* **2021**, *13*, e20010. [CrossRef] [PubMed]
4. O'Brien, A.T.; Deitos, A.; Trinane Pego, Y.; Fregni, F.; Carrillo-de-la-Pena, M.T. Defective Endogenous Pain Modulation in Fibromyalgia: A Meta-Analysis of Temporal Summation and Conditioned Pain Modulation Paradigms. *J. Pain* **2018**, *19*, 819–836. [CrossRef] [PubMed]
5. Treede, R.-D.; Rief, W.; Barke, A.; Aziz, Q.; Bennett, M.I.; Benoliel, R.; Cohen, M.; Evers, S.; Finnerup, N.B.; First, M.B.; et al. Chronic pain as a symptom or a disease: The IASP Classification of Chronic Pain for the International Classification of Diseases (ICD-11). *Pain* **2019**, *160*, 19–27. [CrossRef] [PubMed]
6. Clauw, D.; Sarzi-Puttini, P.; Pellegrino, G.; Shoenfeld, Y. Is fibromyalgia an autoimmune disorder? *Autoimmun. Rev.* **2024**, *23*, 103424. [CrossRef]
7. Vierck, C.J., Jr. Mechanisms underlying development of spatially distributed chronic pain (fibromyalgia). *J. Pain* **2006**, *124*, 242–263. [CrossRef] [PubMed]
8. Meyer, H.P. Myofascial pain syndrome and its suggested role in the pathogenesis and treatment of fibromyalgia syndrome. *Curr. Pain Headache Rep.* **2002**, *6*, 274–283. [CrossRef]
9. Bradley, L.A. Pathophysiology of fibromyalgia. *Am. J. Med.* **2009**, *122* (Suppl. S12), S22–S30. [CrossRef]
10. Gyorfi, M.; Rupp, A.; Abd-Elsayed, A. Fibromyalgia Patophysiology. *Biomedicine* **2022**, *10*, 3070. [CrossRef]
11. Bhargava, J.; Hurley, J.A. *Fibromialgie*; Editura StatPearls: Treasure Island, FL, USA, 2021.
12. Siracusa, R.; Paola, R.D.; Cuzzocrea, S.; Impellizzeri, D. Fibromyalgia: Pathogenesis, Mechanisms, Diagnosis and Treatment Options Update. *Int. J. Mol. Sci.* **2021**, *22*, 3891. [CrossRef]
13. Macfarlane, G.J.; Kronisch, C.; Dean, L.E.; Atzeni, F.; Häuser, W.; Fluß, E.; Choy, E.; Kosek, E.; Amris, K.; Branco, J.; et al. EULAR revised recommendations for the management of fibromyalgia. *Ann. Rheum. Dis.* **2017**, *76*, 318–328. [CrossRef]
14. Jones, E.A.; Asaad, F.; Patel, N.; Jain, E.; Abd-Elsayed, A. Management of Fibromyalgia: An Update. *Biomedicines* **2024**, *12*, 1266. [CrossRef] [PubMed]
15. Alorfi, N.M. Pharmacological treatments of fibromyalgia in adults; overview of phase IV clinical trials. *Front. Pharmacol.* **2022**, *13*, 1017129. [CrossRef] [PubMed]
16. Chen, J.; Han, B.; Wu, C. On the superiority of a combination of aerobic and resistance exercise for fibromyalgia syndrome: A network meta-analysis. *Front. Psychol.* **2022**, *13*, 949256. [CrossRef] [PubMed]
17. Couto, N.; Monteiro, D.; Cid, L.; Bento, T. Effect of different types of exercise in adult subjects with fibromyalgia: A systematic review and meta-analysis of randomised clinical trials. *Sci. Rep.* **2022**, *12*, 10391. [CrossRef]
18. Tangen, S.F.; Helvik, A.S.; Eide, H.; Fors, E.A. Pain acceptance and its impact on function and symptoms in fibromyalgia. *Scand. J. Pain.* **2020**, *20*, 727–736. [CrossRef] [PubMed]
19. Steen, J.P.; Kannan, V.; Zaidi, A.; Cramer, H.; Ng, J.Y. Mind-body therapy for treating fibromyalgia: A sys-tematic review. *Pain Med.* **2024**, *25*, 703–737. [CrossRef]
20. Pieczynski, J.; Cosio, D.; Pierce, W.; Serpa, J.G. Mind-Body Interventions for Rehabilitation Medicine: Promoting Wellness, Healing, and Coping with Adversity. *Phys. Med. Rehabil. Clin. N. Am.* **2020**, *31*, 563–575. [CrossRef]
21. Relaxation Techniques: What You Need To Know [Internet]. National Center for Com-plementary and Integrative Health. 2021. Available online: https://www.nccih.nih.gov/health/relaxation-techniques-what-you-need-to-know (accessed on 17 January 2024).
22. Cohen-Biton, L.; Buskila, D.; Nissanholtz-Gannot, R. Review of Fibromyalgia (FM) Syndrome Treatments. *Int. J. Environ. Res. Public Health* **2022**, *19*, 12106. [CrossRef] [PubMed]
23. Paolucci, T.; de Sire, A.; Ferrillo, M.; di Fabio, D.; Molluso, A.; Patruno, A.; Pesce, M.; Lai, C.; Ciacchella, C.; Saggino, A.; et al. Telerehabilitation proposal of mind-body technique for physical and psychological outcomes in patients with fibromyalgia. *Front. Physiol.* **2022**, *13*, 917956. [CrossRef] [PubMed]
24. Meulenberg, C.J.W.; de Bruin, E.D.; Marusic, U. A perspective on implementation of technology-driven exergames for adults as telerehabilitation services. *Front. Psychol.* **2022**, *13*, 840863. [CrossRef] [PubMed]
25. Theadom, A.; Cropley, M.; Smith, H.E.; Feigin, V.L.; McPherson, K. Mind and body therapy for fibromyalgia. *Cochrane Database Syst. Rev.* **2015**, *2015*, CD001980. [CrossRef] [PubMed]
26. Haugmark, T.; Hagen, K.B.; Smedslund, G.; Zangi, H.A. Mindfulness- and acceptance-based interventions for patients with fibromyalgia—A systematic review and meta-analyses. *PLoS ONE* **2019**, *14*, e0221897. [CrossRef]
27. Agostini, F.; Mangone, M.; Ruiu, P.; Paolucci, T.; Santilli, V.; Bernetti, A. Rehabilitation setting during and after Covid-19: An overview on recommendations. *J. Rehabil. Med.* **2021**, *53*, jrm00141. [CrossRef] [PubMed]
28. Cankurtaran, D.; Tezel, N.; Ercan, B.; Yildiz, S.Y.; Akyuz, E.U. The effects of COVID-19 fear and anxiety on symptom severity, sleep quality, and mood in patients with fibromyalgia: A pilot study. *Adv. Rheumatol.* **2021**, *61*, 41. [CrossRef]

29. Paul, J.K.; Iype, T.; Dileep, R.; Hagiwara, Y.; Koh, J.W.; Acharya, U.R. Characterization of fibromyalgia using sleep EEG signals with nonlinear dynamical features. *Comput. Biol. Med.* **2019**, *111*, 103331. [CrossRef] [PubMed]
30. Haack, M.; Sanchez, E.; Mullington, J.M. Elevated inflammatory markers in response to prolonged sleep restriction are associated with increased pain experience in healthy volunteers. *Sleep* **2007**, *30*, 1145–1152. [CrossRef]
31. Kleinman, L.; Mannix, S.; Arnold, L.M.; Burbridge, C.; Howard, K.; McQuarrie, K.; Pitman, V.; Resnick, M.; Roth, T.; Symonds, T. Assessment of sleep in patients with fibromyalgia: Qualitative development of the fibromyalgia sleep diary. *Health Qual. Life Outcomes* **2014**, *12*, 111. [CrossRef] [PubMed]
32. Wagner, J.-S.; DiBonaventura, M.D.; Chandran, A.B.; Cappelleri, J.C. The association of sleep difficulties with health-related quality of life among patients with fibromyalgia. *BMC Musculoskelet. Disord.* **2012**, *13*, 199. [CrossRef] [PubMed]
33. Kline, C. Sleep Quality. In *Encyclopedia of Behavioral Medicine*; Gellman, M.D., Turner, J.R., Eds.; Springer International Publishing: Cham, Switzerland, 2013; pp. 1811–1813. [CrossRef]
34. Mannerkorpi, K.; Gard, G. Hinders for continued work among persons with fibromyalgia. *BMC Musculoskelet. Disord.* **2012**, *13*, 96. [CrossRef] [PubMed]
35. Lawson, K. Sleep Dysfunction in Fibromyalgia and Therapeutic Approach Options. *OBM Neurobiol.* **2020**, *4*, 49. [CrossRef]
36. Okifuji, A.; Bradshaw, D.H.; Donaldson, G.W.; Turk, D.C. Sequential analyses of daily symptoms in women with fibromyalgia syndrome. *J. Pain* **2011**, *12*, 84–93. [CrossRef] [PubMed]
37. Wu, Y.L.; Chang, L.Y.; Lee, H.C.; Fang, S.C.; Tsai, P.S. Sleep disturbances in fibromyalgia. A meta-analysis of case-control studies. *J. Psychosom. Res.* **2017**, *96*, 89–97. [CrossRef]
38. Bennett, R.M.; Jones, J.; Turk, D.C.; Russell, I.J.; Matallana, L. An internet survey of 2,596 people with fibromyalgia. *BMC Musculoskelet. Disord.* **2007**, *8*, 27. [CrossRef] [PubMed]
39. Finan, P.H.; Goodin, B.R.; Smith, M.T. The association of sleep and pain: An update and a path forward. *J. Pain* **2013**, *14*, 1539–1552. [CrossRef] [PubMed]
40. Clauw, D.J. Fibromyalgia and related conditions. *Mayo Clin. Proc.* **2015**, *90*, 680–692. [CrossRef] [PubMed]
41. Sañudo, B.; Galiano, D.; Carrasco, L.; Blagojevic, M.; Hoyo, M.; Saxton, J. Aerobic Exercise Versus Combined Exercise Therapy in Women With Fibromyalgia Syndrome: A Randomized. *Arch. Phys. Med. Rehabil.* **2010**, *91*, 1838–1843. [CrossRef]
42. Assumpçao, A.; Matsutani, L.A.; Yuan, S.L.; Santo, A.S.; Sauer, J.; Mango, P.; Marques, A.P. Muscle stretching exercises and resistance training in fibromyalgia: Which is better? *A three-arm randomized controlled trial. Eur. J. Phys. Rehabil. Med.* **2017**, *54*, 663–670.
43. Jones, K.D.; Burckhardt, C.S.; Clark, S.R.; Bennett, R.M.; Potempa, K.M. A randomized controlled trial of muscle strengthening versus flexibility training in fibromyalgia. *J. Rheumatol.* **2002**, *29*, 1041–1048.
44. Maindet, C.; Maire, A.; Vermorel, C.; Cracowski, C.; Rolland, C.; Forestier, R.; Comte, A.; Roques, C.F.; Serra, E.; Bosson, J.L. Spa Therapy for the Treatment of Fibromyalgia: An Open, Randomized Multicenter Trial. *J. Pain* **2021**, *22*, 940–951. [CrossRef] [PubMed]
45. Neelapala, Y.V.R.; Mercuri, D.; Macedo, L.; Hanna, S.; Kobsar, D.; Carlesso, L. Mechanisms hypothesized for pain-relieving effects of exercise in fibromyalgia: A scoping review. *Ther. Adv. Musculoskelet. Dis.* **2023**, *15*, 1759720X231182894. [CrossRef]
46. Bidonde, J.; Busch, A.J.; Schachter, C.L.; Overend, T.J.; Kim, S.Y.; Góes, S.M.; Boden, C.; Foulds, H.J.; Cochrane Musculoskeletal Group. Mixed exercise training for adults with fibromyalgia. *Cochrane Database Syst. Rev.* **2019**, *5*, CD013340. [CrossRef]
47. Kalichman, L. Massage therapy for fibromyalgia symptoms. *Rheumatol. Int.* **2010**, *30*, 1151–1157. [CrossRef]
48. Bidonde, J.; Busch, A.J.; Webber, S.C.; Schachter, C.L.; Danyliw, A.; Overend, T.J.; Richards, R.S.; Rader, T. Aquatic exercise training for fibromyalgia. *Cochrane Database Syst. Rev.* **2014**, *2014*, CD011336. [CrossRef] [PubMed]
49. Bungau, S.G.; Popa, V.-C. Between religion and science: Some aspects: Concerning illness and healing in antiquity. *Transylv. Rev.* **2015**, *26*, 3–19.
50. de Silva Salazar, A.P.; Stein, C.; Marchese, R.R.; Plentz, R.D.M.; Pagnussat, A.D.S. Electric Stimulation for Pain Relief in Patients with Fibromyalgia: A Systematic Review and Meta-analysis of Randomized Controlled Trials. *Pain Physician.* **2017**, *20*, 15–25. [CrossRef]
51. Krupp, L.B.; LaRocca, N.G.; Muir-Nash, J.; Steinberg, A.D. The fatigue severity scale: Application to patients with multiple sclerosis and systemic lupus erythematosus. *Arch. Neurol.* **1989**, *46*, 1121–1123. [CrossRef]
52. Nelson, K.L.; Davis, J.E.; Corbett, C.F. Sleep quality: An evolutionary concept analysis. *Nurs. Forum* **2022**, *57*, 144–151. [CrossRef] [PubMed]
53. Buysse, D.J.; Reynolds, C.F., 3rd; Monk, T.H.; Berman, S.R.; Kupfer, D.J. The Pittsburgh Sleep Quality Index: A new instrument for psychiatric practice and research. *Psychiatry Res.* **1989**, *28*, 193–213. [CrossRef] [PubMed]
54. Gerdle, B.; Bjork, J.; Coster, L.; Henriksson, K.; Henriksson, C.; Bengtsson, A. Prevalence of widespread pain and associations with work status: A population study. *BMC Musculoskelet. Disord.* **2008**, *9*, 102. [CrossRef]
55. Andrade, C.P.; Zamunér, A.R.; Forti, M.; Tamburús, N.Y.; Silva, E. Effects of aquatic training and detraining on women with fibromyalgia: Controlled randomized clinical trial. *Eur. J. Phys. Rehabil. Med.* **2019**, *55*, 79–88. [CrossRef]

56. Häuser, W.; Klose, P.; Langhorst, J.; Moradi, B.; Steinbach, M.; Schiltenwolf, M.; Busch, A. Efficacy of different types of aerobic exercise in fibromyalgia syndrome: A systematic review and meta-analysis of randomised controlled trials. *Arthritis Res. Ther.* **2010**, *12*, R79. [CrossRef] [PubMed]
57. Steffens, R.D.; Andrade, A.; Grisard, F.; Dominski, F.H.; de Orleans Casagrande, P. Efeitos dos exercícios físicos no sono de pacientes com síndrome da fibromialgia: Revisao sistematica. *ConScientiae Saúde* **2014**, *13*, 298–304. [CrossRef]
58. Kundakci, B.; Kaur, J.; Goh, S.L.; Hall, M.; Doherty, M.; Zhang, W.; Abhishek, A. Efficacy of nonpharmacological interventions for individual features of fibromyalgia: A systematic review and meta-analysis of randomised controlled trials. *Pain* **2022**, *163*, 1432–1445. [CrossRef] [PubMed]
59. Busch, A.J.; Schachter, C.L.; Overend, T.J.; Peloso, P.M.; Barber, K.A.R. Exercise for Fibromyalgia: A systematic review. *J. Rheumatol.* **2008**, *35*, 1130–1144.
60. Cuenca-Martínez, F.; Suso-Martí, L.; Fernández-Carnero, J.; Muñoz-Alarcos, V.; Sempere-Rubio, N. Exercise-based interventions on sleep quality in patients with fibromyalgia syndrome: An umbrella and mapping review with meta-analysis. *Semin. Arthritis Rheum.* **2023**, *61*, 152216. [CrossRef]
61. Nadal-Nicolás, Y.; Rubio-Arias, J.Á.; Martínez-Olcina, M.; Reche-García, C.; Hernández-García, M.; Martínez-Rodríguez, A. Effects of Manual Therapy on Fatigue, Pain, and Psychological Aspects in Women with Fibromyalgia. *Int. J. Environ. Res. Public Health* **2020**, *17*, 4611. [CrossRef] [PubMed]

medicina

Article

Evaluation of Hypertension-Related Knowledge, Medication Adherence, and Associated Factors Among Hypertensive Patients in the Aljouf Region, Saudi Arabia: A Cross-Sectional Study

Bashayer Farhan ALruwaili

Department of Family and Community Medicine, College of Medicine, Jouf University, Sakaka 72388, Saudi Arabia; bfalrwili@ju.edu.sa; Tel.: +966-551913665

Abstract: *Background and Objectives:* Hypertensive patients' knowledge and adherence to prescribed medicines are critical in managing their condition, as poor adherence may lead to adverse cardiac and cerebrovascular events. The present study assessed hypertension-related knowledge and medication adherence among hypertensive patients attending primary health centers (PHCs) in the Aljouf Province, Saudi Arabia. *Materials and Methods:* Using a cross-sectional design, we conducted this survey on 390 patients. Self-reported hypertension knowledge was assessed using the Hypertension Knowledge Level Scale (HK-LS), and medication adherence was determined using the Hill–Bone Medication Adherence Scale. We used binomial regression analysis (adjusted with other variables) to find the associated factors of medication adherence. *Results:* This study found that nearly half (49.2%) of the participants had inadequate knowledge, and poor medication adherence was noted in 40.8% of the participants. We found a positive correlation between HK-LS and the Hill–Bone Medication Adherence Scale scores (Spearman's rho = 0.312, p = 0.002). Medication adherence was significantly associated with job status (private sector (ref: public sector, adjusted odds ratio [AOR] = 2.02, 95% CI = 1.18–3.62, p = 0.005)), living in an urban region (ref: rural, AOR = 3.61, 95% CI = 1.85–5.72, p = 0.002), and duration since diagnosis of more than 5 years (ref: $\leq$1 year, AOR = 3.53, 95% CI = 2.36–4.95, p = 0.001). *Conclusions:* The present study findings indicate that there is still a critical gap in managing hypertension at the PHCs in this region, and this may lead to poor health outcomes among the patients and burden the healthcare system. Hence, continuous patient education and targeted counseling are recommended for those with poor medication adherence.

Keywords: adherence; diet; knowledge; hypertension; patient education

1. Introduction

Globally, hypertension remains an important public health problem, and about 1.3 billion adults suffer from this chronic condition [1,2]. Nevertheless, the prevalence rate varies across countries, with a higher rate in low- and middle-income nations [3,4]. This scenario is further worsened by the persistent concepts of the "rule of halves" in hypertension [5]. Additionally, this chronic condition is one of the major modifiable risk factors (preventable) for adverse cardiac and cerebrovascular events in adults [6,7]. Similar to the current global situation, this chronic condition is highly prevalent in the Kingdom of Saudi Arabia (KSA); a recent study by Alshammari SA et al. documented that hypertension is highly prevalent (above 22%) among Saudi adults [8].

The management, diagnosis, and prevention of hypertension are influenced by several factors. A lack of understanding and awareness of hypertension and its implications is the main barrier to diagnosis and adequate treatment [9,10]. The existing literature indicates that patients play vital roles in managing hypertension through a holistic approach, including lifestyle changes, regular follow-up, and compliance with the physician's recommendations [11,12]. According to the International Society of Hypertension and the National Institute for Health and Care Excellence (NICE) in London, adhering to prescribed anti-hypertensive drugs is essential for achieving appropriate hypertension control, which lowers healthcare expenditures and reduces cardiovascular morbidity and mortality [13,14].

Adherence to prescribed hypertensive medication is facilitated by numerous factors [15]. These factors are generally divided into sociodemographic, patient-related (such as knowledge), and available healthcare facilities. In the context of health literacy, patients' knowledge plays a central role in hypertension control, including medication adherence [16,17]. Numerous authors have used different methods to explore hypertension-related knowledge among patients. However, culturally suitable scales have yielded valid and reliable results [18,19]. A comparative study conducted by Eshah N F et al. among Jordanian participants showed that good knowledge was observed in the majority of their participants [20]. However, their participants showed inadequate knowledge in some domains, such as diet and lifestyle. Similarly, a study conducted by Abu H et al. in two primary clinics found that patients lacked knowledge about the lifelong condition of hypertension [21]. A recent study in 2024 conducted in the southern region of the KSA found that most of the hypertensive patients had poor knowledge overall in several domains, including medication compliance [22]. Health promotion and disease prevention are emphasized as crucial areas to enhance treatment quality and control costs in the Arab world in hypertension awareness campaigns [8]. According to research conducted in Poland, about 85% of patients correctly identified high blood pressure, but over two-thirds did not know that once diagnosed, hypertension is lifelong, and one-third did not know that hypertension can cause kidney impairment [23].

Healthcare related to hypertension has achieved significant advancement with different strategies of screening programs, the availability of new-generation anti-hypertensive medications, and personalized care [24,25]. Nonetheless, medication adherence remains a critical unresolved issue in hypertension control and improving patients' health outcomes. As mentioned earlier, researchers have noted several barriers and facilitators. Globally, different tools were used to assess the medication adherence among the patients. These tools are either generic or hypertension-specific [26–28].

Regardless of the tools used by different authors, the proportion of adherence among hypertensive patients is low across the different countries, and there is a wide variation. This warrants the necessity of region-specific data related to these aspects, which is crucial. Furthermore, due to the dynamic nature of the influencing factors of adherence, it is highly relevant to assess the medication adherence practice and influencing factors regularly to guide practitioners and policymakers in implementing necessary programs or amending existing programs according to the latest available data. In this context, the present study aimed to assess hypertension-related disease knowledge, medication adherence, and associated influencing factors among patients from the Aljouf region, the KSA. Moreover, we determined the correlation between hypertension-related disease knowledge and medication adherence using appropriate statistical tests.

2. Materials and Methods

2.1. Study Design and Setting

This cross-sectional survey was conducted in the Aljouf Province, the KSA, from May 2024 to September 2024. This province has four main regions: Sakaka, Dwamat Aljindal, Tabarjil, and Qurrayat. According to KSA's statistics, about half a million people live in this region. The present study includes adult (18 years and above) primary hypertensive patients of Saudi nationals from all the primary health centers (PHCs) of the two regions (Sakaka and Dwamat Aljindal). The survey excluded those who had known secondary hypertension, pediatric hypertensive patients, hospitalized patients, unwilling (to participate) patients, and known psychiatric patients. Furthermore, the author excluded those who managed their hypertension only through lifestyle modifications.

2.2. Sampling Description

The author calculated the sample size using an online calculator that followed the principles of standard sample size protocols ($n = z^2pq/e^2$) [29]. In this formula, n = the minimum required sample size. Considering that half of the patients (50%) have good adherence (p = 0.5, and q = 0.5 [1 − p]), 80% power of the study, 95% confidence interval, and 5% margin of error), the authors concluded that to obtain conclusive evidence, there must be a minimum of 384 hypertensive patients participating in the survey. Moreover, this formula was applied to an infinite population. The 50% expected proportion was taken as a standard method to obtain the highest number of samples. We used the convenience sampling method to recruit the study participants. In this method, the patients visiting the selected PHCs were asked to participate in the survey after the follow-up checkup. To ensure that the participants were distributed over the study period, this survey included only five participants per day in one PHC.

2.3. Data Collection Procedures

Data collection started after clearance from the Local Committee for Bioethics, Jouf University (No. 13-09-45, dated 12 May 2024). For data collection, the author coordinated with the concerned family physicians from the selected PHCs. For this study, the data collectors were given standardized training to collect data from hypertensive patients. This study followed all the ethical guidelines according to the Declaration of Helinski. After receiving the patients' informed consent, we requested that they complete the survey through a Google form on data collectors' electronic devices. The data collection form included three sections. The first section asked for the hypertensive patients' background information. The second section included 22 hypertension-related questions (ranging from etiology to complication) using a hypertension knowledge level scale (HK-LS) that assessed the patient's knowledge [20]. The author obtained permission to use the Arabic tool from the corresponding author of the published manuscript. The participants responded to each item as "correct/wrong/not sure". The correct answers were given as one mark. For further analysis, the total score was summed and converted into a number out of 100. A higher score in the knowledge section indicated better knowledge.

The final section determined the patients' medication adherence and refill practices. To determine these aspects, we used the Hill–Bone Medication Adherence Scale (9-item). This tool was created by the National Institute of Health and is freely available [30]. Previous studies that used this tool for assessing medication adherence among hypertensive patients stated that this tool is valid and reliable [30,31]. This tool was originally prepared in English. Using appropriate measures, we translated this tool into Arabic. Regarding the questions posed to the patients involved in this section, we asked them to respond on a four-point Likert scale with the following responses: all the time (1 mark), most of the time (2 marks), sometimes (3 marks), and not at all (4 marks). Like the knowledge section, the total marks were added and then transformed into a number within 100. The higher the score, the better the medication adherence practice. The present study's data collection tool was pre-tested on 31 hypertensive patients to determine cultural adaptability. The Cronbach's alpha values for the knowledge and medication adherence sections were 0.83 and 0.89, respectively. The knowledge scores were categorized into low (<median) and high (≥median). Regarding adherence, we categorized the scores into poor (less than 80% of the overall score) and good adherence (80% or more of the overall score) [32,33].

2.4. Data Analysis

This study's data were analyzed with the statistical package of social sciences (SPSS V. 21.0). The descriptive data are shown in frequencies and proportions for categorical variables, and the mean and standard deviation (SD) are used to depict the continuous data. The correlation between HK-LS and Hill–Bone Medication Adherence Scale scores was determined using Spearman's correlation analysis. The predictors of medication adherence (poor vs. good) were evaluated using binomial regression analysis, which is inherently a multivariate analysis method. In this method, the author attempted to evaluate the predictors after adjusting with the covariables of this study. The statistically significant value (alpha) was set as less than 0.05. Furthermore, binomial regression results are depicted as the adjusted odds ratio (AOR), 95% confidence interval (CI) of AOR, and p-values.

3. Results

During data collection, we asked 446 hypertensive patients to obtain the minimum required participants (390) for this survey (response rate: 87.4%). The background characteristics of the patients are shown in Table 1. Among 390 hypertensive patients, the majority (48.7%) belonged to the age bracket of 46 to 60 years (mean ± SD = 49.5 ± 11.2), were male (55.9%), worked in the public sector (47.2%), were from the urban side (76.7%), were non-smokers (63.3%), had an income from SAR 5000 to 10,000 (36.4%), and had hypertension diagnosed for 2 to 5 years (42.1%).

Table 1. Background characteristics of the patients (n = 390).

Variables	Frequency	Proportion
Age (mean ± SD)	49.5 ± 11.2	
Age group		
≤45 years	116	29.7
46 to 60 years	190	48.7
>60 years	84	21.5
Sex		
Male	218	55.9
Female	172	44.1
Education level		
Up to high school	175	44.9
Graduate and above	215	55.1
Job status		
Public sector	184	47.2
Private sector	124	31.8
Unemployed	33	8.5
Retired	49	12.6
Residence		
Urban	299	76.7
Rural	91	23.3
Monthly income *		
<5000	116	29.7
5000 to 10,000	142	36.4
>10,000	132	33.8
Smoking status		
Yes	143	36.7
No	247	63.3
Presence of other chronic diseases		
Yes	139	35.6
No	251	64.4
Duration since diagnosis (years)		
≤1	68	17.4
2 to 5	164	42.1
>5	158	40.5
Number of medications		
≤2	175	44.9
>2	215	55.1

* Data mentioned here are shown in Saudi Riyals (SAR) (USD 1 = SAR 3.75).

Participants' responses in HK-LS and the overall knowledge score are shown in Table 2. The highest proportion of participants responded correctly to the item related to cardiac complications associated with inadequate treatment (93.8%), followed by the necessity of lifelong anti-hypertensive medicine for most cases (89.7%) and cerebrovascular accident (stroke) risk of untreated hypertension (85.6%). However, the highest number of wrong answers were observed in the meat of choice (red meat—54.6% and white meat—52.3%) and the significance of a regular intake of fruits and vegetables (40.5%). The overall mean ± SD of the HK-LS was 15.56 ± 2.28. Of the studied patients, 49.2% had inadequate knowledge.

Table 2. Participants' responses according to the hypertension knowledge level scale (HK-LS) (n = 390).

Items	Correct Response n (%)	Wrong Response n (%)
An elevated diastolic pressure value denotes high blood pressure	293 (75.1)	97 (24.9)
Either systolic or diastolic pressure implies high blood pressure	309 (79.2)	81 (20.8)
Anti-hypertensive pills should be taken every day	317 (81.3)	73 (18.7)
High blood pressure medicines should be taken only when patients feel sick	235 (60.3)	155 (39.7)
In many cases, anti-hypertensive medicines should be taken for life	350 (89.7)	40 (10.3)
People with high blood pressure should take their medication to feel better	266 (68.2)	124 (31.8)
Lifestyle modifications are not required for patients with anti-hypertensive pills	292 (74.9)	98 (25.1)
Hypertension occurs due to growing old. Therefore, pills are not required	217 (55.6)	173 (44.4)
In many cases, if hypertensive patients adopt healthier lifestyle changes, medical treatment may not be necessary	268 (68.7)	122 (31.3)
Hypertensive patients can eat a salt-rich diet if they take medicines as prescribed	308 (79.0)	82 (21.0)
Smoking is not allowed for hypertensive patients	227 (58.2)	163 (41.8)
Hypertensive patients can drink alcohol regularly	300 (76.9)	90 (23.1)
Hypertensive patients must eat fruits and vegetables regularly	232 (59.5)	158 (40.5)
The best way to cook food is frying for patients with high blood pressure	324 (83.1)	66 (16.9)
The ideal cooking choice is boiling or grilling for patients	223 (57.2)	167 (42.8)
The ideal meat variety for high blood pressure patients is lean meat, such as chicken	186 (47.7)	204 (52.3)
The ideal meat option for patients with high blood pressure is red meat, such as beef	177 (45.4)	213 (54.6)
If we do not treat patients properly, they may die earlier due to complications	292 (74.9)	98 (25.1)
If we do not treat patients properly, patients may experience heart disease, such as heart attacks	366 (93.8)	24 (16.4)
If we do not treat patients properly, hypertensive patients may experience renal problems	326 (83.6)	64 (16.4)
If we do not treat patients properly, hypertensive patients may experience strokes (a cerebrovascular accident)	334 (85.6)	56 (14.4)
If we do not treat patients properly, patients may experience vision complications	227 (58.2)	163 (41.8)
Overall score: mean ± SD, median (IQR)	15.56 ± 2.28, 16 (3)	

Participants' responses to the Hill–Bone Medication Adherence Scale are presented in Table 3. The highest proportion of "not at all" (desired responses) observed was missed in taking anti-hypertensive medicines while feeling better (40.8%) and sick (40.5%). We observed that a sizable proportion of the participants missed their medications (all the time and most of the time) due to forgetfulness (8.2%) and running out of medication (8.2%). The overall mean ± SD of the HK-LS was 28.74 ± 4.46.

Table 3. Participant responses to the Hill–Bone Medication Adherence Scale (n = 390).

	All the Time n (%)	Most of the Time n (%)	Sometime n (%)	Not at All n (%)
Forgot to take anti-hypertensive tablets	16 (4.1)	16 (4.1)	289 (74.1)	69 (17.7)
Chose not to take blood pressure medicine	24 (6.2)	8 (2.1)	264 (67.7)	94 (24.1)
Forgot to refill anti-hypertensive medications	8 (2.1)	17 (4.4)	289 (74.1)	76 (19.5)
Ran out of blood pressure tablets	16 (4.1)	16 (4.1)	265 (67.9)	93 (23.8)
Skipped blood pressure medication before a doctor's visit	8 (2.1)	16 (4.1)	256 (65.6)	110 (28.2)
Missed taking blood pressure medicine while feeling better	8 (2.1)	8 (2.1)	215 (55.1)	159 (40.8)
Missed taking blood pressure medicine while feeling sick	16 (4.1)	8 (2.1)	208 (53.3)	158 (40.5)
Missed taking blood pressure medicine due to carelessness	24 (6.2)	8 (2.1)	231 (59.2)	127 (32.6)
Overall score: mean ± SD, median (IQR)	28.74 ± 4.66, 28 (4)			

According to the cut-off described in the methods, 40.8% of the participants had inadequately (poor) adhered to the prescribed anti-hypertensive medications.

The Spearman's correlation test revealed that HK-LS and Hill–Bone Medication Adherence Scale scores were positively correlated (rho = 0.314, p = 0.002) (Table 4).

Table 4. Spearman analysis results of HK-LS and Hill–Bone Medication Adherence Scale scores.

Correlation Variables	Spearman's Rho	p-Value (Two-Tailed)
HK-LS vs. Hill–Bone Medication Adherence Scale	0.314	0.002

The associated factors for medication adherence that were determined using the binomial logistic regression analysis are depicted in Table 5. After adjusting for other covariables of this study, we found that working in private sectors (AOR = 2.02, 95% CI = 1.18–3.62, p = 0.005), employment status (AOR = 1.42, 95% CI = 1.25–2.73, p = 0.017) (ref: public sector), urban living (ref: rural, AOR = 3.61, 95% CI = 1.85–5.72, p = 0.002), smoking status (ref: smokers, AOR = 0.45, 95% CI = 0.32–0.69, p = 0.015), duration since diagnosis of more than 5 years (ref: ≤1 year, AOR = 3.53, 95% CI = 2.36–4.95, p = 0.001), and adequate knowledge (ref: inadequate, AOR = 2.93, 95% CI = 1.88–4.09, p = 0.003) were significant associated factors (predictors) for medication adherence among hypertensive patients.

Table 5. Factors associated with medication adherence: test applied—binomial logistic regression (multivariate regression analysis) (n = 390).

Variables	Overall	Good (n = 231)	Poor (n = 159)	Binomial Regression Analysis Findings	
				Adjusted Odds Ratio ** (95% Confidence Interval)	p-Value
Age group					
≤45 years	116	57	59	Ref	
46 to 60 years	190	107	83	1.09 (0.48–2.18)	0.149
>60 years	84	67	17	2.31 (0.91–3. 25)	0.074
Sex					
Male	218	117	101	Ref	
Female	172	114	58	0.82 (0.43–1.69)	0.595

Table 5. *Cont.*

Variables	Overall	Good (n = 231)	Poor (n = 159)	Binomial Regression Analysis Findings	
				Adjusted Odds Ratio ** (95% Confidence Interval)	*p*-Value
Education level					
Up to high school	175	112	63	Ref	
Graduate and above	215	119	96	0.47 (0.23–1.27)	0.091
Job status					
Public sector	184	104	80	Ref	
Private sector	124	83	41	2.02 (1.18–3.62)	0.005
Unemployed	33	17	16	1.41 (1.25–2.73)	0.017
Retired	49	27	22	0.87 (0.63–1.57)	0.203
Residence					
Rural	91	54	37	Ref	
Urban	299	177	122	3.61 (1.85–5.72)	0.002
Monthly income *					
<5000	116	74	42	Ref	
5000 to 10,000	142	83	59	1.78 (0.76–3.12)	0.181
>10,000	132	74	58	2.13 (0.85–4.32)	0.103
Smoking status					
Yes	143	68	75	Ref	
No	247	163	84	0.45 (0.32–0.69)	0.015
Presence of other chronic diseases					
Yes	139	106	33	Ref	
No	251	125	126	1.35 (0.66–2.76)	0.412
Duration since diagnosis (years)					
≤1	68	33	35	Ref	
2 to 5	164	89	75	1.77 (0.83–3.91)	0.537
>5	158	109	49	3.53 (2.36–4.95)	0.001
Knowledge category					
Inadequate	192	98	94	Ref	
Adequate	198	133	65	2.93 (1.88–4.09)	0.003
Number of medications					
≤2	175	110	65	Ref	
>2	215	121	94	1.41 (0.87–3.30)	0.217

* USD 1 = SAR 3.75. ** Adjusted variables in the multivariate analysis: age group, sex, education level, job status, residence, monthly income, smoking status, presence of another chronic disease, duration since hypertension diagnosis, knowledge category, and number of anti-hypertensive medications.

4. Discussion

Hypertension continues to be one of the most significant public health problems worldwide and in the KSA. In addition to appropriate treatment, it is very important for the patients to have extensive knowledge and high adherence to the prescribed medications [1] so that an effective reduction in morbidity and mortality associated with hypertension can be achieved as a part of sustainable development goal 3 (target 3.4) [34]. In this context, this study aimed to assess the level of disease knowledge in various aspects, medication adherence to the prescribed pills, and factors influencing medication adherence in the Aljouf region, the KSA.

Adequate knowledge of all domains of any chronic disease is essential, as the patients are required to manage these conditions for life [16,35]. The present study demonstrated that a higher proportion of correct answers were observed in domains related to complications (such as cardiac, about 94%, and cerebrovascular (stroke risk), about 86%) that may occur for untreated or inadequately managed hypertensive patients. Similar to our findings, some studies from the KSA and other countries, such as Malaysia, found that a higher level of knowledge of the complications was associated with hypertension [20,36,37]. For instance, Alshammari SA et al. reported that their participants provided more than 80% correct responses for both cerebrovascular and cardiac complications [36]. The possible high awareness of complications among patients could be due to sufficient emphasis given by the family physicians on follow-up visits at the PHCs. However, this study found that there was a lower level of correct responses in the domains related to the importance of lifestyle changes, including diet, such as the best choice of meat and the importance of a regular intake of adequate fruits and vegetables. These findings are critical to policymakers' decisions to consider implementing counseling sessions for patients regarding diet and other lifestyle changes. It is also worth mentioning that Dash S et al. reported that there are numerous barriers to physicians delivering dietary advice to patients [38]. This further supports the present study's implications on the need for exclusive counseling sessions regarding diet and other lifestyle changes for patients. In contrast to the present study, some other studies have found different findings in assessing the dietary habits required for hypertension patients [38,39]. The possibility of these differences across the study could be differences in cultural settings, the tools used, and the availability of specific healthcare services at the PHCs.

Regarding medication adherence, we found that 6 to 8% of participants responded that they forget "all the time" about most of the items of the Hill–Bone Medication Adherence Scale. Similarly, less than half of the participants responded in all the domains of the scale as "not at all", which is the desired response for better adherence to the prescribed medicines. This finding is very critical for the family physicians at the primary health centers to ensure the highest proportion of desired responses in medication adherence domains. This can be achieved not only at the time of medical consultation at the clinics but also through teleconsultation as a part of follow-up and continuous patient education. Studies that used the same scale from different regions found varying findings [32,33,40]. Furthermore, using a cut-off value of 80%, we found that about 41% of the participants had poor medication adherence practices. The present survey's results are similar to those of some studies and contrast with others. For instance, a study by Stanikzai M H et al. found only a slightly higher proportion of non-adherence among their participants [33]. In contrast, Thirunavukkarasu A et al. [41], Khayyat SM et al. [42] from the KSA, Pan J et al. from China [40], and a critical review from the USA [15] found much higher non-adherence among hypertensive patients. These contrasting results across countries and within the regions of the KSA indicate that one size does not fit all, and tailored, region-specific interventions are required to enhance medication adherence. It is worth noting that similar to non-adherence to hypertension, poor medication adherence for diabetes mellitus patients was also observed by some authors [43,44].

The present study highlighted a positive correlation between HK-LS and medication adherence scores. This positive correlation emphasizes the direct and positive effect of enhancing medication that can contribute to better health outcomes among hypertensive patients and decrease the burden on the existing healthcare system. However, patient education must be continuous. This can be achieved through telehealth services, especially in countries like the KSA, where telehealth services are free for citizens [45–47]. Similar to our study, a significant association between higher knowledge and better medication adherence was observed in the studies by Farah RI et al. [48] and Abdisa L et al. [49].

Regarding factors associated with medication adherence, the present study observed that those working in the private sector, those living in urban areas, and those who had hypertension had significantly higher levels of medication adherence than others. The possible explanation for the results could be that private sector workers might have continuous health monitoring, the availability of additional incentives, and more commitment to keeping their health in a better position. However, in contrast to this study, some authors found a non-significant association between adherence and residence status [48,49]. Similar to a recent study in the KSA, we found a positive association between medication adherence and residence status [41]. The higher level of adherence among the participants from the urban side could be due to the availability and accessibility of health information resources. The duration of illness is another important factor to be considered in chronic diseases such as hypertension and diabetes, as they might have significant roles in initiating medications, health outcomes, and medication adherence [41,50]. Interestingly, the present study did not find a significant association with age, gender, and education status. However, existing studies have documented differences in influencing factors; some depicted significant associations, and others did not. These differences further emphasize that medication adherence and associated factors are widely varied, and region-specific policies and guidelines are required.

This study used a validated HK-LS and the Hill–Bone Medication Adherence Scale in a unique sociocultural setting. Nonetheless, like any other research, this study also has some limitations. First, hypertensive patients from a single KSA province were included in this study. Therefore, the present study's conclusions cannot be extrapolated to patients in other provinces of the KSA. This is particularly because variances in knowledge about hypertension and adherence behaviors could be expected due to sociocultural contexts, education, and regional differences in access to healthcare services. Moreover, differences in healthcare providers' practices across the different facilities (primary health centers and hospitals) and resources across facilities may contribute to patient compliance with prescribed medications, making it difficult to generalize these results. Next, the research participants were sourced from PHCs belonging to the Ministry of Health. Hence, the adherence practices in other healthcare facilities, such as general hospitals and tertiary care centers, may differ. Additionally, due to reliance on self-administered questionnaires, this study could not analyze adherence levels based on specific types of anti-hypertensive medications. Finally, restrictions related to the study design, such as a lack of the ability to identify a temporal association, self-selection bias, and exaggerated responses, must be kept in mind while interpreting the findings.

5. Conclusions

The present study observed that more than 40% of hypertensive patients who attended PHCs in the Aljouf region, the KSA, had poor medication adherence. We also found a positive correlation between patients' hypertension-related knowledge and medication adherence. Medication adherence was significantly higher among certain categories of patients. The present study's findings indicate that there is still a critical gap in managing hypertension at the PHCs in this region, and this may lead to poor health outcomes among patients and burden the healthcare system. Hence, continuous patient education and targeted counseling for those with poor medication adherence are recommended. This can be achieved not only during medical consultations at clinics but also through teleconsultation as a part of follow-up and continuous patient education. Multi-regional studies should be conducted that explore the qualitative components that lead to poor medication adherence to recognize region-specific variations and explore medication adherence patterns based on anti-hypertensive drug types.

Funding: This research is funded by the Deanship of Graduate Studies and Scientific Research at Jouf University through the Fast-Track Research Funding Program.

Institutional Review Board Statement: This study was conducted in accordance with the Declaration of Helsinki and approved by the Institutional Review Board, Jouf University (No. 13-09-45, dated 12 May 2024).

Informed Consent Statement: Informed consent was obtained from all subjects involved in this study.

Data Availability Statement: The raw data supporting the conclusions of this article will be made available by the authors upon request.

Acknowledgments: The author would like to thank the primary care physicians working in the primary health centers of these regions for their immense support in data collection. Additionally, the author extends her sincere thanks to Aliyah Muteb AL-Ruwaili for her immense contribution to this research paper. Finally, we thank Getsy Hannah Bijoy for creating a graphical abstract for the research.

Conflicts of Interest: The authors declare no conflicts of interest.

References

1. WHO. Hypertension. Available online: https://www.who.int/news-room/fact-sheets/detail/hypertension (accessed on 18 January 2024).
2. Mills, K.T.; Stefanescu, A.; He, J. The global epidemiology of hypertension. *Nat. Rev. Nephrol.* **2020**, *16*, 223–237. [CrossRef] [PubMed]
3. NCD-RisC. Worldwide trends in hypertension prevalence and progress in treatment and control from 1990 to 2019: A pooled analysis of 1201 population-representative studies with 104 million participants. *Lancet* **2021**, *398*, 957–980. [CrossRef] [PubMed]
4. Kario, K.; Okura, A.; Hoshide, S.; Mogi, M. The WHO Global report 2023 on hypertension warning the emerging hypertension burden in globe and its treatment strategy. *Hypertens. Res.* **2024**, *47*, 1099–1102. [CrossRef] [PubMed]
5. Wu, A.S.; Dodhia, H.; Whitney, D.; Ashworth, M. Is the rule of halves still relevant today? A cross-sectional analysis of hypertension detection, treatment and control in an urban community. *J. Hypertens.* **2019**, *37*, 2470–2480. [CrossRef]
6. Fuchs, F.D.; Whelton, P.K. High Blood Pressure and Cardiovascular Disease. *Hypertension* **2020**, *75*, 285–292. [CrossRef]
7. Sabih, A.; Tadi, P.; Kumar, A. Stroke Prevention. In *StatPearls*; StatPearls Publishing: Treasure Island, FL, USA, 2024.
8. Alshammari, S.A.; Alshammari, A.S.; Alshammari, H.S.; Ahamed, S.S. Overview of hypertension in Saudi Arabia: A systematic review and meta-analysis. *Saudi Med. J.* **2023**, *44*, 951–964. [CrossRef]
9. Tailakh, A.; Evangelista, L.S.; Mentes, J.C.; Pike, N.A.; Phillips, L.R.; Morisky, D.E. Hypertension prevalence, awareness, and control in Arab countries: A systematic review. *Nurs. Health Sci.* **2014**, *16*, 126–130. [CrossRef] [PubMed]
10. Chimberengwa, P.T.; Naidoo, M. Knowledge, attitudes and practices related to hypertension among residents of a disadvantaged rural community in southern Zimbabwe. *PLoS ONE* **2019**, *14*, e0215500. [CrossRef]
11. Andersson, U.; Bengtsson, U.; Ranerup, A.; Midlöv, P.; Kjellgren, K. Patients and Professionals as Partners in Hypertension Care: Qualitative Substudy of a Randomized Controlled Trial Using an Interactive Web-Based System Via Mobile Phone. *J. Med. Internet Res.* **2021**, *23*, e26143. [CrossRef]
12. Londoño Agudelo, E.; Battaglioli, T.; Díaz Piñera, A.; Rodríguez Salvá, A.; Smekens, T.; Achiong Estupiñán, F.; Carbonell García, I.; Van der Stuyft, P. Effectiveness of a provider and patient-focused intervention to improve hypertension management and control in the primary health care setting in Cuba: A controlled before-after study. *BMC Prim. Care* **2023**, *24*, 10. [CrossRef]
13. Charchar, F.J.; Prestes, P.R.; Mills, C.; Ching, S.M.; Neupane, D.; Marques, F.Z.; Sharman, J.E.; Vogt, L.; Burrell, L.M.; Korostovtseva, L.; et al. Lifestyle management of hypertension: International Society of Hypertension position paper endorsed by the World Hypertension League and European Society of Hypertension. *J. Hypertens.* **2024**, *42*, 23–49. [CrossRef] [PubMed]
14. National Institute for Health and Care Excellence: Guidelines. In *Hypertension in Adults: Diagnosis and Management*; National Institute for Health and Care Excellence (NICE): London, UK, 2023.
15. Hamrahian, S.M.; Maarouf, O.H.; Fülöp, T. A Critical Review of Medication Adherence in Hypertension: Barriers and Facilitators Clinicians Should Consider. *Patient Prefer. Adherence* **2022**, *16*, 2749–2757. [CrossRef] [PubMed]
16. Mohd Isa, D.; Shahar, S.; He, F.J.; Majid, H.A. Associations of Health Literacy with Blood Pressure and Dietary Salt Intake among Adults: A Systematic Review. *Nutrients* **2021**, *13*, 4534. [CrossRef]
17. Du, S.; Zhou, Y.; Fu, C.; Wang, Y.; Du, X.; Xie, R. Health literacy and health outcomes in hypertension: An integrative review. *Int. J. Nurs. Sci.* **2018**, *5*, 301–309. [CrossRef] [PubMed]
18. Ernawati, I.; Fandinata, S.S.; Permatasari, S.N. Translation and validation of the indonesian version of the hypertension knowledge-level scale. *Open Access Maced. J. Med. Sci.* **2020**, *8*, 630–637. [CrossRef]
19. Andrew, A.; Hariharan, M.; Monteiro, S.R.; Padhy, M.; Chivukula, U. Enhancing adherence and management in patients with hypertension: Impact of form and frequency of knowledge intervention. *Indian Heart J.* **2022**, *74*, 302–306. [CrossRef] [PubMed]
20. Eshah, N.F.; Al-Daken, L.I. Assessing Public's Knowledge About Hypertension in a Community-Dwelling Sample. *J. Cardiovasc. Nurs.* **2016**, *31*, 158–165. [CrossRef] [PubMed]
21. Abu, H.; Aboumatar, H.; Carson, K.A.; Goldberg, R.; Cooper, L.A. Hypertension knowledge, heart healthy lifestyle practices and medication adherence among adults with hypertension. *Eur. J. Pers. Cent. Healthc.* **2018**, *6*, 108–114. [CrossRef]
22. Alhazmi, A.; Moafa, H.N.; Kotb, M.; Sayegh, L.; Baydhi, H.; Hazzazi, A.; Moafa, H.; Hakami, A. Assessing knowledge about hypertension and identifying predictors of inadequate knowledge in Saudi Arabia: A cross-sectional study. *PLoS ONE* **2024**, *19*, e0299745. [CrossRef]
23. Paczkowska, A.; Hoffmann, K.; Kus, K.; Kopciuch, D.; Zaprutko, T.; Ratajczak, P.; Michalak, M.; Nowakowska, E.; Bryl, W. Impact of patient knowledge on hypertension treatment adherence and efficacy: A single-centre study in Poland. *Int. J. Med. Sci.* **2021**, *18*, 852–860. [CrossRef]

24. Hunter, P.G.; Chapman, F.A.; Dhaun, N. Hypertension: Current trends and future perspectives. *Br. J. Clin. Pharmacol.* **2021**, *87*, 3721–3736. [CrossRef] [PubMed]
25. Jin, J. Screening for Hypertension in Adults. *JAMA* **2021**, *325*, 1688. [CrossRef] [PubMed]
26. Alammari, G.; Alhazzani, H.; AlRajhi, N.; Sales, I.; Jamal, A.; Almigbal, T.H.; Batais, M.A.; Asiri, Y.A.; AlRuthia, Y. Validation of an Arabic Version of the Adherence to Refills and Medications Scale (ARMS). *Healthcare* **2021**, *9*, 1430. [CrossRef] [PubMed]
27. Shakya, R.; Shrestha, R.; Shrestha, S.; Sapkota, P.; Gautam, R.; Rai, L.; Khatiwada, A.P.; Ranabhat, K.; Kc, B.; Sapkota, B.; et al. Translation, Cultural Adaptation and Validation of the Hill Bone Compliance to High Blood Pressure Therapy Scale to Nepalese Language. *Patient Prefer. Adherence* **2022**, *16*, 957–970. [CrossRef] [PubMed]
28. De Las Cuevas, C.; Peñate, W. Psychometric properties of the eight-item Morisky Medication Adherence Scale (MMAS-8) in a psychiatric outpatient setting. *Int. J. Clin. Health Psychol.* **2015**, *15*, 121–129. [CrossRef] [PubMed]
29. Calculator.net. Sample Size Calculator. Available online: https://www.calculator.net/sample-size-calculator.html (accessed on 18 January 2024).
30. Kim, M.T.; Hill, M.N.; Bone, L.R.; Levine, D.M. Development and testing of the Hill-Bone Compliance to High Blood Pressure Therapy Scale. *Prog. Cardiovasc. Nurs.* **2000**, *15*, 90–96. [CrossRef]
31. Commodore-Mensah, Y.; Delva, S.; Ogungbe, O.; Smulcer, L.A.; Rives, S.; Dennison Himmelfarb, C.R.; Kim, M.T.; Bone, L.; Levine, D.; Hill, M.N. A Systematic Review of the Hill-Bone Compliance to Blood Pressure Therapy Scale. *Patient Prefer. Adherence* **2023**, *17*, 2401–2420. [CrossRef] [PubMed]
32. Uchmanowicz, B.; Chudiak, A.; Uchmanowicz, I.; Rosińczuk, J.; Froelicher, E.S. Factors influencing adherence to treatment in older adults with hypertension. *Clin. Interv. Aging* **2018**, *13*, 2425–2441. [CrossRef]
33. Stanikzai, M.H.; Wafa, M.H.; Tawfiq, E.; Jafari, M.; Le, C.N.; Wasiq, A.W.; Rahimi, B.A.; Baray, A.H.; Ageru, T.A.; Suwanbamrung, C. Predictors of non-adherence to antihypertensive medications: A cross-sectional study from a regional hospital in Afghanistan. *PLoS ONE* **2023**, *18*, e0295246. [CrossRef]
34. UN. Goal 3: Ensure Healthy Lives and Promote Well-Being for All at All Ages. Available online: https://sdgs.un.org/goals/goal3 (accessed on 22 August 2024).
35. Vainauskienė, V.; Vaitkienė, R. Enablers of Patient Knowledge Empowerment for Self-Management of Chronic Disease: An Integrative Review. *Int. J. Environ. Res. Public Health* **2021**, *18*, 2247. [CrossRef]
36. Alshammari, S.A.; Alshathri, A.H.; Alshathri, A.H.; Aleban, S.A.; Alabdullah, D.W.; Abukhlaled, J.K.; Aldharman, S.S. Assessment of Public Knowledge of Hypertension Among the Saudi Population. *Cureus* **2023**, *15*, e37649. [CrossRef] [PubMed]
37. Buang, N.F.B.; Rahman, N.A.A.; Haque, M. Knowledge, attitude and practice regarding hypertension among residents in a housing area in Selangor, Malaysia. *Med. Pharm. Rep.* **2019**, *92*, 145–152. [CrossRef] [PubMed]
38. Dash, S.; Delibasic, V.; Alsaeed, S.; Ward, M.; Jefferson, K.; Manca, D.P.; Arcand, J. Knowledge, Attitudes and Behaviours Related to Physician-Delivered Dietary Advice for Patients with Hypertension. *J. Community Health* **2020**, *45*, 1067–1072. [CrossRef] [PubMed]
39. Geaney, F.; Fitzgerald, S.; Harrington, J.M.; Kelly, C.; Greiner, B.A.; Perry, I.J. Nutrition knowledge, diet quality and hypertension in a working population. *Prev. Med. Rep.* **2015**, *2*, 105–113. [CrossRef]
40. Pan, J.; Hu, B.; Wu, L.; Li, Y. The Effect of Social Support on Treatment Adherence in Hypertension in China. *Patient Prefer. Adherence* **2021**, *15*, 1953–1961. [CrossRef] [PubMed]
41. Thirunavukkarasu, A.; Naser Abdullah Alshahrani, A.; Mazen Abdel-Salam, D.; Homoud Al-Hazmi, A.; Farhan, A.B.; Awad Alsaidan, A.; Narapureddy, B.R.; Muteb Al-Ruwaili, A.; Ghuwayli Aljabri, F.; Khalaf Albalawi, R.; et al. Medication Adherence Among Hypertensive Patients Attending Different Primary Health Centers in Abha, Saudi Arabia: A Cross-Sectional Study. *Patient Prefer. Adherence* **2022**, *16*, 2835–2844. [CrossRef] [PubMed]
42. Khayyat, S.M.; Khayyat, S.M.; Hyat Alhazmi, R.S.; Mohamed, M.M.; Abdul Hadi, M. Predictors of Medication Adherence and Blood Pressure Control among Saudi Hypertensive Patients Attending Primary Care Clinics: A Cross-Sectional Study. *PLoS ONE* **2017**, *12*, e0171255. [CrossRef]
43. Alsaidan, A.A.; Alotaibi, S.F.; Thirunavukkarasu, A.; Alruwaili, B.F.; Alharbi, R.H.; Arnous, M.M.; Alsaidan, O.A.; Alduraywish, A.S.; Alwushayh, Y.A. Medication Adherence and Its Associated Factors among Patients with Type 2 Diabetes Mellitus Attending Primary Health Centers of Eastern Province, Saudi Arabia. *Medicina* **2023**, *59*, 989. [CrossRef]
44. Alosaimi, K.; Alwafi, H.; Alhindi, Y.; Falemban, A.; Alshanberi, A.; Ayoub, N.; Alsanosi, S. Medication Adherence among Patients with Chronic Diseases in Saudi Arabia. *Int. J. Environ. Res. Public Health* **2022**, *19*, 10053. [CrossRef]
45. Yukselen, Z.; Singh, Y.; Malempati, S.; Dasari, M.; Arun Kumar, P.; Ramsaran, E. Virtual patient education for hypertension: The truth about behavioral change. *World J. Cardiol.* **2023**, *15*, 324–327. [CrossRef]
46. Idris, H.; Nugraheni, W.P.; Rachmawati, T.; Kusnali, A.; Yulianti, A.; Purwatiningsih, Y.; Nuraini, S.; Susianti, N.; Faisal, D.R.; Arifin, H.; et al. How Is Telehealth Currently Being Utilized to Help in Hypertension Management within Primary Healthcare Settings? A Scoping Review. *Int. J. Environ. Res. Public Health* **2024**, *21*, 10090. [CrossRef] [PubMed]
47. MOH. Telemedicine in Saudi Arabia. Available online: https://www.moh.gov.sa/en/Ministry/Information-and-services/Pages/Telemedicine.aspx (accessed on 19 August 2024).
48. Farah, R.I.; Alawwa, I.A.; Khateeb, D.Q.; Hwidi, B.E.; Albdour, K.M.; Bani Monia, O.G.; Assaf, R.N.; Aldabaibah, A.A.; Alsaket, G.I.J.; Alshrouf, M.A. Factors Affecting the Level of Adherence to Hypertension Medications: A Cross-Sectional Study Using the Hill-Bone Questionnaire. *Patient Prefer. Adherence* **2024**, *18*, 893–904. [CrossRef] [PubMed]

49. Abdisa, L.; Alemu, A.; Heluf, H.; Sertsu, A.; Dessie, Y.; Negash, B.; Ayana, G.M.; Letta, S. Factors associated with poor medication adherence during COVID-19 pandemic among hypertensive patients visiting public hospitals in Eastern Ethiopia: A cross-sectional study. *BMJ Open* **2022**, *12*, e064284. [CrossRef] [PubMed]
50. Wong, M.C.S.; Tam, W.W.S.; Wang, H.H.X.; Cheung, C.S.K.; Tong, E.L.H.; Cheung, N.T.; Leeder, S.R.; Griffiths, S.M. Duration of initial antihypertensive prescription and medication adherence: A cohort study among 203,259 newly diagnosed hypertensive patients. *Int. J. Cardiol.* **2015**, *182*, 503–508. [CrossRef]

medicina

MDPI

Article

Relationship between Cancer and Intention to Leave Work among Older Workers: A Cross-Sectional Internet-Based Study

Ryutaro Matsugaki [1,*], Shinya Matsuda [2] and Akira Ogami [1]

1 Department of Work Systems and Health, Institute of Industrial Ecological Sciences, University of Occupational and Environmental Health, Kitakyushu 807-8555, Japan
2 Department of Preventive Medicine and Community Health, University of Occupational and Environmental Health, Kitakyushu 807-8555, Japan
* Correspondence: pt-matsugaki@med.uoeh-u.ac.jp; Tel.: +81-93-603-4307

Abstract: *Background and Objectives*: Limited research has focused on the relationship between cancer, job loss, and factors associated with job loss among older workers. Therefore, in this study, we aimed to examine the relationship between cancer and intention to leave and between physical-health-related issues, mental-health-related issues, and cancer-related symptoms and intention to leave among older workers with cancer. *Materials and Methods*: This cross-sectional internet-based study included 4498 workers aged 60–75 years. Intention to leave was assessed based on whether individuals considered quitting their current jobs in the near future. *Results*: A multivariate logistic regression analysis showed a significant association between cancer and intention to leave (adjusted odds ratio [aOR]: 1.42, 95% confidence interval [CI]: 1.01–2.00, $p = 0.045$). In addition, physical-health-related issues (aOR: 2.33, 95% CI: 1.10–4.92, $p = 0.026$) and mental-health-related issues (aOR: 4.44, 95% CI: 1.80–10.98, $p = 0.001$) were significantly associated with the intention to leave. *Conclusions:* Healthcare providers and employers must address the physical- and mental-health-related issues facing older workers with cancer to help them secure their employment.

Keywords: cancer; intention to leave; older worker; unemployment

1. Introduction

The diagnosis and treatment of cancer significantly impact individuals' lives. Recent advances in medicine, especially in high-income countries, have improved the survival rates of patients with cancer [1–3], highlighting the importance of research on the social and occupational challenges faced by survivors of cancer. Unemployment is a critical issue among survivors of cancer. Survivors of cancer have a higher rate of job loss than the general population [4–6], and unemployment can lead to financial toxicity [7–9] and a reduction in quality of life [10–14]. Therefore, the demand for strategies to avoid unemployment among patients with cancer is increasing.

Notably, several factors have been associated with unemployment among survivors of cancer. Personal factors include older age [6,14–17], female sex [6,18], low educational level [6,19], lower income level [18,19], physically or mentally demanding work [17,19], clinical stage [15,16,19], and type of treatment [15–17,19]. The modifiable factors include physical-health-related issues such as low fitness levels and poor physical function [17], mental-health-related issues such as depression [20], and cancer-related symptoms such as fatigue and pain [21–25]. Therefore, healthcare providers, employers, and occupational health staff should address these physical- and mental-health-related issues and cancer-related symptoms to prevent job loss among patients with cancer.

The incidence of cancer is closely associated with aging, peaking in the population in their 60s and 70s [26,27]. Furthermore, the rise in the aging population and retirement-age groups in developed countries has led to a corresponding increase in the proportion of older workers in the labor market [28]. At the intersection of these trends, the employment challenges faced by older survivors of cancer are expected to become increasingly significant. However, limited research has focused on the relationship between cancer, job loss, and factors associated with job loss among older workers. In the present study, we aimed to (1) clarify whether cancer is associated with intentions to leave work among older workers and (2) identify whether physical- and mental-health-related issues and cancer-related symptoms are associated with intentions to leave work among workers with cancer.

2. Materials and Methods

2.1. Study Design and Participants

This cross-sectional internet-based study was conducted to explore the employment and health challenges faced by older workers [29]. The survey targeted workers aged 60–75 years who were employed in the tertiary sector and registered with Cross Marketing Inc. (Tokyo, Japan).

On 1 September 2022, invitations were sent via email or other methods to those panelists who, at the time of their registration, indicated they were employed. The criteria for exclusion included (1) unemployment at the time of the survey, (2) being younger than 60 years or older than 75 years, (3) being self-employed or a family member actively participating in a family business, (4) not working in the tertiary sector as defined by the Indices of Tertiary Industry Activity in Japan, and (5) incorrect answers to a control question designed to filter out unreliable data: "Identify the third largest number from a list of five numbers". The recruitment process concluded on 9 September 2022, with the target of 5000 participants met. Fifty-two individuals who anticipated imminent retirement due to reasons such as reaching retirement age or contract termination for the purposes of this research were excluded, resulting in a final sample size of 4948 participants. All the participants provided informed consent online through a survey interface. The study protocol was approved by the Ethics Committee of the University of Occupational and Environmental Health, Japan (R4-031).

2.2. Assessment of the Prevalence of Cancer

All participants were asked the question, "What illnesses do you have that require outpatient visits or treatment?". Those who responded "yes" to the option for cancer were considered diagnosed with cancer.

2.3. Assessment of Physical, Mental, and Symptomatic Health-Related Issues

In this study, we investigated the health-related problems faced by the participants that prevented them from continuing their current employment. Notably, we focused on physical- and mental-health-related issues and cancer-related symptoms. The participants were asked the question, "What kind of problems are you encountering in order to continue your current job?". Subsequently, the participants were presented with three items: "physical fitness-related problems", "mental health-related problems", and "problems associated with cancer-related symptoms". For each item, the participants were required to respond with either "Yes" or "No". This approach allowed for ascertaining the various health-related challenges encountered by survivors of cancer in their workplace and quantitatively assessing these barriers to sustained employment.

2.4. Assessment of Intention to Leave Work

We assessed the participants' intention to leave using the question "Do you intend to leave your current job in the near future?" with the following response options: "Sure", "I think so", or "Definitely yes". If the participants answered, "I think so" or "definitely yes", they were deemed to have the intention to leave.

2.5. Assessment of Other Variables

The following variables were considered as covariates and were adjusted for in the analysis: age, gender, educational background (junior high school/high school, vocational school/junior college/technical college, and university/graduate school), employment status (regular or non-regular employment), job description (mainly or not mainly manual work), work frequency (≤3, 4, and ≥5 days/week), and company size (<10, 10–99, 100–999, ≥1000 employees).

2.6. Statistical Analysis

All data were expressed as categorical variables using numerical values and percentages. First, a logistic regression analysis involving all participants was performed, with the intention to leave as the dependent variable and the prevalence of cancer as the independent variable. Age, gender, educational background, employment status, job description, work frequency, and company size were used as covariates to adjust for potential confounders. Next, a subsequent logistic regression analysis involving participants with cancer, with the intention to leave as the dependent variable and each health-related problem as the independent variable, was performed. Age, gender, educational background, employment status, job description, work frequency, and company size were used as covariates to adjust for potential confounders. All statistical analyses were performed using Stata version 18.0 (StataCorp LLC, College Station, TX, USA). Statistical significance was set at $p < 0.05$.

3. Results

Table 1 presents the participants' characteristics. The prevalence of cancer was 59.1% (154/4948). The cancer group had a higher proportion of individuals aged >70 years (12.3% vs. 9.5%) and a higher percentage of those with non-regular employment (63.0% vs. 58.2%) than the non-cancer group. Table 2 presents the proportion of participants with intentions to leave their jobs according to their cancer status, along with the adjusted odds ratio (aOR) and 95% confidence interval (95% CI) for the association between cancer and the intention to leave a job. The proportion of participants who intended to leave was higher in the cancer group than in the non-cancer group (33.1% vs. 26.2%). The multivariate logistic regression analysis results indicated that cancer was significantly associated with the intentions to leave (aOR: 1.42, 95% CI: 1.01–2.00, $p = 0.045$).

Table 1. Participants' characteristics.

	Total (n = 4948)	Cancer	
		Without (n = 4794)	With (n = 154)
Age			
60–64	3348 (67.7%)	3257 (67.9%)	91 (59.1%)
65–69	1127 (22.8%)	1083 (22.6%)	44 (28.6%)
70–75	473 (9.6%)	454 (9.5%)	19 (12.3%)
Gender			
Men	2474 (50.0%)	2399 (50.0%)	75 (48.7%)
Women	2474 (50.0%)	2395 (50.0%)	79 (51.3%)
Educational background			
Junior high school/high school	1432 (28.9%)	1387 (28.9%)	45 (29.2%)
Vocational school/college	1107 (22.4%)	1069 (22.3%)	38 (24.7%)
University	2409 (48.7%)	2338 (48.8%)	71 (46.1%)
Employment status			
Regular employment	2060 (41.6%)	2003 (41.8%)	57 (37.0%)
Non-regular employment	2888 (58.4%)	2791 (58.2%)	97 (63.0%)
Job description			
Not mainly manual work	3374 (68.2%)	3271 (68.2%)	103 (66.9%)
Mainly manual work	1574 (31.8%)	1523 (31.8%)	51 (33.1%)
Work frequency (day/week)			
≤3	889 (18.0%)	862 (18.0%)	27 (17.5%)
4	722 (14.6%)	699 (14.6%)	23 (14.9%)
≥5	3337 (67.4%)	3233 (67.4%)	104 (67.5%)
Company size (employees)			
Micro-scale (<10)	686 (13.9%)	665 (13.9%)	21 (13.6%)
Small-scale (10–49)	1044 (21.1%)	1012 (21.1%)	32 (20.8%)
Medium-scale (50–999)	2018 (40.8%)	1956 (40.8%)	62 (40.3%)
Large-scale (≥1000)	1200 (24.3%)	1161 (24.2%)	39 (25.3%)

Table 2. Association between cancer and intention to leave (n = 4948).

	Intention to Leave	Age and Gender Adjusted				Multivariate Adjusted *			
		aOR	95% CI		*p*-Value	aOR	95% CI		*p*-Value
Cancer									
Without (n = 4794)	26.2% (1255/4794)	Reference				Reference			
With (n = 154)	33.1% (51/154)	1.42	1.01	2.00	0.043	1.42	1.01	2.00	0.045

* Adjusted for age, gender, educational background, employment status, job description, work frequency, and company size. aOR, adjusted odds ratio; 95% CI, 95% confidence interval.

Table 3 presents the characteristics of the participants with cancer. Of the 154 participants with cancer, 51 (33.1%) intended to leave their jobs. The group with intentions to leave had a higher proportion of workers who worked >5 days weekly than the group without such intentions (70.6% vs. 66.0%). Table 4 presents the prevalence of health-related problems associated with the intention to leave a job and the aOR and 95% CI for the association between each health-related problem and the intention to leave a job. The prevalence of physical (40.7% vs. 24.7%) and mental (62.1% vs. 27.2%) health-related problems was significantly higher in the group with the intention to leave than in the group without this intention. The multivariate logistic regression analysis showed that physical (aOR: 2.33, 95% CI: 1.10–4.92, $p = 0.026$) and mental (aOR: 4.44, 95% CI: 1.80–10.98, $p = 0.001$) health-related problems were significantly associated with the intention to leave. However, problems associated with cancer-related symptoms were not significantly associated with the intention to leave (aOR: 1.01, 95% CI: 0.49–2.11, $p = 0.969$).

Table 3. Characteristics of participants with cancer.

	Total (n = 154)	Intention to Leave	
		No (n = 103)	Yes (n = 51)
Age			
60–64	91 (59.1%)	65 (63.1%)	26 (51.0%)
65–69	44 (28.6%)	26 (25.2%)	18 (35.3%)
70–75	19 (12.3%)	12 (11.7%)	7 (13.7%)
Gender			
Men	75 (48.7%)	50 (48.5%)	25 (49.0%)
Women	79 (51.3%)	53 (51.5%)	26 (51.0%)
Educational background			
Junior high school/high school	45 (29.2%)	29 (28.2%)	16 (31.4%)
Vocational school/college	38 (24.7%)	27 (26.2%)	11 (21.6%)
University	71 (46.1%)	47 (45.6%)	24 (47.1%)
Employment status			
Regular employment	57 (37.0%)	39 (37.9%)	18 (35.3%)
Non-regular employment	97 (63.0%)	64 (62.1%)	33 (64.7%)
Job description			
Not mainly manual work	103 (66.9%)	68 (66.0%)	35 (68.6%)
Mainly manual work	51 (33.1%)	35 (34.0%)	16 (31.4%)
Work frequency (day/week)			
≤ 3	27 (17.5%)	19 (18.4%)	8 (15.7%)
4	23 (14.9%)	16 (15.5%)	7 (13.7%)
≥ 5	104 (67.5%)	68 (66.0%)	36 (70.6%)
Company size (employees)			
Micro-scale (<10)	21 (13.6%)	12 (11.7%)	9 (17.6%)
Small-scale (10–49)	32 (20.8%)	25 (24.3%)	7 (13.7%)
Medium-scale (50–999)	62 (40.3%)	40 (38.8%)	22 (43.1%)
Large-scale ($\geq$1000)	39 (25.3%)	26 (25.2%)	13 (25.5%)

Table 4. Association of physical-health-related issues, mental-health-related issues, and cancer-related symptoms with the intention to leave (n = 154).

	Intention to Leave	Age-Gender Adjusted				Multivariate Adjusted *			
		aOR	95% CI		*p*-Value	aOR	95% CI		*p*-Value
Physical-health-related issue									
Without (n = 73)	24.7% (18/73)	Reference				Reference			
With (n = 81)	40.7% (33/81)	2.09	1.04	4.23	0.039	2.33	1.10	4.92	0.026
Mental-health-related issue									
Without (n = 125)	27.2% (34/125)	Reference				Reference			
With (n = 29)	62.1% (18/29)	3.69	1.59	8.58	0.002	4.44	1.80	10.98	0.001
Cancer-related symptoms									
Without (n = 99)	33.3% (33/99)	Reference				Reference			
With (n = 55)	32.7% (18/55)	1.03	0.51	2.09	0.937	1.01	0.49	2.11	0.969

* Adjusted for age, gender, educational background, employment status, job description, work frequency, and company size. aOR, odds ratio; 95% CI, 95% confidence interval.

4. Discussion

The present cross-sectional study revealed that cancer was associated with the intention to leave work among older workers. Furthermore, physical- and mental-health-related issues were associated with the intention to leave among older workers with cancer. These findings suggest the need for physical and mental health support to facilitate the sustained employment of older workers with cancer. The present study is novel because it examined factors associated with the intention to leave among older workers who are survivors of cancer.

The present study found a significant association between cancer and the intention to leave work among older workers. These results are consistent with those of previous studies indicating a higher risk of job loss among survivors of cancer than among the general population [4–6], supporting the notion that unemployment among survivors of cancer can lead to serious consequences such as financial toxicity and a decline in the quality of life [7–14]. Medical and occupational health interventions are required to mitigate these negative effects in older workers with cancer.

The present study also highlighted a significant relationship between physical- and mental-health-related issues and the intention to leave among older survivors of cancer. Physical limitations may restrict older workers' abilities to meet the physical demands of their workplace, and mental-health-related issues may further impair their adaptability and performance. These factors may be associated with a decrease in cancer survivors' work ability [30–32], potentially triggering the intention to leave. Physical- and mental-health-related issues are not exclusive to older survivors of cancer; however, aging may exacerbate these issues. Preventive measures can include multidisciplinary interventions initiated during cancer treatment [33], such as occupational physical exercise, counseling, and psychosocial support at work to facilitate sustained employment.

In contrast, issues associated with cancer-related symptoms were not associated with the intention to leave among older workers who were survivors of cancer. This finding is inconsistent with that of previous studies, namely that cancer-related symptoms are associated with job loss [21–25]. This discrepancy can be attributed to the healthy worker effect, as our survey targeted employed individuals, possibly underestimating the association between symptoms and the intention to leave. In addition, symptoms such as fatigue may have been perceived as physical weakness rather than cancer-related symptoms, potentially leading to an underestimation of their impact on the intention to leave a job. The association between cancer-related symptoms and the intention to leave work was negative in the present study; however, these symptoms have been associated with work outcomes such as loss of productivity [17,30,32,34–37], emphasizing their importance in the context of sustained employment.

This study has some limitations that warrant further consideration. First, the generalizability of the study findings is limited. We did not consider cancer progression, resulting in the likely underrepresentation of patients with advanced cancer, making the results less applicable to those with severe conditions. This study focused only on tertiary sector workers, so whether these findings apply to those in more physically demanding industries is unclear. Additionally, owing to the recruitment of participants through an internet survey, we could not rule out the possibility that the target population was biased toward relatively well-educated older workers with access to the internet, as well as older adults who are interested in their health. This study targeted only currently employed individuals aged 60–75, who are generally healthier, potentially underestimating the true impact of cancer on employment. Second, this was a cross-sectional study and may not be suitable for drawing causal inferences. However, causal inferences are unlikely to be reversed in the case of the relationship between cancer and intention to leave employment and between physical and mental problems and intention to leave among patients with cancer. In fact, analyses using panel data also suggest that unemployment itself does not affect health, but health problems are associated with unemployment [38]. Third, this study has unmeasured confounding factors. For example, workplaces with good job flexibility and robust occupational health support systems might reduce the impact of cancer and cancer-related health issues on the intention to leave. Conversely, the impact may be more pronounced in workplaces lacking such flexibility and support systems. However, this study does not account for these factors. Future analyses should consider the role of job flexibility and occupational health support systems when examining the effect of cancer and cancer-related health problems on turnover intention. Finally, the results of this study represent the intention to leave, not actual retirement. How many older workers who have the intention to leave the workforce actually leave is unclear, but it is possible that the percentage is small. Therefore, it is not clear how much of an impact a cancer diagnosis or cancer-related health problem has on actual retirement. Future prospective cohort studies are needed to examine the relationship between physical health problems, mental health problems, and cancer-related symptoms and the actual rate of leaving.

5. Conclusions

This study elucidated the impact of cancer on the intention to leave work among older workers, highlighting the pivotal role of physical- and mental-health-related issues. The findings suggest that a comprehensive approach to improving physical and mental health is necessary to support the sustained employment of older survivors of cancer. The development of such a comprehensive approach is urgently needed in many developed countries with aging workforces.

Author Contributions: Conceptualization, R.M.; methodology, R.M. and S.M.; software, R.M.; formal analysis, R.M.; investigation, R.M. and S.M.; resources, R.M. and S.M.; data curation, R.M.; writing—original draft preparation, R.M.; writing—review and editing, R.M., S.M. and A.O.; supervision, S.M.; project administration, R.M.; funding acquisition, R.M. and A.O. All authors have read and agreed to the published version of the manuscript.

Funding: This research was funded by the Japan Small- and Medium-Sized Enterprise Welfare Foundation and the Fukuoka Public Health Promotion Organization Center Research Fund.

Institutional Review Board Statement: This study was approved by the Institutional Review Board of the University of Occupational and Environmental Health, Japan (approval number: R4-031; approval date: 1 September 2022).

Informed Consent Statement: All participants provided informed consent online through the survey interface.

Data Availability Statement: The original contributions presented in the study are included in the article, further inquiries can be directed to the corresponding author.

Conflicts of Interest: The authors declare no conflicts of interest.

References

1. Arnold, M.; Rutherford, M.J.; Bardot, A.; Ferlay, J.; Andersson, T.M.; Myklebust, T.Å.; Tervonen, H.; Thursfield, V.; Ransom, D.; Shack, L.; et al. Progress in cancer survival, mortality, and incidence in seven high-income countries 1995–2014 (ICBP SURVMARK-2): A population-based study. *Lancet Oncol.* **2019**, *20*, 1493–1505. [CrossRef] [PubMed]
2. Allemani, C.; Matsuda, T.; Di Carlo, V.; Harewood, R.; Matz, M.; Nikšić, M.; Bonaventure, A.; Valkov, M.; Johnson, C.J.; Estève, J.; et al. Global surveillance of trends in cancer survival 2000-14 (CONCORD-3): Analysis of individual records for 37,513,025 patients diagnosed with one of 18 cancers from 322 population-based registries in 71 countries. *Lancet* **2018**, *391*, 1023–1075. [CrossRef] [PubMed]
3. De Angelis, R.; Sant, M.; Coleman, M.P.; Francisci, S.; Baili, P.; Pierannunzio, D.; Trama, A.; Visser, O.; Brenner, H.; Ardanaz, E.; et al. Cancer survival in Europe 1999–2007 by country and age: Results of EUROCARE—5-a population-based study. *Lancet Oncol.* **2014**, *15*, 23–34. [CrossRef] [PubMed]
4. de Boer, A.G.; Taskila, T.; Ojajärvi, A.; van Dijk, F.J.; Verbeek, J.H. Cancer survivors and unemployment: A meta-analysis and meta-regression. *JAMA* **2009**, *301*, 753–762. [CrossRef] [PubMed]
5. Mehnert, A. Employment and work-related issues in cancer survivors. *Crit. Rev. Oncol. Hematol.* **2011**, *77*, 109–130. [CrossRef]
6. Chimienti, M.; Morlino, G.; Ingravalle, F.; Vinci, A.; Colarusso, E.; De Santo, C.; Formosa, V.; Gentile, L.; Lorusso, G.; Mosconi, C.; et al. Unemployment status subsequent to cancer diagnosis and therapies: A systematic review and meta-analysis. *Cancers* **2023**, *15*, 1513. [CrossRef]
7. Honda, K.; Gyawali, B.; Ando, M.; Kumanishi, R.; Kato, K.; Sugiyama, K.; Mitani, S.; Masuishi, T.; Narita, Y.; Bando, H.; et al. Prospective survey of financial toxicity measured by the comprehensive score for financial toxicity in Japanese patients with cancer. *J. Glob. Oncol.* **2019**, *5*, 1–8. [CrossRef]
8. Mols, F.; Tomalin, B.; Pearce, A.; Kaambwa, B.; Koczwara, B. Financial toxicity and employment status in cancer survivors. A systematic literature review. *Support Care Cancer* **2020**, *28*, 5693–5708. [CrossRef]
9. Pearce, A.; Tomalin, B.; Kaambwa, B.; Horevoorts, N.; Duijts, S.; Mols, F.; van de Poll-Franse, L.; Koczwara, B. Financial toxicity is more than costs of care: The relationship between employment and financial toxicity in long-term cancer survivors. *J. Cancer Surviv.* **2019**, *13*, 10–20. [CrossRef]
10. Andreu, Y.; Martínez, P.; Soto-Rubio, A.; Pérez-Marín, M.; Cervantes, A.; Arribas, L. Quality of life in cancer survivorship: Sociodemographic and disease-related moderators. *Eur. J. Cancer Care* **2022**, *31*, e13692. [CrossRef]
11. Tamminga, S.J.; Jansen, L.P.; Frings-Dresen, M.H.W.; de Boer, A.G.E.M. Long-term employment status and quality of life after cancer: A longitudinal prospective cohort study from diagnosis up to and including 5 years post diagnosis. *Work* **2020**, *66*, 901–907. [CrossRef] [PubMed]
12. Duijts, S.F.; Kieffer, J.M.; van Muijen, P.; van der Beek, A.J. Sustained employability and health-related quality of life in cancer survivors up to four years after diagnosis. *Acta. Oncol.* **2017**, *56*, 174–182. [CrossRef] [PubMed]
13. Andreu, Y.; Picazo, C.; Murgui, S.; Soto-Rubio, A.; García-Conde, A.; Romero, R. Exploring the independent association of employment status to cancer survivors' health-related quality of life. *Health Qual. Life Outcomes* **2023**, *21*, 44. [CrossRef]
14. Bahlburg, H.; Reike, M.; Tully, K.; Bach, P.; Butea-Bocu, M.C.; Roghmann, F.; Noldus, J.; Müller, G. Return to work improves quality of life and reduces psychosocial distress after radical cystectomy: Data from a contemporary series of 230 German patients. *J. Cancer Surviv.* **2023**, *18*, 1426–1433. [CrossRef]
15. Yang, S.W.; Chen, W.L.; Wu, W.T.; Wang, C.C. Investigation on returning to work in liver cancer survivors in Taiwan: A 5-year follow-up study. *BMC Public Health* **2021**, *21*, 1846. [CrossRef]
16. Yuan, C.M.; Wang, C.C.; Wu, W.T.; Ho, C.L.; Chen, W.L. Risk factors for return to work in colorectal cancer survivors. *Cancer Med.* **2021**, *10*, 3938–3951. [CrossRef] [PubMed]
17. So, S.C.Y.; Ng, D.W.L.; Liao, Q.; Fielding, R.; Soong, I.; Chan, K.K.L.; Lee, C.; Ng, A.W.Y.; Sze, W.K.; Chan, W.L.; et al. Return to work and work productivity during the first year after cancer treatment. *Front. Psychol.* **2022**, *13*, 866346. [CrossRef]
18. Kang, D.; Bae, K.R.; Kim, H.Y.; Ahn, Y.; Kim, N.; Shim, Y.; Sohn, T.S.; Lee, W.Y.; Baek, J.H.; Kweon, S.S.; et al. Changes in working status after cancer diagnosis and socio-demographic, clinical, work-related, and psychological factors associated with it. *BMC Cancer* **2022**, *22*, 917. [CrossRef]
19. Wang, L.; Hong, B.Y.; Kennedy, S.A.; Chang, Y.; Hong, C.J.; Craigie, S.; Kwon, H.Y.; Romerosa, B.; Couban, R.J.; Reid, S.; et al. Predictors of unemployment after breast cancer surgery: A systematic review and meta-analysis of observational studies. *J. Clin. Oncol.* **2018**, *36*, 1868–1879. [CrossRef]
20. Dahl, A.A.; Fosså, S.D.; Lie, H.C.; Loge, J.H.; Reinertsen, K.V.; Ruud, E.; Kiserud, C.E. Employment status and work ability in long-term young adult cancer survivors. *J. Adolesc. Young Adult Oncol.* **2019**, *8*, 304–311. [CrossRef]
21. Alleaume, C.; Bendiane, M.K.; Bouhnik, A.D.; Rey, D.; Cortaredona, S.; Seror, V.; Peretti-Watel, P. Chronic neuropathic pain negatively associated with employment retention of cancer survivors: Evidence from a national French survey. *J. Cancer Surviv.* **2018**, *12*, 115–126. [CrossRef] [PubMed]
22. Behringer, K.; Goergen, H.; Müller, H.; Thielen, I.; Brillant, C.; Kreissl, S.; Halbsguth, T.V.; Meissner, J.; Greil, R.; Moosmann, P.; et al. Cancer-related fatigue in patients with and survivors of hodgkin lymphoma: The impact on treatment outcome and social reintegration. *J. Clin. Oncol.* **2016**, *34*, 4329–4337. [CrossRef] [PubMed]
23. Cox-Martin, E.; Anderson-Mellies, A.; Borges, V.; Bradley, C. Chronic pain, health-related quality of life, and employment in working-age cancer survivors. *J. Cancer Surviv.* **2020**, *14*, 179–187. [CrossRef] [PubMed]

24. Kerns, S.L.; Fung, C.; Fossa, S.D.; Dinh, J.; Paul, C.; Monahan, P.; Sesso, H.D.; Frisina, R.D.; Feldman, D.R.; Hamilton, R.J.; et al. Relationship of cisplatin-related adverse health outcomes with disability and unemployment among testicular cancer survivors. *JNCI Cancer Spectr.* **2020**, *4*, pkaa022. [CrossRef]
25. Lindbohm, M.L.; Kuosma, E.; Taskila, T.; Hietanen, P.; Carlsen, K.; Gudbergsson, S.; Gunnarsdottir, H. Early retirement and non-employment after breast cancer. *Psychooncology* **2014**, *23*, 634–641. [CrossRef] [PubMed]
26. GBD 2019 Asia and All Cancers Collaborators. Temporal patterns of cancer burden in Asia, 1990–2019: A systematic examination for the Global Burden of Disease 2019 study. *Lancet Reg. Health Southeast Asia* **2024**, *21*, 100333. [CrossRef] [PubMed]
27. GBD 2019 Colorectal Cancer Collaborators. Global, regional, and national burden of colorectal cancer and its risk factors, 1990–2019: A systematic analysis for the Global Burden of Disease Study 2019. *Lancet Gastroenterol. Hepatol.* **2022**, *7*, 627–647. [CrossRef]
28. OECD. Pensions at a Glance 2019: OECD and G20 Indicators. 2019. Available online: https://www.oecd-ilibrary.org/sites/b6d3dcfc-en/index.html?itemId=/content/publication/b6d3dcfc-en (accessed on 20 February 2024).
29. Matsugaki, R.; Matsuzaki, H.; Saeki, S.; Fujino, Y.; Matsuda, S. Frailty and occupational falls among older Japanese workers: An Internet-based cross-sectional study. *J. Occup. Health* **2023**, *65*, e12424. [CrossRef]
30. Fardell, J.E.; Tan, S.Y.C.; Kerin-Ayres, K.; Dhillon, H.M.; Vardy, J.L. Symptom clusters in survivorship and their impact on ability to work among cancer survivors. *Cancers* **2023**, *15*, 5119. [CrossRef]
31. Kim, S.; Kissane, D.W.; Richardson, G.; Senior, J.; Morgan, J.; Gregory, P.; Birks, S.; Ooi, C.; Lipton, L.; Antill, Y.; et al. The role of depression and other psychological factors in work ability among breast cancer survivors in Australia. *Psychooncology* **2022**, *31*, 167–175. [CrossRef]
32. Ambali Parambil, N.; Kannan, S. Work ability, anxiety, and depression among long-term breast cancer survivors of Northern Kerala, India; A historical cohort study. *Asian Pac. J. Cancer Prev.* **2024**, *25*, 115–122. [CrossRef] [PubMed]
33. Leensen, M.C.J.; Groeneveld, I.F.; van der Heide, I.; Rejda, T.; van Veldhoven, P.L.J.; Berkel, S.V.; Snoek, A.; Harten, W.V.; Frings-Dresen, M.H.W.; de Boer, A.G.E.M. Return to work of cancer patients after a multidisciplinary intervention including occupational counselling and physical exercise in cancer patients: A prospective study in the Netherlands. *BMJ Open* **2017**, *7*, e014746. [CrossRef] [PubMed]
34. Tan, C.J.; Yip, S.Y.C.; Chan, R.J.; Chew, L.; Chan, A. Investigating how cancer-related symptoms influence work outcomes among cancer survivors: A systematic review. *J. Cancer Surviv.* **2022**, *16*, 1065–1078. [CrossRef] [PubMed]
35. Dorland, H.F.; Abma, F.I.; Van Zon, S.K.R.; Stewart, R.E.; Amick, B.C.; Ranchor, A.V.; Roelen, C.A.M.; Bültmann, U. Fatigue and depressive symptoms improve but remain negatively related to work functioning over 18 months after return to work in cancer patients. *J. Cancer Surviv.* **2018**, *12*, 371–378. [CrossRef]
36. Wolvers, M.D.J.; Leensen, M.C.J.; Groeneveld, I.F.; Frings-Dresen, M.H.W.; De Boer, A.G.E.M. Longitudinal associations between fatigue and perceived work ability in cancer survivors. *J. Occup. Rehabil.* **2019**, *29*, 540–549. [CrossRef]
37. Vandraas, K.; Falk, R.S.; Bøhn, S.K.H.; Kiserud, C.; Lie, H.C.; Smedsland, S.K.; Ewertz, M.; Dahl, S.; Brekke, M.; Reinertsen, K.V. Work ability 8 years after breast cancer: Exploring the role of social support in a nation-wide survey. *Breast Cancer Res. Treat.* **2022**, *193*, 685–694. [CrossRef]
38. Böckerman, P.; Ilmakunnas, P. Unemployment and self-assessed health: Evidence from panel data. *Health Econ.* **2009**, *18*, 161–179. [CrossRef]

medicina

MDPI

Review

Barriers and Facilitators to Artificial Intelligence Implementation in Diabetes Management from Healthcare Workers' Perspective: A Scoping Review

Giovanni Cangelosi [1,†], Andrea Conti [2,†], Gabriele Caggianelli [3], Massimiliano Panella [2,4,*], Fabio Petrelli [1,*], Stefano Mancin [5], Matteo Ratti [2,‡] and Alice Masini [2,‡]

1 School of Pharmacy, Experimental Medicine and "Stefani Scuri" Public Health Department, University of Camerino, 62032 Camerino, Italy; giovanni01.cangelosi@unicam.it
2 Department of Translational Medicine, Università del Piemonte Orientale, 28100 Novara, Italy; andrea.conti@uniupo.it (A.C.); matteo.ratti@uniupo.it (M.R.); alice.masini@uniupo.it (A.M.)
3 Azienda Ospedaliera San Giovanni Addolorata, 00184 Rome, Italy; caggianelligabriele@gmail.com
4 Direzione Medica dei Presidi Ospedalieri, Azienda Ospedaliero-Universitaria di Alessandria, 15121 Alessandria, Italy
5 IRCCS Humanitas Research Hospital, Via Manzoni 56, Rozzano, 20089 Milan, Italy; stefano.mancin@humanitas.it
* Correspondence: massimiliano.panella@med.uniupo.it (M.P.); fabio.petrelli@unicam.it (F.P.)
† These authors contributed equally to this work.
‡ These authors also contributed equally to this work.

Abstract: *Background and Objectives:* Diabetes is a global public health challenge, with increasing prevalence worldwide. The implementation of artificial intelligence (AI) in the management of this condition offers potential benefits in improving healthcare outcomes. This study primarily investigates the barriers and facilitators perceived by healthcare professionals in the adoption of AI. Secondarily, by analyzing both quantitative and qualitative data collected, it aims to support the potential development of AI-based programs for diabetes management, with particular focus on a possible bottom-up approach. *Materials and Methods:* A scoping review was conducted following PRISMA-ScR guidelines for reporting and registered in the Open Science Framework (OSF) database. The study selection process was conducted in two phases—title/abstract screening and full-text review—independently by three researchers, with a fourth resolving conflicts. Data were extracted and assessed using Joanna Briggs Institute (JBI) tools. The included studies were synthesized narratively, combining both quantitative and qualitative analyses to ensure methodological rigor and contextual depth. *Results*: The adoption of AI tools in diabetes management is influenced by several barriers, including perceived unsatisfactory clinical performance, high costs, issues related to data security and decision-making transparency, as well as limited training among healthcare workers. Key facilitators include improved clinical efficiency, ease of use, time-saving, and organizational support, which contribute to broader acceptance of the technology. *Conclusions*: The active and continuous involvement of healthcare workers represents a valuable opportunity to develop more effective, reliable, and well-integrated AI solutions in clinical practice. Our findings emphasize the importance of a bottom-up approach and highlight how adequate training and organizational support can help overcome existing barriers, promoting sustainable and equitable innovation aligned with public health priorities.

Keywords: diabetes; artificial intelligence; healthcare workers; scoping review; public health

1. Introduction

1.1. Prevalence of Diabetes and Social Impact

According to the International Diabetes Federation (IDF), diabetes currently affects approximately 589 million individuals worldwide between the ages of 20 and 79. Among the various forms of diabetes, Type 2 Diabetes (T2D) accounts for the vast majority of cases, with a prevalence estimated between 87% and 91%. Projections for 2050 indicate a substantial increase in global prevalence, expected to reach 853 million cases within the same age range, which will likely be accompanied by a corresponding rise in healthcare costs [1–5]. The majority of individuals with diabetes are obese and physically inactive, particularly within the 45–64 age group (28.9% of males and 32.8% of females) [6–8]. In Italy alone, the prevalence of diabetes was estimated at 4 million individuals in 2023 [9,10]. While genetic predisposition and advancing age are recognized contributors to the pathogenesis of numerous chronic diseases such as diabetes [11,12], it is predominantly unhealthy lifestyle behaviors that significantly influence both the onset and progression of these conditions [13–17]. In particular, dietary patterns characterized by excessive caloric intake, a high consumption of refined grains in place of whole grains, and insufficient physical activity constitute the principal modifiable risk factors [18–20]. These detrimental habits not only facilitate the development of disease but also exacerbate its clinical course, substantially increasing the risk of complications. Such complications include both peripheral vascular disorders and more complex cardiovascular events, with potentially severe outcomes such as acute myocardial infarction and cerebrovascular accidents (stroke), which are associated with increased morbidity and mortality between in T2D and Type 1 Diabetes (T1D) [21–23]. In light of this evidence, the implementation of comprehensive primary and secondary prevention strategies aimed at promoting healthier lifestyles is imperative [24–26]. Emphasis should be placed on balanced nutritional intake, caloric moderation, and the adoption of regular physical activity, with the goal of reducing the global burden of disease and improving population health outcomes in T1D and T2D [27–30].

1.2. Use of Devices and Technology in Diabetes Management

At the same time, with the promotion of healthy lifestyle behaviors, diabetes management—particularly for T1D—has long benefited significantly from technological innovation applied in clinical settings, especially with regard to glucose self-monitoring and insulin delivery. Devices such as continuous glucose monitoring (CGM) systems, insulin pumps (IP), and smart multiple daily injection (MDI) systems, often integrated into hybrid closed-loop systems, have become indispensable supports in daily clinical practice [21,22]. They play a critical role in reducing glycemic variability and preventing hypoglycemic episodes, thereby helping to avert major diabetes-related complications. In the context of T2D as well, digital technologies—including self-management applications and telemonitoring tools—are proving valuable, particularly in the personalization of therapeutic interventions and the optimization of clinical outcomes and complication management [31–34]. In recent years, artificial intelligence (AI) has taken an increasingly prominent role in both diabetes research and clinical practice, owing to its capacity to process and analyze large volumes of clinical and behavioral data efficiently and accurately [35–38]. Predictive models based on AI techniques such as machine learning (ML) and deep learning (DL) are being developed and implemented to support clinical decision-making, enhance the prediction of complication risks, and personalize treatment pathways [39–41]. Applications of AI in diabetes care range from early diagnosis to automated insulin dosing management and the identification of critical glycemic patterns, thereby contributing to the emergence of a new paradigm in precision medicine for diabetes [35–41]. Nonetheless, the issue of potential barriers and facilitators perceived by healthcare professionals in the effective implementation of these AI-based technologies in routine clinical practice remains largely unexplored—a gap this study aims to address in a bottom-up view, defined as "an approach guided by healthcare workers' insights and daily experiences" [42].

1.3. Study Aims

The primary objective of this study was to investigate the main barriers and facilitators perceived by healthcare professionals involved in the implementation of artificial intelligence (AI) in diabetes management:

- What are the barriers and facilitators to the use of AI by healthcare professionals in the management of diabetes?

Secondarily, the study aims to explore and support research through the collection of both quantitative and qualitative data to inform the development and implementation of specific AI-based programs for diabetes management, following a bottom-up approach involving healthcare professionals.

- Which quantitative and qualitative insights, as perceived by healthcare professionals, can most effectively inform the bottom-up implementation of AI in diabetes care?

2. Materials and Methods

2.1. Study Design and Registration

A scoping review was conducted to ensure methodological rigor and the relevance of selected studies. This review followed the Preferred Reporting Items for Systematic reviews and Meta-Analyses extension for Scoping Reviews guidelines (PRISMA-ScR) (PRISMA-ScR checklist available in Supplementary Table S1) [43]. The protocol for this review was registered in the Open Science Framework database (https://osf.io/xgy2z; accessed on 12 June 2025).

2.2. Search Strategy

The search strategy was developed adopting the Population, Concept, Context (PCC) framework (Table 1), without temporal restrictions [44]. The search strategy, updated to 31 January 2025, involved the use of keywords matched using specific Boolean operators such as AND/OR in the databases PubMed Medline, Scopus, CINHAL, and Embase. Search strings are available in Supplementary Table S2.

Table 1. Inclusion and exclusion criteria, described according to the PCC framework.

Parameter	Inclusion Criteria	Exclusion Criteria
Population	Studies involving healthcare professionals (principally doctors, nurses, specialists, technicians) who manage diabetes with AI.	Studies that do not involve healthcare workers.

Table 1. *Cont.*

Parameter	Inclusion Criteria	Exclusion Criteria
Concept	Studies exploring the adoption and implementation of AI in managing diabetes, such as monitoring systems, diagnostics, predictive therapy, and personalized patient management. AI technologies extended in ML or DL use.	Studies that address AI in non-healthcare contexts or those unrelated to managing diabetes; technological interventions that do not use AI, ML or DL.
Context	Barriers and obstacles perceived from healthcare workers in adopting AI (e.g., technological difficulties, cultural challenges, insufficient training, resistance to change). Facilitators and enabling factors from healthcare workers in terms of AI adoption (e.g., organizational support, training, technology accessibility, evidence of effectiveness).	Studies that do not explore barriers or facilitators in AI adoption by healthcare workers; research that only addresses clinical outcomes of diabetes treatment without focusing on perception, implementation science, and attitude.

AI: artificial intelligence; ML: machine learning; DL: deep learning.

2.3. Eligibility Criteria

The inclusion criteria encompassed primary studies published in English without temporal restriction and relevant to the study's objectives and involving healthcare workers in AI processes. All studies that did not meet the stated inclusion criteria were excluded. The authors nevertheless attempted to include studies in Chinese as well, after evaluating the English-language abstract to ensure it met the inclusion criteria.

2.4. Study Selection Process

The study selection process for this review followed a two-phase procedure: an initial screening of titles and abstracts, followed by a detailed evaluation of full-text articles. All potentially relevant articles were imported into the reference manager Ryyan (https://www.rayyan.ai/; accessed on 20 June 2025) for data organization and management. The initial screening was conducted independently and blind by three authors (G.C., A.M., and M.R.), who evaluated titles and abstracts based on their relevance to the study and in accordance with the predefined inclusion criteria. A fourth independent researcher (A.C.) resolved any disagreements at this stage. Following the initial screening, full-text articles meeting the preliminary criteria were independently assessed by the first three researchers, and the fourth still managed conflicts. Any discrepancies were resolved through consensus meetings, with the last researcher (A.C.) acting as an arbitrator to ensure integrity in the selection process. This systematic approach ensured a rigorous and unbiased selection of studies for this review.

2.5. Data Extraction and Quality Appraisal

Data extraction from the included studies was organized into key categories, consistent with the methodological framework [43,44]. This structured categorization facilitated both detailed reporting and thorough analysis. The main categories included intervention, outer setting, inner setting, individual characteristics, and implementation process. This structured approach enhanced the clarity and depth of our analysis, aligning with established methodological standards. The extracted data were presented as a narrative summary, organized according to the review's objectives and supplemented in Table 2. The risk of bias and methodological quality of the included studies were assessed using established guidelines of the JBI framework [43]. Two independent reviewers (A.M. and

A.C.) conducted the evaluation to ensure objectivity. Any disagreements were resolved through discussions with a third researcher (M.R.), ensuring that a consensus was reached. The risk of bias and methodological quality of the included studies were evaluated using JBI checklists for qualitative [45] and cross-sectional studies [46] and the MMAT tool for mixed-methods studies [47]. Decisions regarding methodological quality of the studies included were made, independently, by two reviewers, and any disagreements were resolved by discussion. The sum of the points was classified as the percentage of the items present; thus, a score lower than 70% was classified as low-quality, between 70 and 79% of the checklist criteria was classified as medium–high-quality, between 80 and 90% was assigned high-quality, and a score greater than 90% of the criteria was classified as excellent-quality [48]. However, due to the exploratory nature of the present work, no studies were excluded for insufficient quality.

2.6. Conceptual and Analytical Framework

The synthesis and presentation of study results followed established guidelines [43,44]. The description of the identified barriers and facilitators is structured according to the Consolidated Framework for Implementation Research (CFIR) [49], a comprehensive theoretical framework widely used to guide implementation research. CFIR comprises five major domains—intervention characteristics, outer setting, inner setting, characteristics of individuals, and implementation process—that offer a systematic approach to understanding factors influencing implementation. In this scoping review, CFIR was used as a guiding structure to map and interpret both qualitative and quantitative data extracted from the selected studies, enabling a comprehensive and theory-informed synthesis of the findings. Key statistical measures, including means (M), standard deviations (SD), and p-values, were integral to the analysis. To maintain the integrity of the original studies, statistical significance reporting was preserved as presented in each study. Consistent with scientific conventions, p-values of 0.05 or lower were considered statistically significant, ensuring the inclusion of robust and meaningful findings in the review. In addition to the quantitative synthesis, qualitative data were also systematically extracted and analyzed, where applicable, to capture nuanced insights and contextual dimensions of the study findings. The qualitative synthesis followed established principal thematic frameworks in the study included and to further enhance and complete the analysis conducted.

2.7. Synthesis of the Results

In this review, while the benefits of meta-analysis are acknowledged, a combined quantitative synthesis was deemed not feasible due to the heterogeneity of the included studies. This variability, characterized by differences in intervention types and methodologies for quantifying relationships between variables, led to inconsistencies in both methodological and statistical approaches. As a result, a detailed narrative synthesis was chosen, following established guidelines for synthesis without meta-analysis (SWiM) [50]. This approach was selected for its effectiveness in transparently and rigorously synthesizing diverse quantitative data, aligning with the PRISMA guidelines [43]. Data synthesis was performed based on the CFIR framework [49]. The CFIR is a well-established conceptual model in implementation science, and it is a comprehensive and standardized meta-theoretical framework. The updated version of the framework is organized into five domains: intervention, outer setting, inner setting, individual characteristics, and implementation process [49]. The CFIR served as a foundational structure for the exploratory assessment of barriers and facilitators to implementing imaging-based, AI-assisted diagnostic decision-making. The comprehensive and adaptable use of the updated CFIR throughout data collection, analysis, and reporting aimed to enhance research efficiency, generate generalizable findings to inform AI implementation practices, and contribute to a robust evidence base for tailoring implementation strategies to overcome key barriers.

3. Results

The PRISMA flowchart of the screening process is shown in Figure 1. A total of n = 3451 records were retrieved from the databases, and after carefully removing the duplicates (n = 593), the researchers (GC, AM, AC, and MR) screened a total of n = 3143 for title and abstract. Thirty-two full texts were screened. Finally, a total of n = 7 studies, conducted between 2019 and 2024, were included [51–57].

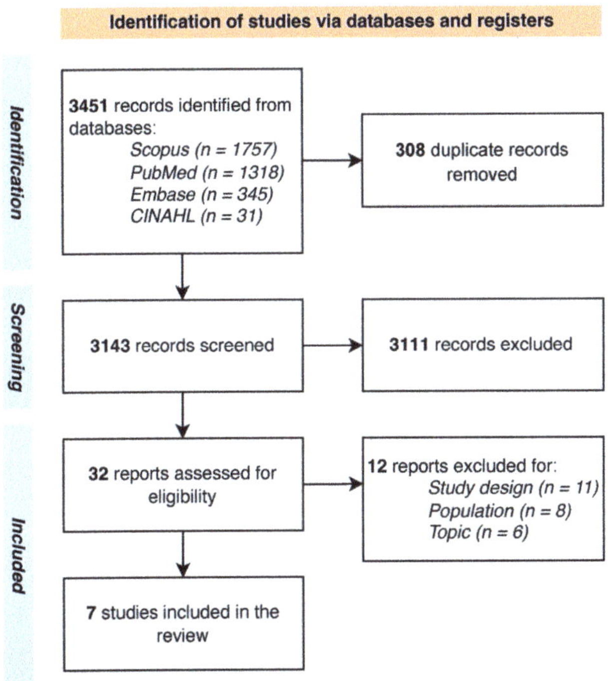

Figure 1. PRISMA flowchart.

Studies' characteristics are shown in Table 2. The population varied from 10 participants to 207, with a range of ages from 40 to 60 years. The involved healthcare professionals were mainly nurses, healthcare assistants, and doctors (i.e., ophthalmologists, diabetologists, endocrinologists, physicians, and general practitioners).

Table 2. Summary of the included studies.

Study	Country	Study Design	Setting	Sample Size (N, % Female)	AI Type
Held et al., 2022 [51]	Germany	Qualitative	Primary care	24 (42)	Smartphone-based and AI-supported diagnosis tools for the screening of diabetic retinopathy
Liao et al., 2024 [52]	China	Qualitative	Hospital and community healthcare center	40 (42.5)	AI-assisted system for diabetic retinopathy screening

Table 2. *Cont.*

Study	Country	Study Design	Setting	Sample Size (N, % Female)	AI Type
Petersen et al., 2024 [53]	Denmark	Qualitative	Hospital	18 (61)	AI-assisted system for diabetic retinopathy screening
Romero et al., 2019 [55]	United States	Mixed -methods	Primary care outpatient clinics	83 (N/A)	AI-powered clinical decision support system for identifying diabetes patients at risk of poor glycemic control
Roy et al., 2024 [54]	India	Cross-sectional	Physicians in clinical practice	202 (N/A)	AI-based diabetes diagnostic interventions
Wahlich et al., 2024 [57]	United Kingdom	Qualitative	Hospital and community healthcare center	98 (N/A)	AI-assisted system for diabetic retinopathy screening
Wewetzer et al., 2023 [56]	Germany	Cross-sectional	Primary care	209 (107)	AI-assisted system for diabetic retinopathy screening

AI: artificial intelligence; N: number; N/A: not applicable; %: percentage.

The study conducted by Liao et al. also included healthcare administrative staff and information technology experts [52]. The majority of the included studies were focused on the use of AI for diabetic retinopathy screening [51–53,56,57], with only two studies focused on AI as a tool for glycemic control and AI as a general tool for diagnostic intervention [54,55].

Most of the studies adopted a qualitative design (n = 4) that used semi-structured interviews [51–53,57]. Two quantitative cross-sectional studies were based on surveys [54,56], and finally, one study adopted a mixed-methods design [55].

All the included studies described research conducted in primary care settings, with the exception of the study conducted by Roy et al. [54], which was conducted in a clinic. Notably, two studies were performed inside community healthcare centers [52,57].

3.1. Quality Appraisal

Table 3 shows the overall quality of the included studies according to the JBI framework [44]. Complete quality appraisal is available in Supplementary Tables S3–S5.

Table 3. Results of quality appraisal.

Study	Checklist	Overall Quality
Held et al., 2022 [51]	JBI for qualitative studies	Medium
Liao et al., 2024 [52]	JBI for qualitative studies	Excellent
Petersen et al., 2024 [53]	JBI for qualitative studies	High
Romero et al., 2019 [55]	MMAT	High
Roy et al., 2024 [54]	JBI for analytical cross-sectional studies	Low
Wahlich et al., 2024 [57]	JBI for qualitative studies	Medium
Wewetzer et al., 2023 [56]	JBI for analytical cross-sectional studies	Medium

MMAT: Mixed-Methods Appraisal Tool; JBI: Joanna Briggs Institute.

Regarding the four qualitative studies, Whalich et al. [57] and Held et al. [51] were rated as medium-quality due to the absence of statements addressing the researchers' cultural positions and the mutual influence between the researchers and the research process. The studies by Liao et al. [52] and Peterson et al. [53] were well designed.

The two studies with a cross-sectional design presented as low-quality due to the lack of information during the description of the inclusion and exclusion criteria [54] and the setting of the study, while the study by Wewetzer et al. [56] was reported as medium-quality owing to the lack of managing confounding factors.

Finally, the mixed-methods study performed by Romero et al. [55] all was well designed and conducted, with a high-quality rating.

3.2. Barriers and Facilitators Identified According to the CFIR Framework

The following sections present findings according to the CFIR framework domains, and Figure 2 illustrates the main identified barriers and facilitators. Comprehensive data extraction is shown in Supplementary Table S6.

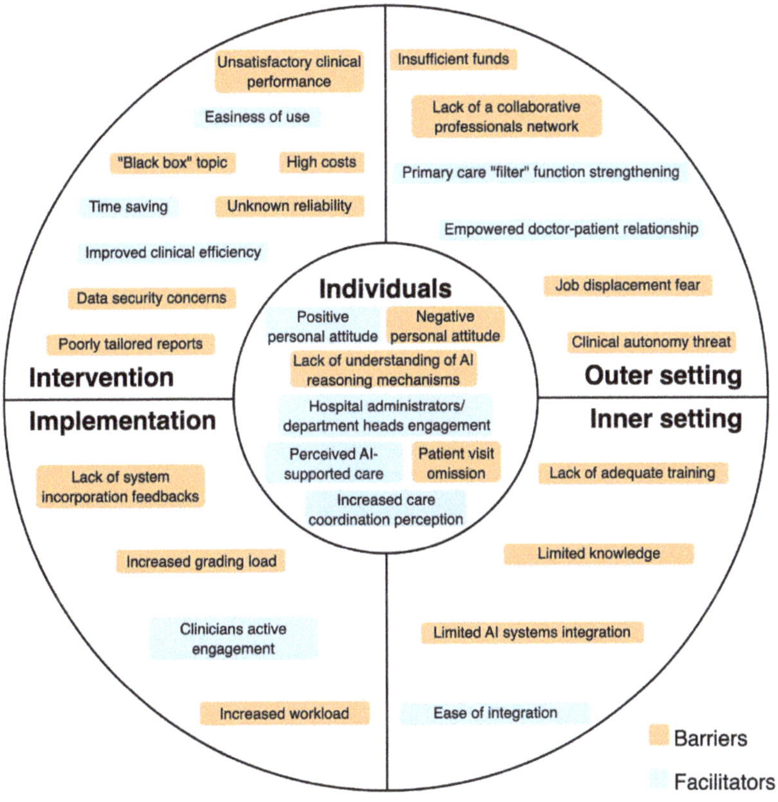

Figure 2. Barriers and facilitators of AI implementation for diabetes management reported by healthcare professionals.

3.2.1. Individuals Domain

The principal barrier is the negative personal attitude towards AI systems, with associated skepticism [51], incompetence in understanding the AI reasoning mechanisms [52], or forgetfulness to visit the patient [53].

The facilitators belonging to this domain are engagement of hospital administrators or department heads [52], positive attitude towards the future of AI technology [57], perception of increased care coordination [55], or perception of AI as a support [57].

3.2.2. Intervention Domain

The relevant barrier under this domain is the unsatisfactory clinical performance of the AI system. This aspect is related to image recognition, time (duration of examination and latency of results), validity (AI system may miss some retinopathy changes), and uncertainty about the accuracy and trustworthiness of AI outputs [51–54]. Also, Romero et al. [55] reported as a barrier the high false positive rate in patient risk classification, whereas the studies of Wewetzer et al. [56] and Wahlich et al. [57] highlighted diagnostic limitations of AI systems (they may not detect other conditions besides the one for which they have been designed for, leading to incomplete diagnosis). Finally, doubts about reliability and accuracy may negatively impact physician confidence in the system [56,57]. Another common barrier is related to the financial burden of AI software/high acquisition costs [52,53,56].

Another fundamental barrier to consider is the concern about data security, liability, and how the system made the decision (black box problem) [54,55,57]. Romero et al. [55] and Liao et al. [52] also reported the poorly tailored reporting of AI systems.

The identified facilitators are an improved clinical efficiency [52,54,55], easiness of use [52,54], and the time sparing effect, both for the patient and for the physician [53,56,57]. Only one study reported a financial facilitator [51].

3.2.3. Implementation Process Domain

The principal barriers are the lack of feedback in incorporation of the system [52], the increased workload due to extra steps outside the routine workflow [55], and the impact of a grading workload [57].

The only facilitator identified in the implementation process is the successful active engagement of the clinicians [52].

3.2.4. Inner Setting Domain

The principal barrier related to the inner setting is the lack of adequate training or limited knowledge and training on the AI system [52,54,55]. Also, the lack of integration of the AI system into the hospital/facility information system is another relevant concern that acts as a barrier [54–56].

The only inner setting facilitator identified under this domain is the ease of integration, with the associated simple installation [51,52].

3.2.5. Outer Setting Domain

For the outer setting domain, the crucial emerging barrier is the lack of a collaborative network between primary, secondary, and tertiary hospitals, which includes the related tensions between GPs and specialists with the concern of a lower referral rate [51,52]. Also, the fear of job displacement or changes in clinical autonomy is another concern that is reported as a barrier [54]. A study also reported that insufficient reimbursement by health care systems may act as a significant barrier [56].

The facilitators reported that can be classified under this domain are the development of national guidelines related to AI [52], the strengthening of the primary doctor filter function, and an associated closer relationship between patient and GP [51].

4. Discussion

The implementation of AI systems in healthcare represents one of the most significant challenges of the coming decade, not only for daily clinical practice but also for public health systems as a whole. The findings of this study, interpreted through the CFIR framework [49], clearly show that the barriers and facilitators to AI adoption operate on multiple levels, reflecting organizational, technological, individual, and systemic dynamics that influence full implementation and value realization.

4.1. Innovation, Effectiveness, and Trust in Technology

The most critical issue that emerged relates to the perceived unsatisfactory clinical performance—an aspect with profound implications for public health [58,59]. If AI systems are unable to ensure adequate levels of sensitivity and specificity—or if their reliability is perceived as uncertain—they risk undermining the quality of care and increasing the chances of missed or inappropriate diagnoses [60]. In the context of population screening (such as diabetic retinopathy), a high number of false positives or false negatives could either overload the system or falsely reassure patients. This confirms what has already been observed in international studies, which emphasize the need for rigorous clinical validation before the large-scale deployment of AI systems [61,62]. Furthermore, the lack of transparency in AI's decision-making processes undermines the trust of healthcare professionals and patients, posing an ethical and regulatory challenge essential for the sustainable development of the technology [60,63]. This issue is currently the focus of attention within the European Health Data Space and the EU Artificial Intelligence Act, which introduces strict requirements for the "explainability" and traceability of collected data [64]. These concerns are rooted primarily in the CFIR domain of intervention, where the perceived evidence strength, complexity, and relative advantage of the AI tools are critical to their adoption. Additionally, elements from the individuals domain emerge, particularly regarding trust and acceptance by healthcare professionals.

4.2. Equity and Sustainability: AI Costs, Access, and Integration

The barrier represented by the costs of acquiring and managing AI can also be interpreted in terms of equity in access to healthcare innovations [65]. This economic barrier was identified within the CFIR domain of intervention characteristics, highlighting the perceived complexity and resource intensity associated with adopting AI-based tools. Mainly in publicly funded universal healthcare systems, the adoption of expensive technologies risks creating territorial inequalities, where larger or better-funded facilities can afford to implement AI, while peripheral or resource-limited ones risk being effectively excluded [66]. This issue was already highlighted by the World Health Organization (WHO) in the 2021 report "Ethics and Governance of Artificial Intelligence for Health", which urges careful evaluation of AI's redistributive impact in public health contexts [67]. Adding to this is the poor integration with existing information systems, which are often not designed to accommodate supplementary technologies, thereby hindering true interoperability. Without full connectivity between AI, electronic health records, and healthcare management systems, AI risks remaining an isolated technology, incapable of delivering real value to patient care [68,69]. These considerations also align with the principles of the United Nations Sustainable Development Goals (SDGs), particularly those promoting health, innovation, and equity in access to care [70].

4.3. Healthcare System and Multilevel Governance

In terms of governance and shared decision-making, it becomes clear that the lack of coordination between levels of care (e.g., primary care, specialists, hospitals) and potential communication difficulties among professionals represent critical barriers to AI implementation. This issue is part of a broader challenge in healthcare governance, which calls for dynamic and modern models of both vertical and horizontal service integration [71–73]. Technology alone does not solve these problems; on the contrary, it can amplify them if introduced without a clear and shared organizational framework. The concern, particularly regarding the potential loss of clinical autonomy—clearly emerging from the data reviewed—is a key issue for the "social" legitimacy of digital innovations in healthcare [74,75]. According to Greenhalgh et al. (2017), the adoption of new technologies requires a co-construction of change, in which professionals are actively involved not only in the use but also in the design and evaluation of the tools to be implemented in clinical practice [76]. These barriers align with the CFIR domains of *inner setting* and *implementation process*, emphasizing organizational coordination gaps and limited stakeholder engagement in technology adoption.

4.4. Training, Digital Literacy, and Empowerment

These issues fall within the CFIR domain of characteristics of individuals, particularly focusing on knowledge, self-efficacy, and the need for ongoing professional development to support effective AI adoption. From an internal perspective, the lack of adequate training on AI tools is a systemic barrier that must be urgently addressed—especially if the goal is to adopt AI-based care systems across multiple levels of healthcare delivery [77]. Structured pathways for continuous education are therefore essential, integrating "AI literacy" into university curriculum, ongoing professional development programs, and career advancement tracks. This ensures they do not become mere executors but rather informed actors who use technology as an extension of their clinical skill expertise [78,79].

4.5. Opportunities for Public Health

Despite the critical issues that have emerged, the identified facilitators show significant transformative potential. Time savings, increased clinical efficiency, the perception of greater care coordination and positive acceptance by some operators are valuable elements for the success of public policies that aim at the equitable and sustainable digitalization of healthcare [80–82].

The presence of possible national and international guidelines to support health professionals is perceived as an enabling element, and in this scenario, AI could represent a turning point if integrated with global implementation strategies, clinical audits, and impact assessment [64]. It is desirable that an international public control room is created to guarantee the implementation of AI, capable of providing technical standards, ethical assessments, and support to local decision makers and organizers of health services in general that meet all the quality standards necessary for the use of AI in clinical practice [67,83]. These facilitators reflect the CFIR domains of *outer setting* and *implementation process*, particularly highlighting the role of policy support, external incentives, and structured strategies to guide effective and equitable AI integration.

4.6. Barriers and Facilitators in a Bottom-Up Perspective

The introduction of AI and other technological tools into clinical settings—particularly for the management of chronic diseases—represents a significant opportunity to rethink traditional models of care and transition toward a more predictive, proactive, and personalized approach [84–89]. Chronic conditions such as diabetes, hypertension, cardiovascular, and respiratory diseases represent a substantial burden for public healthcare systems and require coordinated, continuous, and patient-centered management strategies [90,91]. In this context, AI can serve as a catalyst for innovation, provided that it is embedded in a well-structured and responsive clinical and organizational ecosystem [92]. Building on the CFIR framework, our analysis identified key barriers and facilitators across its five domains: characteristics of the intervention, outer setting, inner setting, individual characteristics, and implementation process. These domains provided the foundation for a structured and theory-informed classification of the data, while the discussion reframed these results in light of a bottom-up perspective—that is, how professionals working within healthcare systems perceive, experience, and respond to the integration of AI in their clinical practice [49,93,94]. From a practical standpoint, AI-based systems—such as those used for diabetic retinopathy screening or cardiovascular risk stratification [95,96]—can support the early detection of complications, thereby reducing the need for hospital-based interventions and enabling more timely, preventive care. This dual benefit supports both patients, who receive appropriate interventions sooner, and healthcare systems, which benefit from improved outcomes and resource efficiency [97]. However, integrating AI into routine clinical practice necessitates parallel transformations in organizational routines, workforce training, and digital competencies among healthcare professionals [98]. Rather than framing AI as a substitute for human expertise, it is essential to foster a collaborative model in which technology enhances the clinical judgment and skills of professionals. This reframing can help overcome cultural resistance to adoption, often rooted in concerns about professional identity and loss of autonomy [99,100]. Among the barriers, frontline professionals reported challenges such as poor interoperability of AI with existing electronic health records, lack of shared implementation strategies, and insufficient digital literacy. These aspects reflect issues related to the CFIR domains of intervention characteristics, inner setting, and outer setting. Additionally, fragmented care coordination and lack of shared governance structures were seen as limiting factors in the effective deployment of AI across healthcare levels [101,102]. Conversely, several facilitators emerged from a bottom-up viewpoint, highlighting how AI adoption can be positively influenced by perceived improvements in workflow efficiency, time savings, and greater integration between primary and specialty care. Professionals also reported a willingness to engage with new tools in general technology devices when training is adequate and when they are actively involved in implementation decisions in clinical and social decision [103–105].

4.7. A Public Health View on AI in Clinical Practice

For chronic disease management, where continuity and coordination of care are essential, AI systems can support transitions between care settings, enhance remote monitoring, and offer predictive insights that guide therapeutic decisions [106–108]. However, without appropriate regulation and inclusive planning, the risk of exacerbating health inequities remains high—particularly in underserved or digitally marginalized populations [109,110]. To prevent such disparities, healthcare professionals must be empowered not only as end users but also as digital mediators and educators, helping to guide patients and caregivers in the effective and ethical use of AI technologies [111–115]. Their proximity to patients and deep understanding of local care pathways position them as crucial actors in fostering responsible innovation. Finally, the development of AI for chronic care must be embedded in a broader cultural and ethical framework that views data as a collective asset and public health as the primary driver for technological development. This shift is necessary to ensure that data-driven medicine evolves in a fair, sustainable, and inclusive direction [116,117].

4.8. Strengths and Limitations

The study's strengths include its solid methodological framework, facilitated by the adoption of the JBI methodology, the PRISMA-ScR guidelines for reporting [43,44], and the registration of the protocol on the OSF database, elements that ensure transparency and international rigor. The use of the CFIR framework [49] allowed for an in-depth analysis of the factors influencing AI adoption by healthcare workers, facilitating a coherent and useful classification from a public health perspective. However, some limitations should be considered. The exploratory nature of the scoping review did not allow for a quantitative synthesis of data due to the methodological heterogeneity of the included studies and the cohorts considered. Additionally, many findings are based on subjective perceptions of the involved workers in the studies included, which requires caution in interpreting the collected data and highlights the need for future integration with objective data and evidence-driven research. For these elements, future studies aimed at addressing these gaps are required. In particular, it is suggested to develop longitudinal research and randomized studies that evaluate not only perceptions but also the real effectiveness and efficiency of AI in managing diabetes and chronic diseases in general from a healthcare worker's point of view. This approach would help build more comprehensive and useful evidence for the sustainable implementation of technological innovation in public health perspectives.

5. Conclusions

The adoption of AI in chronic care, particularly in diabetes management, is shaped by a dynamic interplay of perceived barriers and facilitators among healthcare professionals. Their active and continuous involvement represents a key opportunity to develop more effective, reliable, and context-aware AI solutions that are better integrated into everyday clinical workflows. Promoting targeted training programs and sustained organizational support for healthcare workers involved in the complex management of diabetes may help overcome current challenges, advancing more equitable and sustainable innovation. Crucially, these findings point toward the value of a bottom-up approach—one that prioritizes the perspectives and practical needs of frontline professionals—as a promising pathway to support the successful implementation of AI in clinical practice. Framing AI adoption within a broader public health perspective, attentive to systemic readiness and social equity, can guide more inclusive strategies that align innovation with real-world healthcare priorities.

Supplementary Materials: The following supporting information can be downloaded at: https://www.mdpi.com/article/10.3390/medicina61081403/s1, Table S1: PRISMA-ScR checklist; Table S2: Search strategy; Table S3: Cross-sectional studies quality appraisal; Table S4: Qualitative studies quality appraisal; Table S5: Mixed-methods studies quality appraisal; Table S6: Complete data extraction.

Author Contributions: Conceptualization, G.C. (Giovanni Cangelosi), A.M., M.R., A.C., M.P. and F.P.; methodology, M.P., F.P., A.M. and G.C. (Giovanni Cangelosi); validation, M.P. and F.P.; formal analysis, G.C. (Giovanni Cangelosi), A.M., A.C., M.R., G.C. (Gabriele Caggianelli) and S.M.; investigation, G. Cangelosi, A.M., A.C., M.R., G.C. (Gabriele Caggianelli) and S.M.; data curation, A.M., M.R., G.C. (Giovanni Cangelosi), G.C. (Gabriele Caggianelli) and S.M.; writing—original draft preparation, A.C., G.C. (Giovanni Cangelosi), G.C. (Gabriele Caggianelli) and S.M.; writing—review and editing, A.M., M.R., M.P., F.P., A.C., G.C. (Giovanni Cangelosi) and G.C. (Gabriele Caggianelli); visualization, A.C.; supervision, M.P. and F.P. All authors have read and agreed to the published version of the manuscript.

Funding: This research received no external funding.

Institutional Review Board Statement: Not applicable.

Informed Consent Statement: Not applicable.

Data Availability Statement: Data is contained within the article or Supplementary Material.

Acknowledgments: Any use of artificial intelligence in the preparation of this manuscript was exclusively for final linguistic editing, supported by a native English-speaking author of the study. The content of this article is entirely the result of the original intellectual effort and research of the authors.

Conflicts of Interest: The authors declare no conflicts of interest.

Abbreviations

The following abbreviations are used in this manuscript:

AI	Artificial Intelligence
IDF	International Diabetes Foundation
T2D	Type 2 Diabetes
T1D	Type 1 Diabetes
CGM	Continuous Glucose Monitoring
IP	Insulin Pump
MDI	Multiple Daily Injection
ML	Machine Learning
DL	Deep Learning
PRISMA-ScR	Preferred Reporting Items for Systematic reviews and Meta-Analyses extension for Scoping Reviews
OSF	Open Science Foundation
PCC	Population, Concept, Context
JBI	Joanna Briggs Institute
MMAT	Mixed-Methods Appraisal Tool
CFIR	Consolidated Framework for Implementation Research
SD	Standard Deviation
SWIM	Synthesis Without Meta-Analysis
GP	General Practitioner
WHO	World Health Organization
EU	European Union

References

1. Aschner, P.; Karuranga, S.; James, S.; Simmons, D.; Basit, A.; Shaw, J.E.; Wild, S.H.; Ogurtsova, K.; Saeedi, P. The International Diabetes Federation's Guide for Diabetes Epidemiological Studies. *Diabetes Res. Clin. Pract.* **2021**, *172*, 108630. [CrossRef] [PubMed]
2. World Health Organization Diabetes—Fact Sheets. Available online: https://www.who.int/news-room/fact-sheets/detail/diabetes (accessed on 13 June 2025).
3. Chen, X.; Zhang, L.; Chen, W. Global, Regional, and National Burdens of Type 1 and Type 2 Diabetes Mellitus in Adolescents from 1990 to 2021, with Forecasts to 2030: A Systematic Analysis of the Global Burden of Disease Study 2021. *BMC Med.* **2025**, *23*, 48. [CrossRef] [PubMed]
4. Saeedi, P.; Petersohn, I.; Salpea, P.; Malanda, B.; Karuranga, S.; Unwin, N.; Colagiuri, S.; Guariguata, L.; Motala, A.A.; Ogurtsova, K.; et al. Global and Regional Diabetes Prevalence Estimates for 2019 and Projections for 2030 and 2045: Results from the International Diabetes Federation Diabetes Atlas, 9th Edition. *Diabetes Res. Clin. Pract.* **2019**, *157*, 107843. [CrossRef] [PubMed]
5. Nguyen, P.; Le, L.K.-D.; Ananthapavan, J.; Gao, L.; Dunstan, D.W.; Moodie, M. Economics of Sedentary Behaviour: A Systematic Review of Cost of Illness, Cost-Effectiveness, and Return on Investment Studies. *Prev. Med.* **2022**, *156*, 106964. [CrossRef]
6. Alkaf, B.; Blakemore, A.I.; Järvelin, M.-R.; Lessan, N. Secondary Analyses of Global Datasets: Do Obesity and Physical Activity Explain Variation in Diabetes Risk across Populations? *Int. J. Obes.* **2021**, *45*, 944–956. [CrossRef]
7. Komuro, K.; Kaneko, H.; Komuro, J.; Suzuki, Y.; Okada, A.; Mizuno, A.; Fujiu, K.; Takeda, N.; Morita, H.; Node, K.; et al. Differences in the Association of Lifestyle-Related Modifiable Risk Factors with Incident Cardiovascular Disease between Individuals with and without Diabetes. *Eur. J. Prev. Cardiol.* **2025**, *32*, 376–383. [CrossRef]
8. Chimoriya, R.; Rana, K.; Adhikari, J.; Aitken, S.J.; Poudel, P.; Baral, A.; Rawal, L.; Piya, M.K. The Association of Physical Activity With Overweight/Obesity and Type 2 Diabetes in Nepalese Adults: Evidence From a Nationwide Non-Communicable Disease Risk Factor Survey. *Obes. Sci. Pract.* **2025**, *11*, e70046. [CrossRef]
9. Istituto Superiore di Sanità Giornata Mondiale Diabete: Dalla Prevalenza All'accesso Alle Cure, I Numeri Della Sorveglianza Passi. Available online: https://www.iss.it/-/giornata-mondiale-diabete-da-prevalenza-ad-accesso-cure-i-numeri-del-sistema-passi (accessed on 13 June 2025).
10. Istituto Nazionale di Statistica Il Diabete in Italia. Available online: https://www.istat.it/it/files/2017/07/REPORT_DIABETE.pdf (accessed on 13 June 2025).

11. Jiang, Y.; Hu, J.; Chen, F.; Liu, B.; Wei, M.; Xia, W.; Yan, Y.; Xie, J.; Du, S.; Tian, X.; et al. Comprehensive Systematic Review and Meta-Analysis of Risk Factors for Childhood Obesity in China and Future Intervention Strategies. *Lancet Reg. Health-West. Pac.* **2025**, *58*, 101553. [CrossRef]
12. Blanken, C.P.S.; Bayer, S.; Buchner Carro, S.; Hauner, H.; Holzapfel, C. Associations Between *TCF7L2*, *PPARγ*, and *KCNJ11* Genotypes and Insulin Response to an Oral Glucose Tolerance Test: A Systematic Review. *Mol. Nutr. Food Res.* **2025**, *69*, e202400561. [CrossRef]
13. Wang, Y.; Cao, P.; Liu, F.; Chen, Y.; Xie, J.; Bai, B.; Liu, Q.; Ma, H.; Geng, Q. Gender Differences in Unhealthy Lifestyle Behaviors among Adults with Diabetes in the United States between 1999 and 2018. *IJERPH* **2022**, *19*, 16412. [CrossRef]
14. Teck, J. Diabetes-Associated Comorbidities. *Prim. Care Clin. Off. Pract.* **2022**, *49*, 275–286. [CrossRef]
15. Pearson-Stuttard, J.; Holloway, S.; Polya, R.; Sloan, R.; Zhang, L.; Gregg, E.W.; Harrison, K.; Elvidge, J.; Jonsson, P.; Porter, T. Variations in Comorbidity Burden in People with Type 2 Diabetes over Disease Duration: A Population-Based Analysis of Real World Evidence. *eClinicalMedicine* **2022**, *52*, 101584. [CrossRef]
16. Yu, M.G.; Gordin, D.; Fu, J.; Park, K.; Li, Q.; King, G.L. Protective Factors and the Pathogenesis of Complications in Diabetes. *Endocr. Rev.* **2024**, *45*, 227–252. [CrossRef] [PubMed]
17. Bech, A.A.; Madsen, M.D.; Kvist, A.V.; Vestergaard, P.; Rasmussen, N.H. Diabetes Complications and Comorbidities as Risk Factors for MACE in People with Type 2 Diabetes and Their Development over Time: A Danish Registry-Based Case–Control Study. *J. Diabetes* **2025**, *17*, e70076. [CrossRef] [PubMed]
18. Henney, A.E.; Gillespie, C.S.; Alam, U.; Hydes, T.J.; Boyland, E.; Cuthbertson, D.J. Ultra-processed Food and Non-communicable Diseases in the United Kingdom: A Narrative Review and Thematic Synthesis of Literature. *Obes. Rev.* **2024**, *25*, e13682. [CrossRef] [PubMed]
19. Chen, Z.; Khandpur, N.; Desjardins, C.; Wang, L.; Monteiro, C.A.; Rossato, S.L.; Fung, T.T.; Manson, J.E.; Willett, W.C.; Rimm, E.B.; et al. Ultra-Processed Food Consumption and Risk of Type 2 Diabetes: Three Large Prospective U.S. Cohort Studies. *Diabetes Care* **2023**, *46*, 1335–1344. [CrossRef]
20. Dai, W.; Albrecht, S.S. Sitting Time and Its Interaction With Physical Activity in Relation to All-Cause and Heart Disease Mortality in U.S. Adults with Diabetes. *Diabetes Care* **2024**, *47*, 1764–1768. [CrossRef]
21. Rafiei, S.K.S.; Fateh, F.; Arab, M.; Espanlo, M.; Dahaghin, S.; Gilavand, H.K.; Shahrokhi, M.; Fallahi, M.S.; Zardast, Z.; Ansari, A.; et al. Weight Change and the Risk of Micro and Macro Vascular Complications of Diabetes: A Systematic Review. *MJMS* **2024**, *31*, 18–31. [CrossRef]
22. Costa Hoffmeister, M.; Hammel Lovison, V.; Priesnitz Friedrich, E.; Da Costa Rodrigues, T. Ambulatory Blood Pressure Monitoring and Vascular Complications in Patients with Type 1 Diabetes Mellitus—Systematic Review and Meta-Analysis of Observational Studies. *Diabetes Res. Clin. Pract.* **2024**, *217*, 111873. [CrossRef]
23. Perais, J.; Agarwal, R.; Evans, J.R.; Loveman, E.; Colquitt, J.L.; Owens, D.; Hogg, R.E.; Lawrenson, J.G.; Takwoingi, Y.; Lois, N. Prognostic Factors for the Development and Progression of Proliferative Diabetic Retinopathy in People with Diabetic Retinopathy. *Cochrane Database Syst. Rev.* **2023**, *2023*, CD013775. [CrossRef]
24. Cangelosi, G.; Grappasonni, I.; Nguyen, C.T.T.; Acito, M.; Pantanetti, P.; Benni, A.; Petrelli, F. Mediterranean Diet (MedDiet) and Lifestyle Medicine (LM) for Support and Care of Patients with Type II Diabetes in the COVID-19 Era: A Cross-Observational Study. *Acta Biomed. Atenei Parm.* **2023**, *94*, e2023189. [CrossRef]
25. Kanbour, S.; Ageeb, R.A.; Malik, R.A.; Abu-Raddad, L.J. Impact of Bodyweight Loss on Type 2 Diabetes Remission: A Systematic Review and Meta-Regression Analysis of Randomised Controlled Trials. *Lancet Diabetes Endocrinol.* **2025**, *13*, 294–306. [CrossRef]
26. Petrelli, F.; Cangelosi, G.; Scuri, S.; Cuc Thi Thu, N.; Debernardi, G.; Benni, A.; Vesprini, A.; Rocchi, R.; De Carolis, C.; Pantanetti, P.; et al. Food Knowledge of Patients at the First Access to a Diabetology Center: Food Knowledge of Patients at the First Access to a Diabetology Center. *Acta Biomed. Atenei Parm.* **2020**, *91*, 160–164. [CrossRef]
27. Aljawarneh, Y.M.; Wardell, D.W.; Wood, G.L.; Rozmus, C.L. A Systematic Review of Physical Activity and Exercise on Physiological and Biochemical Outcomes in Children and Adolescents with Type 1 Diabetes. *J. Nurs. Scholarsh.* **2019**, *51*, 337–345. [CrossRef]
28. Steiman De Visser, H.; Fast, I.; Brunton, N.; Arevalo, E.; Askin, N.; Rabbani, R.; Abou-Setta, A.M.; McGavock, J. Cardiorespiratory Fitness and Physical Activity in Pediatric Diabetes: A Systemic Review and Meta-Analysis. *JAMA Netw. Open* **2024**, *7*, e240235. [CrossRef]
29. Santos, L. The Impact of Nutrition and Lifestyle Modification on Health. *Eur. J. Intern. Med.* **2022**, *97*, 18–25. [CrossRef] [PubMed]
30. Amerkamp, J.; Benli, S.; Isenmann, E.; Brinkmann, C. Optimizing the Lifestyle of Patients with Type 2 Diabetes Mellitus—Systematic Review on the Effects of Combined Diet-and-Exercise Interventions. *Nutr. Metab. Cardiovasc. Dis.* **2025**, *35*, 103746. [CrossRef] [PubMed]
31. Mannoubi, C.; Kairy, D.; Menezes, K.V.; Desroches, S.; Layani, G.; Vachon, B. The Key Digital Tool Features of Complex Telehealth Interventions Used for Type 2 Diabetes Self-Management and Monitoring with Health Professional Involvement: Scoping Review. *JMIR Med. Inf.* **2024**, *12*, e46699. [CrossRef] [PubMed]

32. Jancev, M.; Vissers, T.A.C.M.; Visseren, F.L.J.; Van Bon, A.C.; Serné, E.H.; DeVries, J.H.; De Valk, H.W.; Van Sloten, T.T. Continuous Glucose Monitoring in Adults with Type 2 Diabetes: A Systematic Review and Meta-Analysis. *Diabetologia* **2024**, *67*, 798–810. [CrossRef]
33. Ferreira, R.O.M.; Trevisan, T.; Pasqualotto, E.; Chavez, M.P.; Marques, B.F.; Lamounier, R.N.; Van De Sande-Lee, S. Continuous Glucose Monitoring Systems in Noninsulin-Treated People with Type 2 Diabetes: A Systematic Review and Meta-Analysis of Randomized Controlled Trials. *Diabetes Technol. Ther.* **2024**, *26*, 252–262. [CrossRef]
34. Saetang, T.; Greeviroj, P.; Thavaraputta, S.; Santisitthanon, P.; Houngngam, N.; Laichuthai, N. The Effectiveness of Telemonitoring and Integrated Personalized Diabetes Management in People with Insulin-treated Type 2 Diabetes Mellitus. *Diabetes Obes. Metab.* **2024**, *26*, 5233–5238. [CrossRef] [PubMed]
35. Kiran, M.; Xie, Y.; Anjum, N.; Ball, G.; Pierscionek, B.; Russell, D. Machine Learning and Artificial Intelligence in Type 2 Diabetes Prediction: A Comprehensive 33-Year Bibliometric and Literature Analysis. *Front. Digit. Health* **2025**, *7*, 1557467. [CrossRef] [PubMed]
36. Yang, Z.; Tian, D.; Zhao, X.; Zhang, L.; Xu, Y.; Lu, X.; Chen, Y. Evolutionary Patterns and Research Frontiers of Artificial Intelligence in Age-Related Macular Degeneration: A Bibliometric Analysis. *Quant. Imaging Med. Surg.* **2025**, *15*, 813–830. [CrossRef] [PubMed]
37. Yang, Q.; Bee, Y.M.; Lim, C.C.; Sabanayagam, C.; Yim-Lui Cheung, C.; Wong, T.Y.; Ting, D.S.W.; Lim, L.-L.; Li, H.; He, M.; et al. Use of Artificial Intelligence with Retinal Imaging in Screening for Diabetes-Associated Complications: Systematic Review. *eClinicalMedicine* **2025**, *81*, 103089. [CrossRef]
38. Elmotia, K.; Abouyaala, O.; Bougrine, S.; Ouahidi, M.L. Effectiveness of AI-Driven Interventions in Glycemic Control: A Systematic Review and Meta-Analysis of Randomized Controlled Trials. *Prim. Care Diabetes* **2025**, *19*, 345–354. [CrossRef]
39. Yismaw, M.B.; Tafere, C.; Tefera, B.B.; Demsie, D.G.; Feyisa, K.; Addisu, Z.D.; Zeleke, T.K.; Siraj, E.A.; Worku, M.C.; Berihun, F. Artificial Intelligence Based Predictive Tools for Identifying Type 2 Diabetes Patients at High Risk of Treatment Non-Adherence: A Systematic Review. *Int. J. Med. Inform.* **2025**, *198*, 105858. [CrossRef]
40. Usman, T.M.; Saheed, Y.K.; Nsang, A.; Ajibesin, A.; Rakshit, S. A Systematic Literature Review of Machine Learning Based Risk Prediction Models for Diabetic Retinopathy Progression. *Artif. Intell. Med.* **2023**, *143*, 102617. [CrossRef]
41. Khokhar, P.B.; Gravino, C.; Palomba, F. Advances in Artificial Intelligence for Diabetes Prediction: Insights from a Systematic Literature Review. *Artif. Intell. Med.* **2025**, *164*, 103132. [CrossRef]
42. Senot, C.; Chandrasekaran, A.; Ward, P.T. Role of Bottom-Up Decision Processes in Improving the Quality of Health Care Delivery: A Contingency Perspective. *Prod. Oper. Manag.* **2016**, *25*, 458–476. [CrossRef]
43. Tricco, A.C.; Lillie, E.; Zarin, W.; O'Brien, K.K.; Colquhoun, H.; Levac, D.; Moher, D.; Peters, M.D.J.; Horsley, T.; Weeks, L.; et al. PRISMA Extension for Scoping Reviews (PRISMA-ScR): Checklist and Explanation. *Ann. Intern. Med.* **2018**, *169*, 467–473. [CrossRef]
44. Pollock, D.; Peters, M.D.J.; Khalil, H.; McInerney, P.; Alexander, L.; Tricco, A.C.; Evans, C.; De Moraes, É.B.; Godfrey, C.M.; Pieper, D.; et al. Recommendations for the Extraction, Analysis, and Presentation of Results in Scoping Reviews. *JBI Evid. Synth.* **2023**, *21*, 520–532. [CrossRef]
45. Lockwood, C.; Munn, Z.; Porritt, K. Qualitative Research Synthesis: Methodological Guidance for Systematic Reviewers Utilizing Meta-Aggregation. *Int. J. Evid.-Based Healthc.* **2015**, *13*, 179–187. [CrossRef] [PubMed]
46. Moola, S.; Munn, Z.; Tufanaru, C.; Aromataris, E.; Sears, K.; Sfetcu, R.; Currie, M.; Qureshi, R.; Mattis, P.; Lisy, K.; et al. Chapter 7: Systematic Reviews of Etiology and Risk. In *Joanna Briggs Institute Reviewer's Manual*; Aromataris, E., Munn, Z., Eds.; The Joanna Briggs Institute: North Adelaide, Australia, 2017.
47. Hong, Q.N.; Fàbregues, S.; Bartlett, G.; Boardman, F.; Cargo, M.; Dagenais, P.; Gagnon, M.-P.; Griffiths, F.; Nicolau, B.; O'Cathain, A.; et al. The Mixed Methods Appraisal Tool (MMAT) Version 2018 for Information Professionals and Researchers. *EFI* **2018**, *34*, 285–291. [CrossRef]
48. Camp, S.; Legge, T. Simulation as a Tool for Clinical Remediation: An Integrative Review. *Clin. Simul. Nurs.* **2018**, *16*, 48–61. [CrossRef]
49. Damschroder, L.J.; Aron, D.C.; Keith, R.E.; Kirsh, S.R.; Alexander, J.A.; Lowery, J.C. Fostering Implementation of Health Services Research Findings into Practice: A Consolidated Framework for Advancing Implementation Science. *Implement. Sci.* **2009**, *4*, 50. [CrossRef]
50. Campbell, M.; McKenzie, J.E.; Sowden, A.; Katikireddi, S.V.; Brennan, S.E.; Ellis, S.; Hartmann-Boyce, J.; Ryan, R.; Shepperd, S.; Thomas, J.; et al. Synthesis without Meta-Analysis (SWiM) in Systematic Reviews: Reporting Guideline. *BMJ* **2020**, *368*, l6890. [CrossRef]
51. Held, L.A.; Wewetzer, L.; Steinhäuser, J. Determinants of the Implementation of an Artificial Intelligence-Supported Device for the Screening of Diabetic Retinopathy in Primary Care—A Qualitative Study. *Health Inform. J.* **2022**, *28*, 14604582221112816. [CrossRef]

52. Liao, X.; Yao, C.; Jin, F.; Zhang, J.; Liu, L. Barriers and Facilitators to Implementing Imaging-Based Diagnostic Artificial Intelligence-Assisted Decision-Making Software in Hospitals in China: A Qualitative Study Using the Updated Consolidated Framework for Implementation Research. *BMJ Open* **2024**, *14*, e084398. [CrossRef]
53. Petersen, G.B.; Joensen, L.E.; Kristensen, J.K.; Vorum, H.; Byberg, S.; Fangel, M.V.; Cleal, B. How to Improve Attendance for Diabetic Retinopathy Screening: Ideas and Perspectives From People with Type 2 Diabetes and Health-Care Professionals. *Can. J. Diabetes* **2024**, *49*, 121–127. [CrossRef]
54. Roy, M.; Jamwal, M.; Vasudeva, S.; Singh, M. Physicians Behavioural Intentions towards AI-Based Diabetes Diagnostic Interventions in India. *J. Public Health* **2024**. [CrossRef]
55. Romero-Brufau, S.; Wyatt, K.D.; Boyum, P.; Mickelson, M.; Moore, M.; Cognetta-Rieke, C. A Lesson in Implementation: A Pre-Post Study of Providers' Experience with Artificial Intelligence-Based Clinical Decision Support. *Int. J. Med. Inform.* **2020**, *137*, 104072. [CrossRef]
56. Wewetzer, L.; Held, L.A.; Goetz, K.; Steinhäuser, J. Determinants of the Implementation of Artificial Intelligence-Based Screening for Diabetic Retinopathy-a Cross-Sectional Study with General Practitioners in Germany. *Digit. Health* **2023**, *9*, 20552076231176644. [CrossRef]
57. Wahlich, C.; Chandrasekaran, L.; Chaudhry, U.A.R.; Willis, K.; Chambers, R.; Bolter, L.; Anderson, J.; Shakespeare, R.; Olvera-Barrios, A.; Fajtl, J.; et al. Patient and Practitioner Perceptions around Use of Artificial Intelligence within the English NHS Diabetic Eye Screening Programme. *Diabetes Res. Clin. Pract.* **2025**, *219*, 111964. [CrossRef]
58. Lucero-Prisno, D.E.; Shomuyiwa, D.O.; Kouwenhoven, M.B.N.; Dorji, T.; Odey, G.O.; Miranda, A.V.; Ogunkola, I.O.; Adebisi, Y.A.; Huang, J.; Xu, L.; et al. Top 10 Public Health Challenges to Track in 2023: Shifting Focus beyond a Global Pandemic. *Public Health Chall.* **2023**, *2*, e86. [CrossRef] [PubMed]
59. Lucero-Prisno, D.E.; Shomuyiwa, D.O.; Kouwenhoven, M.B.N.; Dorji, T.; Adebisi, Y.A.; Odey, G.O.; George, N.S.; Ajayi, O.T.; Ekerin, O.; Manirambona, E.; et al. Top 10 Public Health Challenges for 2024: Charting a New Direction for Global Health Security. *Public Health Chall.* **2025**, *4*, e70022. [CrossRef]
60. Balasubramaniam, N.; Kauppinen, M.; Rannisto, A.; Hiekkanen, K.; Kujala, S. Transparency and Explainability of AI Systems: From Ethical Guidelines to Requirements. *Inf. Softw. Technol.* **2023**, *159*, 107197. [CrossRef]
61. Rajesh, A.E.; Davidson, O.Q.; Lee, C.S.; Lee, A.Y. Artificial Intelligence and Diabetic Retinopathy: AI Framework, Prospective Studies, Head-to-Head Validation, and Cost-Effectiveness. *Diabetes Care* **2023**, *46*, 1728–1739. [CrossRef]
62. Hasan, S.U.; Siddiqui, M.A.R. Diagnostic Accuracy of Smartphone-Based Artificial Intelligence Systems for Detecting Diabetic Retinopathy: A Systematic Review and Meta-Analysis. *Diabetes Res. Clin. Pract.* **2023**, *205*, 110943. [CrossRef] [PubMed]
63. Jha, D.; Durak, G.; Das, A.; Sanjotra, J.; Susladkar, O.; Sarkar, S.; Rauniyar, A.; Kumar Tomar, N.; Peng, L.; Li, S.; et al. Ethical Framework for Responsible Foundational Models in Medical Imaging. *Front. Med.* **2025**, *12*, 1544501. [CrossRef]
64. European Commission Regulation (EU) 2024/1689 of the European Parliament and of the Council of 13 June 2024 Laying down Harmonised Rules on Artificial Intelligence and Amending Regulations (EC) No 300/2008, (EU) No 167/2013, (EU) No 168/2013, (EU) 2018/858, (EU) 2018/1139 and (EU) 2019/2144 and Directives 2014/90/EU, (EU) 2016/797 and (EU) 2020/1828 (Artificial Intelligence Act) (Text with EEA Relevance) 2024. Available online: https://eur-lex.europa.eu/eli/reg/2024/1689/oj/eng (accessed on 28 July 2025).
65. Ahmad, Z.; Rahim, S.; Zubair, M.; Abdul-Ghafar, J. Artificial Intelligence (AI) in Medicine, Current Applications and Future Role with Special Emphasis on Its Potential and Promise in Pathology: Present and Future Impact, Obstacles Including Costs and Acceptance among Pathologists, Practical and Philosophical Considerations. A Comprehensive Review. *Diagn. Pathol.* **2021**, *16*, 24. [CrossRef]
66. Wilkinson, D.; Savulescu, J. Cost-Equivalence and Pluralism in Publicly-Funded Health-Care Systems. *Health Care Anal.* **2018**, *26*, 287–309. [CrossRef]
67. World Health Organization Ethics and Governance of Artificial Intelligence for Health. WHO Guidance. Available online: https://www.who.int/publications/i/item/9789240029200 (accessed on 5 June 2025).
68. Walker, D.M.; Tarver, W.L.; Jonnalagadda, P.; Ranbom, L.; Ford, E.W.; Rahurkar, S. Perspectives on Challenges and Opportunities for Interoperability: Findings From Key Informant Interviews with Stakeholders in Ohio. *JMIR Med. Inf.* **2023**, *11*, e43848. [CrossRef]
69. Garabedian, P.; Kain, J.; Emani, S.; Singleton, S.; Rozenblum, R.; Samal, L.; Mueller, S. User Requirements and Conceptual Design for an Electronic Data Platform for Interhospital Transfer Between Acute Care Hospitals: User-Centered Design Study. *JMIR Hum. Factors* **2025**, *12*, e67884. [CrossRef] [PubMed]
70. United Nations Sustainable Development Goals. Available online: https://sdgs.un.org/goals (accessed on 21 July 2025).
71. Gordon, D.; McKay, S.; Marchildon, G.; Bhatia, R.S.; Shaw, J. Collaborative Governance for Integrated Care: Insights from a Policy Stakeholder Dialogue. *Int. J. Integr. Care* **2020**, *20*, 3. [CrossRef]

72. Faijue, D.D.; Segui, A.O.; Shringarpure, K.; Razavi, A.; Hasan, N.; Dar, O.; Manikam, L. Constructing a One Health Governance Architecture: A Systematic Review and Analysis of Governance Mechanisms for One Health. *Eur. J. Public Health* **2024**, *34*, 1086–1094. [CrossRef] [PubMed]
73. Wagner, J.K.; Doerr, M.; Schmit, C.D. AI Governance: A Challenge for Public Health. *JMIR Public Health Surveill.* **2024**, *10*, e58358. [CrossRef] [PubMed]
74. Sharma, M.; Savage, C.; Nair, M.; Larsson, I.; Svedberg, P.; Nygren, J.M. Artificial Intelligence Applications in Health Care Practice: Scoping Review. *J Med. Internet Res.* **2022**, *24*, e40238. [CrossRef]
75. Hassan, M.; Kushniruk, A.; Borycki, E. Barriers to and Facilitators of Artificial Intelligence Adoption in Health Care: Scoping Review. *JMIR Hum Factors* **2024**, *11*, e48633. [CrossRef]
76. Greenhalgh, T.; Wherton, J.; Papoutsi, C.; Lynch, J.; Hughes, G.; A'Court, C.; Hinder, S.; Fahy, N.; Procter, R.; Shaw, S. Beyond Adoption: A New Framework for Theorizing and Evaluating Nonadoption, Abandonment, and Challenges to the Scale-Up, Spread, and Sustainability of Health and Care Technologies. *J Med. Internet Res.* **2017**, *19*, e367. [CrossRef]
77. Ahmed, M.I.; Spooner, B.; Isherwood, J.; Lane, M.; Orrock, E.; Dennison, A. A Systematic Review of the Barriers to the Implementation of Artificial Intelligence in Healthcare. *Cureus* **2023**, *15*, e46454. [CrossRef]
78. Han, S.; Kang, H.S.; Gimber, P.; Lim, S. Nursing Students' Perceptions and Use of Generative Artificial Intelligence in Nursing Education. *Nurs. Rep.* **2025**, *15*, 68. [CrossRef]
79. Chew, B.-H.; Ngiam, K.Y. Artificial Intelligence Tool Development: What Clinicians Need to Know? *BMC Med.* **2025**, *23*, 244. [CrossRef]
80. Alowais, S.A.; Alghamdi, S.S.; Alsuhebany, N.; Alqahtani, T.; Alshaya, A.I.; Almohareb, S.N.; Aldairem, A.; Alrashed, M.; Bin Saleh, K.; Badreldin, H.A.; et al. Revolutionizing Healthcare: The Role of Artificial Intelligence in Clinical Practice. *BMC Med. Educ.* **2023**, *23*, 689. [CrossRef]
81. Singh, K.; Prabhu, A.; Kaur, N. The Impact and Role of Artificial Intelligence (AI) in Healthcare: Systematic Review. *CTMC* **2025**, *25*. [CrossRef]
82. Aravazhi, P.S.; Gunasekaran, P.; Benjamin, N.Z.Y.; Thai, A.; Chandrasekar, K.K.; Kolanu, N.D.; Prajjwal, P.; Tekuru, Y.; Brito, L.V.; Inban, P. The Integration of Artificial Intelligence into Clinical Medicine: Trends, Challenges, and Future Directions. *Dis.-a-Mon.* **2025**, *71*, 101882. [CrossRef] [PubMed]
83. Corrêa, N.K.; Galvão, C.; Santos, J.W.; Del Pino, C.; Pinto, E.P.; Barbosa, C.; Massmann, D.; Mambrini, R.; Galvão, L.; Terem, E.; et al. Worldwide AI Ethics: A Review of 200 Guidelines and Recommendations for AI Governance. *Patterns* **2023**, *4*, 100857. [CrossRef]
84. Ratti, M.; Ceriotti, D.; Rescinito, R.; Bibi, R.; Panella, M. Does Robotic Assisted Technique Improve Patient Utility in Total Knee Arthroplasty? A Comparative Retrospective Cohort Study. *Healthcare* **2024**, *12*, 1650. [CrossRef] [PubMed]
85. Uwimana, A.; Gnecco, G.; Riccaboni, M. Artificial Intelligence for Breast Cancer Detection and Its Health Technology Assessment: A Scoping Review. *Comput. Biol. Med.* **2025**, *184*, 109391. [CrossRef] [PubMed]
86. Sguanci, M.; Mancin, S.; Gazzelloni, A.; Diamanti, O.; Ferrara, G.; Morales Palomares, S.; Parozzi, M.; Petrelli, F.; Cangelosi, G. The Internet of Things in the Nutritional Management of Patients with Chronic Neurological Cognitive Impairment: A Scoping Review. *Healthcare* **2024**, *13*, 23. [CrossRef]
87. Sguanci, M.; Palomares, S.M.; Cangelosi, G.; Petrelli, F.; Sandri, E.; Ferrara, G.; Mancin, S. Artificial Intelligence in the Management of Malnutrition in Cancer Patients: A Systematic Review. *Adv. Nutr.* **2025**, *16*, 100438. [CrossRef]
88. Hosain, M.N.; Kwak, Y.-S.; Lee, J.; Choi, H.; Park, J.; Kim, J. IoT-Enabled Biosensors for Real-Time Monitoring and Early Detection of Chronic Diseases. *Phys. Act. Nutr.* **2024**, *28*, 60–69. [CrossRef]
89. Pantanetti, P.; Cangelosi, G.; Morales Palomares, S.; Ferrara, G.; Biondini, F.; Mancin, S.; Caggianelli, G.; Parozzi, M.; Sguanci, M.; Petrelli, F. Real-World Life Analysis of a Continuous Glucose Monitoring and Smart Insulin Pen System in Type 1 Diabetes: A Cohort Study. *Diabetology* **2025**, *6*, 7. [CrossRef]
90. Global Burden of Disease Collaborative Network Global. Burden of Disease Study 2021 (GBD 2021) Results. 2024. Available online: https://www.healthdata.org/sites/default/files/2024-05/GBD_2021_Booklet_FINAL_2024.05.16.pdf (accessed on 5 June 2025).
91. Subramanian, M.; Wojtusciszyn, A.; Favre, L.; Boughorbel, S.; Shan, J.; Letaief, K.B.; Pitteloud, N.; Chouchane, L. Precision Medicine in the Era of Artificial Intelligence: Implications in Chronic Disease Management. *J. Transl. Med.* **2020**, *18*, 472. [CrossRef] [PubMed]
92. Shao, H.; Shi, L.; Lin, Y.; Fonseca, V. Using Modern Risk Engines and Machine Learning/Artificial Intelligence to Predict Diabetes Complications: A Focus on the BRAVO Model. *J. Diabetes Its Complicat.* **2022**, *36*, 108316. [CrossRef] [PubMed]

93. Rodrigues, I.B.; Fahim, C.; Garad, Y.; Presseau, J.; Hoens, A.M.; Braimoh, J.; Duncan, D.; Bruyn-Martin, L.; Straus, S.E. Developing the Intersectionality Supplemented Consolidated Framework for Implementation Research (CFIR) and Tools for Intersectionality Considerations. *BMC Med. Res. Methodol.* **2023**, *23*, 262. [CrossRef]
94. Wienert, J.; Zeeb, H. Implementing Health Apps for Digital Public Health—An Implementation Science Approach Adopting the Consolidated Framework for Implementation Research. *Front. Public Health* **2021**, *9*, 610237. [CrossRef]
95. Scanzera, A.C.; Beversluis, C.; Potharazu, A.V.; Bai, P.; Leifer, A.; Cole, E.; Du, D.Y.; Musick, H.; Chan, R.V.P. Planning an Artificial Intelligence Diabetic Retinopathy Screening Program: A Human-Centered Design Approach. *Front. Med.* **2023**, *10*, 1198228. [CrossRef]
96. Pan, M.; Li, R.; Wei, J.; Peng, H.; Hu, Z.; Xiong, Y.; Li, N.; Guo, Y.; Gu, W.; Liu, H. Application of Artificial Intelligence in the Health Management of Chronic Disease: Bibliometric Analysis. *Front. Med.* **2025**, *11*, 1506641. [CrossRef]
97. Serin, O.; Yıldırım, B.F.; Duman, F.; Ercorumlu, K.; Yavas, R.; Tasar, M.A.; Celik, M. Physician Perspectives on Artificial Intelligence in Healthcare: A Cross-Sectional Study of Child-Focused Care in a Turkish Tertiary Hospital. *Int. J. Med. Inform.* **2025**, *203*, 106003. [CrossRef]
98. Gumus, E.; Alan, H. Perspectives of Physicians, Nurses, and Patients on the Use of Artificial Intelligence and Robotic Nurses in Healthcare. *Int. Nurs. Rev.* **2025**, *72*, e70017. [CrossRef]
99. Vanamali, D.R.; Gara, H.K.; Dronamraju, V.A.C. Evaluation of Knowledge, Attitudes, and Practices among Healthcare Professionals toward Role of Artificial Intelligence in Healthcare. *J. Assoc. Phys. India* **2025**, *73*, e6–e12.
100. Singareddy, S.; Sn, V.P.; Jaramillo, A.P.; Yasir, M.; Iyer, N.; Hussein, S.; Nath, T.S. Artificial Intelligence and Its Role in the Management of Chronic Medical Conditions: A Systematic Review. *Cureus* **2023**, *15*, e46066. [CrossRef]
101. Nair, P.M.; Silwal, K.; Kodali, P.B.; Fogawat, K.; Binna, S.; Sharma, H.; Tewani, G.R. Impact of Holistic, Patient-Centric Yoga & Naturopathy-Based Lifestyle Modification Program in Patients with Musculoskeletal Disorders: A Quasi-Experimental Study. *Adv. Integr. Med.* **2023**, *10*, 184–189. [CrossRef]
102. Baines, R.; Bradwell, H.; Edwards, K.; Stevens, S.; Prime, S.; Tredinnick-Rowe, J.; Sibley, M.; Chatterjee, A. Meaningful Patient and Public Involvement in Digital Health Innovation, Implementation and Evaluation: A Systematic Review. *Health Expect.* **2022**, *25*, 1232–1245. [CrossRef] [PubMed]
103. Wong, A.; Berenbrok, L.A.; Snader, L.; Soh, Y.H.; Kumar, V.K.; Javed, M.A.; Bates, D.W.; Sorce, L.R.; Kane-Gill, S.L. Facilitators and Barriers to Interacting with Clinical Decision Support in the ICU: A Mixed-Methods Approach. *Crit. Care Explor.* **2023**, *5*, e0967. [CrossRef] [PubMed]
104. Scuri, S.; Tesauro, M.; Petrelli, F.; Argento, N.; Damasco, G.; Cangelosi, G.; Nguyen, C.T.T.; Savva, D.; Grappasonni, I. Use of an Online Platform to Evaluate the Impact of Social Distancing Measures on Psycho-Physical Well-Being in the COVID-19 Era. *IJERPH* **2022**, *19*, 6805. [CrossRef] [PubMed]
105. Trinh, S.; Skoll, D.; Saxon, L.A. Health Care 2025: How Consumer-Facing Devices Change Health Management and Delivery. *J. Med. Internet Res.* **2025**, *27*, e60766. [CrossRef]
106. Awad, A.; Trenfield, S.J.; Pollard, T.D.; Ong, J.J.; Elbadawi, M.; McCoubrey, L.E.; Goyanes, A.; Gaisford, S.; Basit, A.W. Connected Healthcare: Improving Patient Care Using Digital Health Technologies. *Adv. Drug. Deliv. Rev.* **2021**, *178*, 113958. [CrossRef]
107. Neborachko, M.; Pkhakadze, A.; Vlasenko, I. Current Trends of Digital Solutions for Diabetes Management. *Diabetes Metab. Syndr. Clin. Res. Rev.* **2019**, *13*, 2997–3003. [CrossRef]
108. Yang, J.; Amrollahi, A.; Marrone, M. Harnessing the Potential of Artificial Intelligence: Affordances, Constraints, and Strategic Implications for Professional Services. *J. Strateg. Inf. Syst.* **2024**, *33*, 101864. [CrossRef]
109. Castiello, T. The Benefits and Challenges of Digitally-Enabled Cardiology. *Br. J. Hosp. Med.* **2025**, *86*, 1–6. [CrossRef]
110. Warraich, H.J.; Tazbaz, T.; Califf, R.M. FDA Perspective on the Regulation of Artificial Intelligence in Health Care and Biomedicine. *JAMA* **2025**, *333*, 241. [CrossRef]
111. Geukes Foppen, R.J.; Gioia, V.; Gupta, S.; Johnson, C.L.; Giantsidis, J.; Papademetris, M. Methodology for Safe and Secure AI in Diabetes Management. *J. Diabetes Sci. Technol.* **2025**, *19*, 620–627. [CrossRef] [PubMed]
112. Gundlack, J.; Negash, S.; Thiel, C.; Buch, C.; Schildmann, J.; Unverzagt, S.; Mikolajczyk, R.; Frese, T.; PEAK Consortium. Artificial Intelligence in Medical Care—Patients' Perceptions on Caregiving Relationships and Ethics: A Qualitative Study. *Health Expect.* **2025**, *28*, e70216. [CrossRef] [PubMed]
113. Gundlack, J.; Thiel, C.; Negash, S.; Buch, C.; Apfelbacher, T.; Denny, K.; Christoph, J.; Mikolajczyk, R.; Unverzagt, S.; Frese, T. Patients' Perceptions of Artificial Intelligence Acceptance, Challenges, and Use in Medical Care: Qualitative Study. *J. Med. Internet Res.* **2025**, *27*, e70487. [CrossRef] [PubMed]
114. Witkowski, K.; Okhai, R.; Neely, S.R. Public Perceptions of Artificial Intelligence in Healthcare: Ethical Concerns and Opportunities for Patient-Centered Care. *BMC Med. Ethics* **2024**, *25*, 74. [CrossRef]
115. Alsaleh, A. The Impact of Technological Advancement on Culture and Society. *Sci. Rep.* **2024**, *14*, 32140. [CrossRef]

116. Fatoum, H.; Hanna, S.; Halamka, J.D.; Sicker, D.C.; Spangenberg, P.; Hashmi, S.K. Blockchain Integration With Digital Technology and the Future of Health Care Ecosystems: Systematic Review. *J. Med. Internet Res.* **2021**, *23*, e19846. [CrossRef]
117. Xie, Y.; Zhai, Y.; Lu, G. Evolution of Artificial Intelligence in Healthcare: A 30-Year Bibliometric Study. *Front. Med.* **2025**, *11*, 1505692. [CrossRef]

medicina

MDPI

Review

Integrated Hospital–Territory Organizational Models and the Role of Family and Community Nurses in the Management of Chronic Conditions: A Scoping Review

Gianluca Azzellino [1,2,*], Patrizia Vagnarelli [2], Mauro Passamonti [2], Luca Mengoli [3], Lia Ginaldi [1,4] and Massimo De Martinis [1,3,5,*]

1 Department of Life, Health and Environmental Sciences, University of L'Aquila, 67100 L'Aquila, Italy; lia.ginaldi@univaq.it
2 U.O.C. Adriatic District Area, AUSL 04 Teramo, 64100 Teramo, Italy; patrizia.vagnarelli@aslteramo.it (P.V.); mauro.passamonti@aslteramo.it (M.P.)
3 Long-Term Care Unit, "Maria SS. dello Splendore" Hospital, AUSL 04 Teramo, 64021 Giulianova, Italy; luca.mengoli@aslteramo.it
4 Allergy and Clinical Immunology Unit, Center for the Diagnosis and Treatment of Osteoporosis, AUSL 04 Teramo, 64100 Teramo, Italy
5 UniCamillus-Saint Camillus International University of Health Sciences, 00131 Rome, Italy
* Correspondence: gianluca.azzellino@graduate.univaq.it (G.A.); demartinis@cc.univaq.it (M.D.M.)

Abstract: *Background and Objectives*: One of the challenges of modern healthcare systems, in terms of economic and organizational sustainability and the impact on patients' quality of life, is the progressive increase in chronicity and care complexity. In this scenario, hospital–community integration models represent possible strategies to ensure the continuity of care, reduce readmission rates, and improve clinical outcomes. This study aims to map integrated care models for patients with chronic diseases, with active involvement of the family and community nurse, describing their functions and associated clinical, organizational, and economic outcomes, as well as barriers and facilitators to their implementation. *Materials and Methods*: The review was conducted using the JBI methodology and the PRISMA-ScR protocol and identified 26 studies with a publication range from 2000 to 2025. *Results*: The emerging results highlight the use of integrated and personalized organizational models in the post-discharge phases, with a leading role for the family and community nurse in the assessment, planning, and coordination of various steps. *Conclusions*: The interventions are associated with an increase in patient and caregiver satisfaction, a reduction in outcomes such as the rehospitalization rate, and greater continuity of care.

Keywords: family nurse; community nurse; chronic care; integrated care; hospital discharge; nurse-led; case management

1. Introduction

Aging of the population has led to an increase in the prevalence of multiple diseases, and this represents one of the most significant challenges for modern healthcare systems. Over 50% of adults over 65 live with at least two chronic conditions, a situation that increases the risk of hospital readmissions, loss of autonomy, deterioration in the quality of life, and high healthcare costs [1]. In this new healthcare context, fragmented care models may prove ineffective in ensuring effective, continuous, and patient-centered management [2,3]. Organizational models of hospital–community integration have been developed precisely to respond to this new need. The goal is to make patient care proactive, guiding and facilitating the transition between various care settings, ensuring continuity, coordination, and the personalization of care, especially in such a delicate phase as hospital discharge and returning home [4,5]. In this regard, the literature indicates that these models, especially when they include structured nursing models (e.g., case management and transitional care), can reduce readmission rates, healthcare costs [6], and mortality in elderly patients with chronic diseases [3,7–9]. Recent studies emphasize the importance of territorial reorganization strategies and chronic disease management, such as the adoption of telemedicine and the activation of Territorial Operational Centers, with the aim of strengthening the continuity of care and the coordination of integrated care pathways [7]. As highlighted in a recent scoping review, the use of digital and telemedicine tools in transitional care has shown promising results in enhancing the continuity of care, improving patient outcomes, and supporting healthcare professionals in managing postoperative pain at home [8]. Moreover, protected discharge models with the adoption of combined interventions, including nursing follow-ups and caregiver involvement, have proven to be an effective strategy to improve the care experience of frail and chronic patients while also reducing early readmissions [9]. In particular, the role of the family and community nurse plays a key and strategic role in ensuring care transition, acting as a bridge between various hospital and territorial services.

In several healthcare systems (e.g., Italy and Spain), this role is defined as a distinct professional profile that requires specialized post-graduate training in family or community nursing [10]. It differs from generalist community nursing positions by focusing on longitudinal care, proactive case management, and structured support for patients with chronic and complex conditions. However, its scope and implementation vary by country and organizational context [11]. The coordination of care by a responsible and designated healthcare professional is considered one of the crucial elements in the provision of integrated care [12]. Through assessment, planning, education, psychosocial support, and follow-up activities, the nurse figure can contribute to improving therapeutic adherence and self-care by chronic patients [13,14]. However, despite several international experiences and pilot projects, there is still no complete framework that clearly and concisely describes the characteristics of these integrated models that directly involve the community nurse, nor the resulting outcomes. Even the results of studies in the literature are sometimes heterogeneous or limited to specific pathological contexts, such as heart failure or geriatric frailty [5,15]. Moreover, the literature shows a significant lack of standard definitions in care approaches (e.g., nurse-led care, transitional care, integrated care, geriatric team, etc.), making it difficult to compare and use a uniform approach [1,2]. In light of the above, this scoping review aimed to map hospital–community integrated models in the management of chronic diseases with the active involvement of the family nurse, trying to describe the specificity of their role, identify associated clinical, organizational, economic, and experiential outcomes, explore barriers and facilitators to implementation, and assess the level of diffusion, experimentation, or institutionalization in different international healthcare settings.

2. Materials and Methods

The study was conducted following the PRISMA-ScR checklist and the methodology proposed by the Joanna Briggs Institute (JBI) for scoping reviews. All of the various methodological steps were carried out with rigidity in order to ensure transparency and reproducibility. The research questions addressed in the review are the following:

- What models of integrated hospital-to-community care are used for the management of chronic conditions with nursing involvement?
- What is the role of the family and community nurse within these organizational models?

- What outcomes (clinical, organizational, economic, or experiential) are associated with such models?
- What barriers and facilitators influence the implementation of these models?

The PCC framework (Population, Concept, Context) was used to define the inclusion criteria:

- Population: Nurses who work in community contexts or in integrated care settings, including family and community nurses.
- Concept: Organizational models for the management of chronic conditions that include an active role of nursing care.
- Context: Any health system, national or local, with no geographical restrictions.

2.1. Databases Used and Search Strategy

The bibliographic search was carried out using databases such as PubMed, Scopus, and Web of Science. The search strategy was built using MeSH terms and keywords, combining terms such as "family nurse", "community nurse", "chronic care", "integrated care", "hospital discharge", "nurse-led", and "case management" with Boolean operators.

Articles published from 2000 to the present were included, with the exclusion of letters, editorials, abstracts without full text, and studies focused exclusively on the hospital setting. The complete search strings for each database are available in Supplementary File S1.

2.2. Data Extraction

Referring to the JBI methodology for scoping reviews [16], a data extraction table was created for the included studies. A standardized model was used to create the table. The latter included the following elements: author/year, main theme, geographical context, study design and methods, population and sample characteristics, key findings, and research gaps.

2.3. Study Selection

Studies were excluded if they did not concern integrated hospital-to-community models or were predominantly hospital-based, if they did not include the nurse as an active part, or if they did not describe outcomes or processes relevant to the role of the family and community nurse.

2.4. Screening Process

To ensure the accurate inclusion of studies relevant to the review, the process was divided into two phases. In the first phase, two independent reviewers screened the titles and abstracts of the articles identified through the search strategy, based on the selected inclusion and exclusion criteria. In the second phase, the full texts of the studies were read to confirm their compatibility with the objectives of the review. All studies were managed using Zotero (Corporation for Digital Scholarship, George Mason University, Fairfax, VA, USA), available at: https://www.zotero.org/, last accessed 30 April 2025, which supported the authors in organizing citations and full texts throughout the entire scoping review process. Discrepancies between the two reviewers were resolved with the involvement of three additional reviewers. The selection process is illustrated in the PRISMA 2020 flow diagram (Figure 1), in accordance with the PRISMA-ScR protocol [17].

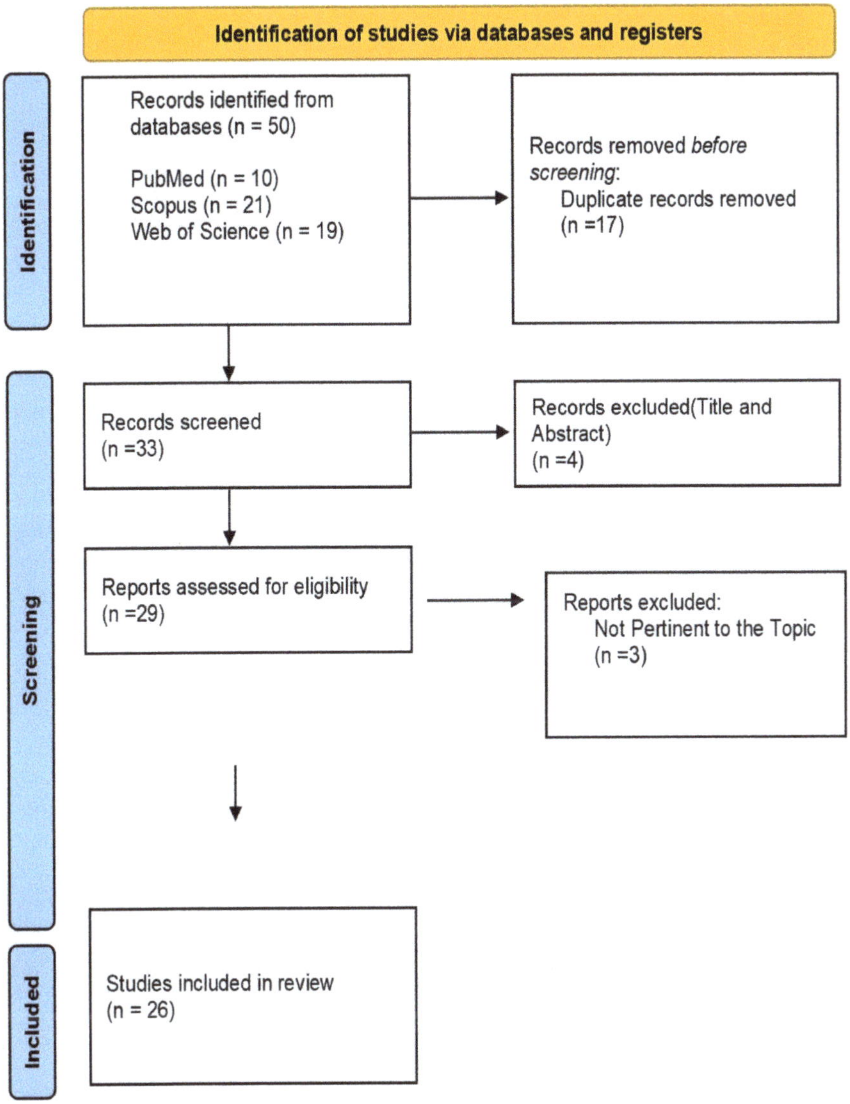

Figure 1. PRISMA 2020 flow diagram illustrating the study selection process. The databases searched were PubMed, Scopus, and Web of Science.

2.5. Quality Assessment and Risk of Bias

The risk of bias assessment was not performed for this study, as it is not required for a scoping review. The aim of this study was to map and analyze the available evidence, rather than to critically evaluate each individual study. The authors' decision is consistent with the methodological guidelines for scoping reviews, as outlined in the *JBI Manual for Evidence Synthesis* and the *PRISMA-ScR*.

2.6. Data Synthesis

The results of the included studies were synthesized following the approach outlined in the *JBI Manual for Evidence Synthesis* (2020) for scoping reviews. A descriptive synthesis, without critical appraisal of methodological quality, was used to extract and organize the data as recommended for this type of review. The synthesis was structured into three phases. In the first phase, after data extraction, two independent reviewers identified key themes by analyzing the content of the studies to determine the characteristics of integrated hospital–community care models, the role of the family and community nurse, and the reported clinical, organizational, and experiential outcomes. In the second phase, the data were grouped thematically, highlighting the following main areas: types of organizational models adopted; functions and competencies assigned to the family and community nurse; reported outcomes (e.g., improved continuity of care, reduced readmissions, and patient and caregiver satisfaction); and barriers and facilitators to implementation.

In the third phase, the results were qualitatively described and synthesized. The authors provided a structured overview of the available evidence, highlighting both the potential and limitations of the analyzed organizational models. Although no formal risk of bias assessment was conducted, the presence of several systematic reviews, randomized controlled trials, and mixed-methods studies suggests a moderate overall strength of evidence. Findings were generally consistent for outcomes such as patient satisfaction and reduced readmissions, while evidence on mortality and cost-effectiveness remained more variable. To support and refine the language and style of the manuscript, the authors used artificial intelligence (AI), specifically ChatGPT-4o (OpenAI, San Francisco, CA, USA), available at: https://openai.com/index/hello-gpt-4o/, last accessed 30 April 2025. All methodological steps and scientific decisions were made solely and exclusively by the authors.

3. Results

3.1. Selection of Studies

The initial search conducted in electronic databases (PubMed, Scopus, and Web of Science) yielded a total of 50 records (PubMed = 10; Scopus = 21; Web of Science = 19). After the removal of 17 duplicates using Zotero, 33 records were screened by title and abstract. This screening led to the exclusion of four studies. Subsequently, 29 full-text articles were assessed for eligibility. Of these, three were excluded for not meeting the review objectives, specifically for not addressing integrated hospital-to-community care models, lacking active nurse involvement, or not reporting relevant outcomes. A total of 26 studies were included in the final analysis (Table 1). The selection process was conducted independently by two reviewers, and any discrepancies were resolved through discussion and consensus, with the support of three additional reviewers.

Table 1. Characteristics of included studies (n = 26).

Author/ Year	Main Theme	Geographical Context	Study Type	Sample/Population	Key Findings	Research Gaps
Endalamaw et al., 2024 [1]	Mapping care models for chronic multimorbidity, with a focus on their components, impacts, implementation barriers, and facilitators, especially relevant for low- and middle-income countries	Multinational	Scoping review	54 studies addressing care models for adults with chronic multimorbidity; models covered included integrated, collaborative, nurse-led, chronic, and geriatric models, among others	Care models have been implemented to improve patient satisfaction, cost efficiency, health outcomes, and the overall quality of care. The analysis highlighted several key elements, including multidisciplinary teams, personalized care plans, follow-up, the use of information and communication technologies (ICTs), the involvement of patients and caregivers, leadership, and funding structures. Some critical issues emerged, such as limited resources, team coordination, communication, and access to technology. Among the models analyzed, nurse-led and integrated models proved to be effective and adaptable to various care settings.	Few studies conducted in low-income countries; limited evidence on implementation feasibility in resource-constrained contexts; lack of standardized evaluation tools; need for culturally adapted models and further testing of models in diverse healthcare systems.
Sargent et al., 2007 [2]	Understanding patient and carer perspectives on nurse-led case management for long-term conditions in community settings	United Kingdom	Qualitative study	72 patients and 52 carers receiving community matron case management across six Primary Care Trusts (PCTs)	Five key areas were identified in care delivery based on the principles of case management: (1) clinical care, (2) care coordination, (3) health education, (4) advocacy, and (5) psychosocial support. Patients and caregivers assigned equal importance to psychosocial support and clinical care, often describing "community matrons" as the only reliable source of emotional support. Their role, in terms of advocacy and psychological support, went beyond the recommendations outlined in the Department of Health guidelines.	Discrepancy between official policy definitions and real-world practice ("implementation surplus"); need for inclusion of psychosocial support as a formal competency domain; limited prior exploration of dual support role for both patients and carers in UK community case management.

Table 1. *Cont.*

Author/ Year	Main Theme	Geographical Context	Study Type	Sample/Population	Key Findings	Research Gaps
Ruikes et al., 2016 [4]	To evaluate the effectiveness of an integrated primary care model based on multidisciplinary case management for frail older adults compared to usual care	Netherlands	Cluster controlled trial	536 frail elderly aged ≥70 years (287 in the intervention group, 249 in the control group); identified using the EASY-Care Two-Step screening tool	The use of the CareWell program, designed for primary care targeting frail older adults, included structured interventions such as proactive care planning, case management, medication review, and multidisciplinary team meetings. However, it did not yield significant results regarding functional status (Katz-15), quality of life (EQ-5D), mental health, social functioning, hospital admissions, institutionalization, or mortality. Subgroup analyses also did not show any relevant differences.	Twelve-month duration may be insufficient to show effects; high heterogeneity and individual tailoring of interventions; need for person-centered outcome measures and further longitudinal research on frailty trajectories and timing of interventions.
Takeda et al., 2012 [5]	Effectiveness of different models of clinical service organization in reducing mortality and hospital readmissions among patients with chronic heart failure	Multinational	Systematic review of 25 RCTs	5942 adult patients with chronic heart failure recently discharged from the hospital; follow-up of at least 6 months	There are three care models analyzed in patients with heart failure: case management, outpatient care, and multidisciplinary interventions. In particular, case management models that included specialist nurses, home visits, and telephone follow-ups consistently showed an association with reduced hospital readmissions and all-cause mortality. Other multidisciplinary approaches were also identified as effective in reducing readmissions. In contrast, interventions delivered exclusively in outpatient settings produced mixed results. Key and recurring components of the most effective care models included patient education, medication review, and support for self-management.	Uncertainty remains regarding the optimal components of each intervention; high heterogeneity across studies; lack of standardization in outcomes and intervention reporting; limited evidence on cost-effectiveness and long-term sustainability.

Table 1. *Cont.*

Author/Year	Main Theme	Geographical Context	Study Type	Sample/Population	Key Findings	Research Gaps
Beaudin et al., 2025 [13]	Factors influencing the integration of self-management support by primary care nurses for patients with coexisting chronic diseases and common mental disorders, and strategies for improvement	Canada	Qualitative interpretive descriptive study	23 primary care nurses with experience in follow-up care for patients with both chronic diseases and common mental disorders	The key determinants influencing the spread of nurse-led self-management support include clinical factors (knowledge, skills, workload, clinical tools, and attitudes), professional factors (roles, interdisciplinary collaboration, and team composition), and regulatory and functional factors (organizational culture and operational mechanisms). Potential improvement strategies include training focused on common mental health disorders, the development of appropriate clinical tools, and clinical support and coaching. All of this requires effective collaboration and cultural change.	Need for targeted training programs and standardized tools for SMS integration; lack of implementation frameworks and cultural safety considerations; future research needed on the effectiveness of digital tools and on the perspectives of other stakeholders including patients.
Shirey et al., 2021 [14]	Development and implementation of a nurse-led, interprofessional collaborative practice (IPCP) model focused on transitional care coordination and chronic disease management for under-served populations	United States	Descriptive implementation study	Uninsured and underinsured adults with diabetes (PATH clinic) and heart failure (HRTSA clinic), mainly African American and low-income, with complex chronic and behavioral health needs	The nurse-led care models analyzed and identified in the included studies showed high heterogeneity in terms of design, target populations, and implementation settings. Key components emerging from the most effective models included multidisciplinary collaboration, person-centered care planning, structured post-discharge follow-up, and support for patient self-management. Nurse-coordinated interventions were associated with improved continuity of care, higher patient satisfaction, and increased self-efficacy. Some studies highlighted a reduction in the unplanned use of healthcare services, such as hospital readmissions and emergency department visits, although with variable evidence. The effectiveness of these models was strongly influenced by contextual factors such as nursing autonomy, interprofessional integration, and system-level support.	Further research needed on scalability, sustainability, and generalizability to other populations and systems; limited empirical evidence linking IPCP to Quadruple Aim outcomes; call for rigorous mixed-methods evaluation and cost-effectiveness analysis across settings.

Table 1. *Cont.*

Author/Year	Main Theme	Geographical Context	Study Type	Sample/Population	Key Findings	Research Gaps
Koontalay et al., 2025 [15]	Codesign and development of a user-centered, nurse-led chronic care model for patients with heart failure in a limited-resource setting	Thailand	A codesign study	19 participants: 1 heart failure patient, 16 clinicians (nurses, cardiologist, pharmacist, and dietitian), and 2 organizational leaders from a tertiary hospital	Nine models aimed at improving continuity of care were identified. Among them, the most effective and suitable for the management of chronic heart failure (CHF) was nurse-led case management, supported by a multidisciplinary team and characterized by strong integration with community-based services.	Need for future testing and evaluation of the prototype's impact on patient outcomes, cost-effectiveness, and scalability in other low- and middle-income countries; limited patient participation due to illness/readmission; potential barriers to implementation include resource constraints and hierarchical cultural norms.
Deschodt et al., 2020 [18]	Core components and effects of nurse-led integrated care models for home-dwelling older people	Europe, North America, New Zealand	Systematic review and meta-analysis	19 studies, 22,168 older adults (mostly ≥65 years) living at home	Most nurse-led models were oriented toward a person-centered approach, with individualized care plans and support from multidisciplinary teams. Although many studies reported positive effects on quality of life, mortality, and hospital and emergency department access, meta-analyses did not show overall statistically significant results.	The meta-analyses did not show significant effects on outcomes. Almost no model used implementation theories to explain how the model should work. Aspects such as reimbursement, costs, and the use of technologies (e.g., telemedicine) were rarely included or described.
Davis et al., 2024 [19]	Feasibility of a nurse-led transitional care intervention via telehealth for adult patients with multimorbidity discharged from an acute care hospital	Australia	Feasibility study using mixed methods	21 adult patients (mean age 78 years) with multimorbidity (3 to 10 chronic conditions), followed for 6–10 weeks post-discharge	The study analyzed a nurse-led intervention for patients with multimorbidity, focused on continuity of care and remote transitional support (telehealth). Patients reported high satisfaction, improved access to services, and a reduced perception of readmission risk. In fact, only 24% were actually readmitted. Furthermore, healthcare professionals played an active role in managing hospital flow through the presence of a Transition Coordinator. The intervention proved to be feasible, practical, and adaptable to the clinical context.	Need for a randomized controlled trial to assess effectiveness and cost-efficiency; absence of systematic hospital readmission risk assessment for patients with multimorbidity; inconsistencies in discharge handover to primary care.

Table 1. *Cont.*

Author/ Year	Main Theme	Geographical Context	Study Type	Sample/Population	Key Findings	Research Gaps
Jepma et al., 2021 [20]	Experiences of frail older cardiac patients with a nurse-coordinated transitional care intervention (Cardiac Care Bridge)	Netherlands	Qualitative study	16 frail cardiac patients aged ≥70 years (mean age: 82.4) who had participated in the intervention arm of a transitional care program	Study participants expressed satisfaction with the active support received through post-discharge home visits, which ensured continuity of care. However, recovery experiences varied: some reported physical improvements, while others faced difficulties due to comorbidities or frailty. Home visits conducted by the community nurse had a positive impact, although their added value is often not fully recognized. Individuals who regularly rely on formal or informal support networks tended to be skeptical about the interventions provided by professionals involved in the continuity-of-care team.	Difficulty distinguishing between usual care and the intervention; uncertainty about which patient subgroups benefit most; need to tailor interventions to frailty level, self-management abilities, and existing care networks.
Uittenbroek et al., 2018 [21]	Experiences and role adaptation of case managers in delivering person-centered and integrated care to older adults through the Embrace model	Netherlands	Qualitative study	11 case managers	Case managers have shifted from a task-based model to a person-centered one, focusing on building trust-based relationships, empowerment, and patient autonomy. The main themes that emerged included a new relational approach with older patients, the introduction of new professional roles, the enhancement of skills and knowledge, and the perceived benefits resulting from case management activities. Despite the role not receiving the recognition it deserves, case managers found this position rewarding both personally and professionally.	Need for clearer support structures, integration of guidelines, and better role definition; issues with combining traditional roles and case management; the importance of continuous training and organizational backing to support long-term implementation and identity development in new care models.

Table 1. *Cont.*

Author/ Year	Main Theme	Geographical Context	Study Type	Sample/Population	Key Findings	Research Gaps
Armold, 2017 [22]	Effectiveness of a nurse-led community case management (CCM) program in reducing healthcare utilization in chronically ill adult patients	United States	Retrospective observational study	307 patients with at least one chronic disease; 151 accepted CCM services, 156 refused	Patients who took part in chronic care management (CCM) services experienced a 55% reduction in emergency department visits and a 61% decrease in hospital admissions compared to those who did not participate. A reduction of 47% in non-urgent visits was also observed, although it was not statistically significant. The CCM services, offered free of charge, were delivered by nurses with advanced training and a master's degree through home visits and care coordination activities.	Lack of demographic data to identify which subgroups benefit most; limited tracking of patients who may have used other health systems or moved; further research needed on the timing and specific interventions that yield the greatest impact.
Davis et al., 2020 [23]	Development of a nurse-led, person-centered care coordination model to improve the continuity of care for people with multimorbidity at the primary–secondary healthcare interface	Australia	Qualitative descriptive	44 stakeholders (nurses, physicians, allied health professionals, consumer advocates, Aboriginal representatives, executives, general practitioners, and academics) participated in forums and a validation workshop	A pragmatic and adaptable nurse-led care coordination model was designed. The model is built around a transversal component (intersectoral multidisciplinary collaboration), four domains (coordination, governance, communication, and culture), and six operational areas. It addresses existing care challenges in light of current models, integrates cultural and governance elements, ensures personalized and person-centered care, and enhances continuity of care across different healthcare settings.	The model's feasibility and impact are yet to be evaluated in practice (to be addressed in Part 2 of the study); future studies should assess its implementation, sustainability, and effect on health outcomes; need for tools to validate stakeholder input and broader application in diverse care settings.

Table 1. *Cont.*

Author/ Year	Main Theme	Geographical Context	Study Type	Sample/Population	Key Findings	Research Gaps
Chow et al., 2008 [24]	Evaluation of the impact of community nursing services (CNSs) on self-reported health and hospital readmission among chronically ill patients after discharge	Hong Kong, China	Secondary analysis of a randomized controlled trial	46 chronically ill patients	Clinical nurse specialists (CNSs) played an important role in improving the perceived health status of patients with cardiac and respiratory conditions. However, no significant reduction in hospital readmissions was observed. The vast majority of identified issues were related to physiological factors and health-related behaviors. The most commonly adopted nursing intervention was surveillance, followed by health education activities and care procedures. For patients with respiratory conditions, greater emphasis was placed on health education.	Home visits led to significant improvements in self-reported health among patients with respiratory and cardiovascular conditions, but no statistically significant effects were found for hospital readmissions. Additionally, age, gender, and financial status were identified as predictors of self-perceived health.
Chow & Wong, 2010 [25]	A nurse-led case management program with motivational telephone follow-up to improve the quality of life of patients undergoing peritoneal dialysis	Hong Kong	Randomized controlled trial with pre- and post-test designs	85 patients with end-stage renal failure (43 in the intervention group, 42 in the control)	The study found that the nurse-led case management model, followed by motivational telephone follow-ups, significantly improved the quality of life in patients undergoing peritoneal dialysis. Improvements were noted in symptoms, the impact of kidney disease, sleep, pain, emotional well-being, social functioning, and patient satisfaction. Additional positive outcomes included perceived support from healthcare staff, sleep quality, and social functioning. However, no significant differences were observed in physical health or in the general perception of overall health status.	Generalizability limited due to recruitment from only two hospitals; control group also had access to hotline services, which may have diluted differences; further studies needed to assess long-term outcomes, cost-effectiveness, and scalability across broader renal populations.

Table 1. *Cont.*

Author/ Year	Main Theme	Geographical Context	Study Type	Sample/Population	Key Findings	Research Gaps
Chow & Wong, 2014 [26]	Effectiveness of a nurse-led case management program using empowerment strategies to improve outcomes in older adults with multiple chronic conditions after hospital discharge	Hong Kong	Randomized controlled trial	281 older adults	Older adults with at least two chronic conditions received case management interventions, specifically home visits and phone calls. They were randomly assigned to two intervention groups and one control group. The results showed that readmission rates in the intervention groups were significantly reduced within 84 days after discharge. Additionally, these patients reported improvements in self-efficacy, perceived health status, and physical quality of life. No significant differences were found in mental health outcomes. Key elements contributing to the success of post-discharge interventions delivered by nurse case managers included personalization, empowerment, and support for self-management.	Unclear long-term impact beyond 12 weeks; further evaluation needed for cost-effectiveness and scalability; results influenced by nurse–patient relationship and intervention fidelity; generalizability may be limited due to local context and inclusion criteria.
Davis et al., 2019 [27]	Design and implementation of a nurse-led model to enhance continuity of care across health sectors for individuals with multimorbidity	Australia	Mixed-methods study protocol	Patients with multimorbidity discharged from a tertiary hospital	The protocol proposes a flexible, person-centered nurse-led care coordination model. It consists of six phases: assessment during hospitalization, identification of an individualized care plan, post-discharge follow-up, communication with general practitioners, coordination of care across different healthcare settings, and evaluation. Particular emphasis is placed on multidisciplinary collaboration and the integration of governance and cultural aspects within the reference model.	As a study protocol, no clinical outcomes have yet been reported. Future work is needed to evaluate the feasibility, effectiveness, and cost-efficiency of the model in real-world practice, especially its impact on patient outcomes and health system integration.

Table 1. *Cont.*

Author/ Year	Main Theme	Geographical Context	Study Type	Sample/Population	Key Findings	Research Gaps
Davis et al., 2021 [28]	Effectiveness of nurse-led services in achieving continuity of care for chronic disease patients across the primary–secondary healthcare interface	Multinational	Quantitative systematic review	14 studies included with a total of 4090 adult patients (aged 29–95) with chronic diseases	Nurse-led services are associated with improved patient outcomes, such as reduced hospitalizations and readmissions, increased patient satisfaction, enhanced quality of life, better self-management, and improved symptom control. All the analyzed models included interventions that ensured continuity of care—relational, informational, and managerial—but only a few measured continuity as a specific outcome using validated tools.	Need for cost-effectiveness studies and validation of continuity measurement tools.
Grimsmo et al., 2018 [29]	Feasibility of implementing disease-specific clinical pathways in primary care settings, with a focus on multimorbidity and care transitions	Norway	Mixed-methods study (qualitative + quantitative)	155 health professionals and managers in two case studies (qualitative); 214,722 adult inhabitants and 6061 home healthcare patients across four municipalities (quantitative)	The structuring of disease-specific clinical pathways is not suitable for managing chronic patients in the context of primary care. An effective approach is person-centered, using flexible and personalized care pathways based on individual needs rather than a single condition. Disease-specific pathways tend to be too complex and rigid to apply in everyday practice, especially in home care settings where time is limited and flexibility is essential.	Insufficient research on the contextual adaptation of clinical guidelines during care transitions from hospital to home.
Harvey et al., 2017 [30]	Design, implementation, and evaluation of a nurse-led, person-centered integrated care model for people living with long-term conditions (LTCs)	New Zealand	Implementation project with mixed-methods evaluation (qualitative, quantitative, and participatory)	Adults with LTCs, particularly those recently discharged from a hospital or newly diagnosed; focus on populations in high-deprivation areas	The model introduced the role of Liaison Nurse Consultants (LNCs) with the aim of coordinating care between primary and secondary services, thereby reducing hospital admissions. Key aspects examined included continuity of care, quality of life, equity, and health literacy. Preliminary analyses showed a reduction in hospital admissions and greater engagement within disadvantaged communities. This model highlighted the importance of cultural competence, intersectoral collaboration, and patient empowerment.	Full outcome data and long-term results pending.

Table 1. *Cont.*

Author/ Year	Main Theme	Geographical Context	Study Type	Sample/Population	Key Findings	Research Gaps
Gonçalves et al., 2022 [31]	Mapping and classification of nurse-led care management models for hospitalized patients with multimorbidity	Multinational	Scoping review	21 included studies	The review identified three categories of nurse-led care models: (1) nurse-led programs (such as discharge planning activities, outpatient clinics, and targeted interventions), (2) case management models (led by clinical nurse specialists, nurse practitioners, etc.), and (3) models with nurse facilitators (e.g., nurse navigators and care coordinators). All these approaches share the goal of delivering patient-centered care, supporting transitions between care settings, and promoting self-management. However, variability was observed in terms of autonomy, roles, and competencies across the different models.	Lack of standardized definitions for nurse-led care models. Need for clarity on the roles and competencies required.
McParland et al., 2022 [32]	Identification and evaluation of nurse-led interventions for people with multimorbidity, and the outcomes these interventions impact	Multinational	Mixed-methods systematic review	20 studies	Most of the interventions reviewed included case management or transitional care models, all led by nurses with advanced competencies. Common features identified included support for self-management, person-centered care planning, and continuity of care. Positive effects were most evident in patient-reported outcomes, such as perceived quality of care, health-related quality of life, and self-efficacy. However, the impact on healthcare service use, costs, and mortality proved to be more variable.	Few studies used standardized definitions or validated tools for continuity and multimorbidity; more robust evaluations needed to assess long-term and cost-related outcomes.
Latour et al., 2007 [33]	Effectiveness of nurse-led case management for complex ambulatory patients in general health care	Multinational	Systematic review	Ambulatory adults (≥18 years) with complex needs (e.g., multimorbidity, psychiatric comorbidity, and social vulnerabilities), not disease-specific	Post-discharge nursing case management shows - Positive effects on patient satisfaction; - No impact on emergency room visits; - Contrasting results on other clinical outcomes.	Greater clarity is needed in the definitions of "complex patient" and in the standardized evaluation of outcomes. High-quality randomized controlled trials (RCTs) are necessary, with sufficiently long follow-up periods and precise indicators of patient complexity.

Table 1. *Cont.*

Author/ Year	Main Theme	Geographical Context	Study Type	Sample/Population	Key Findings	Research Gaps
McGovern et al., 2018 [34]	Evaluation of a multidisciplinary, nurse-led transitional care program (JUMP) for young adults with chronic neurological conditions moving from pediatric to adult healthcare	France	Descriptive observational study with quantitative outcome assessment (satisfaction survey)	111 patients	In relation to the transition processes of patients with chronic neurological conditions, high levels of satisfaction were reported by both patients (89%) and parents (91%). Key factors contributing to these outcomes included a personalized and multidisciplinary approach, along with the role of Coordination Nurse Specialists (CoNSs), who ensured continuity of care by supporting patients before, during, and after the transition.	Limited generalizability due to single-center design; lack of long-term outcome data; response rate of 48% may bias results; further evaluation needed on adherence, quality of life, and engagement post-transition.
O'Connell et al., 2023 [35]	Assessment of the effects of nurse-assisted and multidisciplinary outpatient follow-up interventions for patients with decompensated liver cirrhosis	Multinational (16 studies from Europe, Asia, the USA, and Australia)	Systematic review	1224 adult patients; 16 included studies	Three main types of interventions were identified: (1) Educational interventions; (2) Nurse-led case management; (3) Standardized hospital follow-up. All these approaches demonstrated at least one improvement in various outcomes, such as reduced mortality, decreased readmissions, increased knowledge, greater self-efficacy, and improved quality of life. In some cases, a favorable cost-effectiveness ratio was also observed. However, none of these models proved to be superior to the others.	Significant heterogeneity across interventions and outcomes; most studies had moderate-to-low methodological quality; need for well-designed RCTs to evaluate real-world effectiveness, especially in personalized nurse-led models for liver disease.
Schraeder et al., 2008 [36]	Effectiveness of a collaborative nurse-led case management model in reducing healthcare utilization and costs for chronically ill older adults in primary care	United States	Non-randomized controlled trial	677 community-dwelling adults aged ≥65 years at high risk for mortality, functional decline, or high healthcare use (400 in intervention group, 277 in control)	The integration of nurse case managers into primary care for frail older adults significantly reduced the risk of rehospitalization among hospitalized patients, improved continuity of care, and contributed to a modest reduction in overall healthcare costs.	Generalizability is limited due to regional scope; non-randomized design may introduce bias; future studies should include broader populations, randomized designs, and long-term outcome evaluations to confirm sustainability and effectiveness.

3.2. Main Results

The analysis of the 26 studies showed significant diversity in organizational models, clinical outcomes, and strategies adopted, but at the same time, it also highlighted common patterns attributable to four thematic areas: organizational models, nursing roles and functions, clinical and organizational outcomes, and barriers/facilitators.

- Integrated organizational models

The most widely implemented models are as follows:

- Nurse case management in the post-discharge phase, implemented through tools such as telephone, home, or outpatient follow-up, has shown significant effectiveness in reducing hospital readmissions [5,26,36].
- The transitional care model, led by specialist nurses or community matrons, has been highlighted as effective in ensuring continuity of care after hospital discharge [2,23,34].
- Multidisciplinary team-based care, through the active and coordinated involvement of physicians, social workers, family/community nurses, and psychologists, has proven to be a valuable approach to improving care continuity and patient outcomes [13,14,31].
- Codesigned or patient-centered models, such as those implemented in heart failure care programs [15] or in neurological transitional care pathways [34], have demonstrated the importance of tailoring interventions to individual needs and preferences.

The hospital-to-community transition is commonly implemented through personalized and structured interventions, based on multidimensional and multiprofessional assessment [4,33].

- Role of the Community/Family Nurse

Nurses play a multifunctional and adaptive role in chronic care management. They assess clinical and social needs and identify frail individuals [21,32]. They are responsible for planning care pathways and for the proactive and personalized management of interventions [22,28]. They support self-care, therapeutic education, and motivational coaching, often focused on chronic conditions [13,25]. They also act as clinical leaders within interdisciplinary teams and in coordinating the hospital-to-community transition [14,36].

- Clinical, organizational, and subjective outcomes

Among the most frequently improved outcomes are the reduction in hospital readmissions within 30 to 90 days [5,26,37]. Across the various models applied, improvements were also observed in perceived quality of care, care continuity, and patient and caregiver satisfaction [15,32,34]. Additionally, the studies report an increase in self-care, disease knowledge, and treatment adherence [13,36]. Notably, a positive impact on healthcare costs and a reduction in length of stay were observed in chronic care systems with well-coordinated and effective models [28,33]. However, effectiveness in terms of mortality, functional outcomes (ADL/IADL), or economic indicators remains less consistent and appears to depend on the intensity and continuity of the intervention [4,5].

- Barriers and Facilitators

Among the barriers identified in the studies are the fragmentation of services in chronic disease management and the poor interoperability between different care settings [28,32]. Another barrier is the lack of standardized clinical tools and uniform training on chronic diseases [13,33], combined with nursing workload overload and cultural resistance to integrated approaches [31]. Among the facilitators, nursing leadership stands out, with strong trust in the case manager's role in chronic care management and interprofessional collaboration [14,36]. Early discharge planning and the timely activation of hospital–community integration services are also highlighted as enablers [5]. Additionally, the use of modern digital tools and telemonitoring technologies, although still not widely adopted, emerges as a promising facilitator [1].

4. Discussion

In current international healthcare contexts, one of the most important, complex, and relevant challenges is the management of chronic patients, not only for the economic sustainability of the system, but above all for the social, organizational, and quality-of-life consequences for patients and caregivers. This study acknowledges the effectiveness of hospital–community integration models under the direct guidance of the family and community nurse as a concrete response to the management of chronicity and as a contribution to the improvement of continuity, quality of care, and satisfaction of patients and caregivers. These models rely on proactive patient management, with the aim of anticipating the patient's needs through the construction of a personalized care pathway, avoiding the fragmentation of episodic care. In this scenario, the nurse emerges as a key connector between services, supporting the stages of assessment, therapeutic education, follow-up, and coordination between different care settings. It should also be noted that fragmented and uncoordinated organizational models can increase the phenomenon of missed nursing care, with negative repercussions on care quality and patient safety [38]. The results of this scoping review are aligned with multiple findings from the international literature. The study by Deschodt et al. [18], for example, analyzed studies that confirm the importance of the nursing role in integrated chronic care management models. The study by Counsell et al. [39] is consistent with the results of our work, showing how a nurse-led multidisciplinary approach can improve quality of life by reducing emergency department visits. Other studies, such as that of Suiker et al. [40], highlight an improvement in the quality of life in chronic patients managed through multifactorial nursing models. This confirms what emerged in our review in terms of perceived continuity, empowerment, and satisfaction. Similarly, the study by Imhof et al. [41] demonstrates a significant reduction in hospitalizations at three months in chronic patients managed at home by nurses, a result that reinforces the idea of an effective community care model. Another point of reflection comes from the study by Stijnen et al. [42], documenting the positive impact of home visits on the social dimension, an aspect often overlooked by policy-makers, yet relevant to the well-being of chronic and frail patients. However, the diversity of results, as demonstrated by the study of Boult et al. [43], shows that the effectiveness of integrated models also depends on contextual factors, such as staff training, care pathway personalization, and institutional support. Other reviews in the literature confirm the aforementioned findings. McParland et al. [32], through a review, summarized various nursing interventions aimed at patients with multimorbidity, with positive outcomes on quality of life, satisfaction, and the perception of care, reaffirming the centrality of the nurse-led model. Among the studies included in the review, the Guided Care model demonstrated how the activity of the nurse case manager improves the patient experience, enhances self-care, and reduces the use of healthcare services. Along the same lines is the study by Naylor et al. [44], showing how nurse-led management in the early stages post-discharge allows a significant reduction in hospital readmission rates and length of stay, thanks to effective hospital–community continuity. Studies such as that of Rich et al. [45] confirm the above, highlighting the importance and effectiveness of structured education and follow-up in reducing hospital readmission rates in patients with chronic conditions such as heart failure. However, not all studies in the literature confirm favorable outcomes: Weinberger et al. [46], for example, observe improvements in satisfaction but not in readmission rates, emphasizing the importance of the organizational context for the effectiveness of interventions. Further positive confirmations come from a study by Morilla-Herrara et al. [47], which demonstrates that structured discharge planning with connection to community services through models such as nurse case management leads to improvements. A review by Latour et al. [33] focuses on nurse case management in the post-hospital discharge phases in complex and chronic patients, showing positive clinical outcomes and high satisfaction in patients and caregivers. These findings in the literature are integrated with those of our scoping review, where not only clinical benefits emerged, but also relational and organizational ones. Comparing our study with the systematic review by Deschodt et al. [18], interesting data emerge: although aggregate outcomes (mortality, ADL, and hospitalization rate) are not always statistically significant, the effects in terms of quality reported by patients, caregivers, and professionals indicate added value in educational, relational, and organizational terms. This is highly relevant for chronic care management, where therapeutic adherence, patient decision-making capacity, and long-term support are key elements just as important as traditional clinical indicators. In summary, the review confirms the importance of the nursing contribution in the management of frail and chronic patients, and this is not limited only to clinical surveillance but also to the promotion of empowerment, guidance in decision-making processes, and long-term continuity of care. Personalizing the intervention, adopting constant follow-up, and coordinating resources are factors that make holistic care feasible, centered not only on the disease, but on the person and their life network. In this sense, integrated models not only provide an organizational response but also represent a cultural proposal for rethinking chronicity, based on proximity, relationship, and autonomy of the assisted person.

4.1. Limitations of the Study

This scoping review was based on indexed sources, with the potential risk of excluding unpublished data or policy documents. The descriptive nature of this review does not allow for quantifying the effectiveness of the analyzed interventions. Moreover, the variability in the study designs included, combined with terminological differences, made it difficult to categorize care models uniformly. The use of AI (ChatGPT-4o) supported the linguistic refinement of the manuscript. While the content and methodological decisions were entirely made by the authors, the influence of AI on language style and phrasing should be acknowledged as a minor aspect potentially affecting narrative consistency.

4.2. Future Perspectives

Considering the results that emerged, further studies are needed to deepen the understanding of the effectiveness, sustainability, and transferability of hospital-to-community integrated care models in the management of chronic conditions and frail patients. Longitudinal studies and randomized controlled trials could systematically measure the clinical, economic, and experiential outcomes associated with such models. In the future, it is essential to standardize and develop tools for assessing continuity of care, as well as to define shared roles and nursing competencies across different contexts. Moreover, modern technologies such as telemonitoring, remote monitoring, and the use of artificial intelligence represent a promising perspective that requires further exploration in the context of chronic care management, hospital–community integration processes, and support for patient self-care.

5. Conclusions

The scoping review confirms the need for integrated hospital-to-community care models to support frail and chronically ill patients. A key finding of the study is that the leading role in this process must be played by the family and community nurse. Despite the heterogeneity of the included studies, there is a general agreement that nursing activity provides added value in ensuring continuity of care, promoting self-care, and increasing therapeutic adherence and satisfaction among patients and caregivers. The need for standardized post-discharge pathways, the adoption of case management models, and collaboration with other healthcare professionals emerge as fundamental elements to provide effective chronic care. The presence of a healthcare professional in close contact with families within communities, equipped with clinical, educational, and relational skills, proves to be crucial. In managing chronic conditions, it is essential to rely on a healthcare professional who can oversee the transitional phases across different settings, prevent fragmentation and delays, and ensure a holistic approach—leading to high standards of quality and safety in care. However, the study also identifies challenges that need to be addressed. Among these are the lack of standardized models, limited coordination and integration between hospitals and community services, and the need to enhance training and supportive organizational tools. Further robust experimental studies are necessary to assess long-term outcomes such as economic sustainability and patient empowerment.

In conclusion, reducing the gap and finding an effective organizational solution for managing chronic conditions requires the implementation of integrated care models and, above all, recognition of the central role of the family and community nurse. This, however, calls for a cultural shift among policy-makers towards a proactive, sustainable, and holistic healthcare system capable of providing concrete responses to the complex needs of frail and chronic patients.

Supplementary Materials: The following supporting information can be downloaded at https://www.mdpi.com/article/10.3390/medicina61071175/s1, Table S1: Supplementary File S1.

Author Contributions: Conceptualization, G.A., L.M., M.P., L.G. and M.D.M.; methodology, G.A., L.G. and M.D.M.; software, G.A.; validation, G.A., L.M., L.G. and M.D.M.; formal analysis, G.A. and M.D.M.; investigation, G.A., L.M., M.P., P.V., L.G. and M.D.M.; resources, G.A. and M.D.M.; data curation, G.A. and M.D.M.; writing—original draft preparation, G.A., L.M., L.G. and M.D.M.; writing—review and editing, G.A., L.M., M.P., P.V., L.G. and M.D.M.; visualization, G.A., L.M., M.P., P.V., L.G. and M.D.M.; supervision, G.A., L.G. and M.D.M.; project administration, G.A. and M.D.M. All authors have read and agreed to the published version of the manuscript.

Funding: This research received no external funding.

Institutional Review Board Statement: Ethical review was not required for this study as it is a scoping review that analyzes previously published data.

Informed Consent Statement: Informed consent was not required for this study as it is a scoping review that analyzes previously published data.

Data Availability Statement: No new data were created or analyzed in this study.

Acknowledgments: Artificial intelligence was involved exclusively to enhance the clarity and coherence of the text and language. AI did not contribute to the study design, data collection, or results analysis. The authors acknowledge the use of ChatGPT-4o (OpenAI, San Francisco, CA, USA) solely as support for the purposes mentioned above.

Conflicts of Interest: The authors declare no conflicts of interest.

References

1. Endalamaw, A.; Zewdie, A.; Wolka, E.; Assefa, Y. Care models for individuals with chronic multimorbidity: Lessons for low- and middle-income countries. *BMC Health Serv. Res.* **2024**, *24*, 895. [CrossRef] [PubMed]
2. Sargent, P.; Pickard, S.; Sheaff, R.; Boaden, R. Patient and carer perceptions of case management for long-term conditions. *Health Soc. Care Community* **2007**, *15*, 511–519. [CrossRef]

3. Schraeder, K.; Dimitropoulos, G.; McBrien, K.; Li, J.; Samuel, S. Perspectives from primary health care providers on their roles for supporting adolescents and young adults transitioning from pediatric services. *BMC Fam. Pract.* **2020**, *21*, 140. [CrossRef]
4. Ruikes, F.; Zuidema, S.; Akkermans, R.; Assendelft, W.; Schers, H.; Koopmans, R. Multicomponent Program to Reduce Functional Decline in Frail Elderly People: A Cluster Controlled Trial. *J. Am. BOARD Fam. Med.* **2016**, *29*, 209–217. [CrossRef] [PubMed]
5. Takeda, A.; Taylor, S.; Taylor, R.; Khan, F.; Krum, H.; Underwood, M. Clinical service organisation for heart failure. *Cochrane Database Syst. Rev.* **2012**, *9*, CD002752. [CrossRef]
6. Joo, J.Y.; Liu, M.F. Understanding Nurse-led Case Management in Patients with Chronic Illnesses: A Realist Review. *West. J. Nurs. Res.* **2021**, *43*, 182–195. [CrossRef] [PubMed]
7. Azzellino, G.; De Martinis, M. Territorial reorganization, telemedicine and operative centres: Challenges and opportunities for the nursing profession. *J. Clin. Nurs.* **2024**, *33*, 4518–4519. [CrossRef]
8. Azzellino, G.; Aitella, E.; Ginaldi, L.; Vagnarelli, P.; De Martinis, M. Use of Digital and Telemedicine Tools for Postoperative Pain Management at Home: A Scoping Review of Health Professionals' Roles and Clinical Outcomes. *J. Clin. Med.* **2025**, *14*, 4009. [CrossRef]
9. Azzellino, G.; Aitella, E.; Passamonti, M.; Ginaldi, L.; De Martinis, M. Protected discharge and combined interventions: A viable path to reduce hospital readmissions. *Eur. J. Intern. Med.* 2025; *epub ahead of print*. [CrossRef]
10. Scrimaglia, S.; Ricci, M.; Masini, A.; Montalti, M.; Conti, A.; Camedda, C.; Panella, M.; Dallolio, L.; Longobucco, Y. The Role of Family or Community Nurse in Dealing with Frail and Chronic Patients in Italy: A Scoping Review. *Geriatrics* **2024**, *9*, 81. [CrossRef]
11. Gasperini, G.; Renzi, E.; Longobucco, Y.; Cianciulli, A.; Rosso, A.; Marzuillo, C.; De Vito, C.; Villari, P.; Massimi, A. State of the Art on Family and Community Health Nursing International Theories, Models and Frameworks: A Scoping Review. *Healthcare* **2023**, *11*, 2578. [CrossRef]
12. Leijten, F.R.M.; Struckmann, V.; van Ginneken, E.; Czypionka, T.; Kraus, M.; Reiss, M.; Tsiachristas, A.; Boland, M.; de Bont, A.; Bal, R.; et al. The SELFIE framework for integrated care for multi-morbidity: Development and description. *Health Policy Amst. Neth.* **2018**, *122*, 12–22. [CrossRef]
13. Beaudin, J.; Chouinard, M.-C.; Hudon, É.; Hudon, C. Factors and Strategies Influencing Integrated Self-Management Support for People with Chronic Diseases and Common Mental Disorders: A Qualitative Study of Canadian Primary Care Nurses' Experience. *J. Adv. Nurs.* 2025; *epub ahead of print*. [CrossRef]
14. Shirey, M.; Selleck, C.; White-Williams, C.; Talley, M.; Harper, D. Interprofessional Collaborative Practice Model to Advance Population Health. *Popul. Health Manag.* **2021**, *24*, 69–77. [CrossRef] [PubMed]
15. Koontalay, A.; Botti, M.; Hutchinson, A. Development of a User-Centred Chronic Care Model for Patients with Heart Failure in a Limited-Resource Setting: A Codesign Study. *Health Expect.* **2025**, *28*, e70142. [CrossRef] [PubMed]
16. Peters, M.D.J.; Marnie, C.; Tricco, A.C.; Pollock, D.; Munn, Z.; Alexander, L.; McInerney, P.; Godfrey, C.M.; Khalil, H. Updated methodological guidance for the conduct of scoping reviews. *JBI Evid. Synth.* **2020**, *18*, 2119–2126. [CrossRef]
17. Page, M.J.; McKenzie, J.E.; Bossuyt, P.M.; Boutron, I.; Hoffmann, T.C.; Mulrow, C.D.; Shamseer, L.; Tetzlaff, J.M.; Akl, E.A.; Brennan, S.E.; et al. The PRISMA 2020 statement: An updated guideline for reporting systematic reviews. *BMJ* **2021**, *372*, n71. [CrossRef]
18. Deschodt, M.; Laurent, G.; Cornelissen, L.; Yip, O.; Zúñiga, F.; Denhaerynck, K.; Briel, M.; Karabegovic, A.; De Geest, S.; Blozik, E.; et al. Core components and impact of nurse-led integrated care models for home-dwelling older people: A systematic review and meta-analysis. *Int. J. Nurs. Stud.* **2020**, *105*, 103552. [CrossRef] [PubMed]
19. Davis, K.; Ramsey, I.; Sharplin, G.; Eckert, M.; Shakib, S. A nurse-led, telehealth transitional care intervention for people with multimorbidity: A feasibility study. *Aust. J. Adv. Nurs.* **2024**, *41*, 43–52. [CrossRef]
20. Jepma, P.; Latour, C.H.M.; ten Barge, I.H.J.; Verweij, L.; Peters, R.J.G.; Scholte op Reimer, W.J.M.; Buurman, B.M. Experiences of frail older cardiac patients with a nurse-coordinated transitional care intervention-a qualitative study. *BMC Health Serv. Res.* **2021**, *21*, 786. [CrossRef]
21. Wynia, K.; Uittenbroek, R.J.; van der Mei, S.F.; Slotman, K.; Reijneveld, S.A. Experiences of case managers in providing person-centered and integrated care based on the Chronic Care Model: A qualitative study on embrace. *PLoS ONE* **2018**, *13*, e0207109. [CrossRef]
22. Armold, S. Utilization of the Health Care System of Community Case Management Patients. *Prof. CASE Manag.* **2017**, *22*, 155–162. [CrossRef]
23. Davis, K.; Eckert, M.; Hutchinson, A.; Harmon, J.; Sharplin, G.; Shakib, S.; Caughey, G. Continuity of care for people with multimorbidity: The development of a model for a nurse-led care coordination service. *Aust. J. Adv. Nurs.* **2020**, *37*, 7–19. [CrossRef]

24. Chow, S.K.Y.; Wong, F.K.Y.; Chan, T.M.F.; Chung, L.Y.F.; Chang, K.K.P.; Lee, R.P.L. Community nursing services for postdischarge chronically ill patients. *J. Clin. Nurs.* **2008**, *17*, 260–271. [CrossRef] [PubMed]
25. Chow, S.K.Y.; Wong, F.K.Y. Health-related quality of life in patients undergoing peritoneal dialysis: Effects of a nurse-led case management programme. *J. Adv. Nurs.* **2010**, *66*, 1780–1792. [CrossRef]
26. Chow, S.K.Y.; Wong, F.K.Y. A randomized controlled trial of a nurse-led case management programme for hospital-discharged older adults with co-morbidities. *J. Adv. Nurs.* **2014**, *70*, 2257–2271. [CrossRef]
27. Davis, K.; Eckert, M.; Shakib, S.; Harmon, J.; Hutchinson, A.; Sharplin, G.; Caughey, G. Development and Implementation of a Nurse-Led Model of Care Coordination to Provide Health-Sector Continuity of Care for People with Multimorbidity: Protocol for a Mixed Methods Study. *JMIR Res. Protoc.* **2019**, *8*, e15006. [CrossRef] [PubMed]
28. Davis, K.; Eckert, M.; Hutchinson, A.; Harmon, J.; Sharplin, G.; Shakib, S.; Caughey, G. Effectiveness of nurse-led services for people with chronic disease in achieving an outcome of continuity of care at the primary-secondary healthcare interface: A quantitative systematic review. *Int. J. Nurs. Stud.* **2021**, *121*, 103986. [CrossRef]
29. Grimsmo, A.; Løhre, A.; Røsstad, T.; Gjerde, I.; Heiberg, I.; Steinsbekk, A. Disease-specific clinical pathways-are they feasible in primary care? A mixed-methods study. *Scand. J. Prim. Health Care* **2018**, *36*, 152–160. [CrossRef] [PubMed]
30. Harvey, C.; Sibley, J.; Palmer, J.; Phillips, A.; Willis, E.; Marshall, R.; Thompson, S.; Ward, S.; Forrest, R.; Pearson, M. Development, implementation and evaluation of nurse-led integrated, person-centred care with long-term conditions. *J. Integr. CARE* **2017**, *25*, 186–195. [CrossRef]
31. Gonçalves, M.; Mendes, D.; Caldeira, S.; Jesus, E.; Nunes, E. Nurse-led care management models for patients with multimorbidity in hospital settings: A scoping review. *J. Nurs. Manag.* **2022**, *30*, 1960–1973. [CrossRef]
32. McParland, C.; Johnston, B.; Cooper, M. A mixed-methods systematic review of nurse-led interventions for people with multimorbidity. *J. Adv. Nurs.* **2022**, *78*, 3930–3951. [CrossRef]
33. Latour, C.H.M.; van der Windt, D.A.W.M.; de Jonge, P.; Riphagen, I.I.; de Vos, R.; Huyse, F.J.; Stalman, W.A.B. Nurse-led case management for ambulatory complex patients in general health care: A systematic review. *J. Psychosom. Res.* **2007**, *62*, 385–395. [CrossRef] [PubMed]
34. Mc Govern, E.M.; Maillart, E.; Bourgninaud, M.; Manzato, E.; Guillonnet, C.; Mochel, F.; Bourmaleau, J.; Lubetzki, C.; Baulac, M.; Roze, E. Making a 'JUMP' from paediatric to adult healthcare: A transitional program for young adults with chronic neurological disease. *J. Neurol. Sci.* **2018**, *395*, 77–83. [CrossRef]
35. O'Connell, M.B.; Bendtsen, F.; Nørholm, V.; Brødsgaard, A.; Kimer, N. Nurse-assisted and multidisciplinary outpatient follow-up among patients with decompensated liver cirrhosis: A systematic review. *PLoS ONE* **2023**, *18*, e0278545. [CrossRef]
36. Schraeder, C.; Fraser, C.; Clark, I.; Long, B.; Shelton, P.; Waldschmidt, V.; Kucera, C.; Lanker, W. Evaluation of a primary care nurse case management intervention for chronically ill community dwelling older people. *J. Clin. Nurs.* **2008**, *17*, 407–417. [CrossRef] [PubMed]
37. O'Connell, A.; Petty, J. Preparing young people with complex needs and their families for transition to adult services. *Nurs. Child. Young People* **2019**, *31*, 25–31. [CrossRef] [PubMed]
38. Azzellino, G.; Dante, A.; Petrucci, C.; Caponnetto, V.; Aitella, E.; Lancia, L.; Ginaldi, L.; De Martinis, M. Intention to leave and missed nursing care: A scoping review. *Int. J. Nurs. Stud. Adv.* **2025**, *8*, 100312. [CrossRef] [PubMed]
39. Counsell, S.R.; Callahan, C.M.; Clark, D.O.; Tu, W.; Buttar, A.B.; Stump, T.E.; Ricketts, G.D. Geriatric care management for low-income seniors: A randomized controlled trial. *JAMA* **2007**, *298*, 2623–2633. [CrossRef]
40. Suijker, J.; van Rijn, M.; Buurman, B.; ter Riet, G.; van Charante, E.; de Rooij, S. Effects of Nurse-Led Multifactorial Care to Prevent Disability in Community-Living Older People: Cluster Randomized Trial. *PLoS ONE* **2016**, *11*, e0158714. [CrossRef]
41. Imhof, L.; Naef, R.; Wallhagen, M.I.; Schwarz, J.; Mahrer-Imhof, R. Effects of an advanced practice nurse in-home health consultation program for community-dwelling persons aged 80 and older. *J. Am. Geriatr. Soc.* **2012**, *60*, 2223–2231. [CrossRef]
42. Stijnen, M.M.N.; Jansen, M.W.J.; Vrijhoef, H.J.M.; Duimel-Peeters, I.G.P. Development of a home visitation programme for the early detection of health problems in potentially frail community-dwelling older people by general practices. *Eur. J. Ageing* **2013**, *10*, 49–60. [CrossRef]
43. Boult, C.; Reider, L.; Leff, B.; Frick, K.D.; Boyd, C.M.; Wolff, J.L.; Frey, K.; Karm, L.; Wegener, S.T.; Mroz, T.; et al. The effect of guided care teams on the use of health services: Results from a cluster-randomized controlled trial. *Arch. Intern. Med.* **2011**, *171*, 460–466. [CrossRef] [PubMed]
44. Naylor, M.; Hirschman, K.; Toles, M.; Jarrín, O.; Shaid, E.; Pauly, M. Adaptations of the evidence-based Transitional Care Model in the U.S. *Soc. Sci. Med.* **2018**, *213*, 28–36. [CrossRef] [PubMed]
45. Rich, T.L.; Falbo, K.J.; Phelan, H.; Gravely, A.; Krebs, E.E.; Finn, J.A.; Matsumoto, M.; Muschler, K.; Olney, C.M.; Kiecker, J.; et al. Clinician perspectives on postamputation pain assessment and rehabilitation interventions. *Prosthet. Orthot. Int.* **2024**, *48*, 441–447. [CrossRef]

46. Weinberger, M.; Oddone, E.Z.; Henderson, W.G. Does increased access to primary care reduce hospital readmissions? Veterans Affairs Cooperative Study Group on Primary Care and Hospital Readmission. *N. Engl. J. Med.* **1996**, *334*, 1441–1447. [CrossRef] [PubMed]
47. Morilla-Herrera, J.C.; Garcia-Mayor, S.; Martín-Santos, F.J.; Kaknani Uttumchandani, S.; Leon Campos, Á.; Caro Bautista, J.; Morales-Asencio, J.M. A systematic review of the effectiveness and roles of advanced practice nursing in older people. *Int. J. Nurs. Stud.* **2016**, *53*, 290–307. [CrossRef]

medicina

MDPI

Systematic Review

Vitamin D Deficiency in Kazakhstani Children: Insights from a Systematic Review and Meta-Analysis

Indira Karibayeva [1,*], Galiya Bilibayeva [2], Assiya Iglikova [2], Aya Yerzhanova [2], Roza Alekesheva [2], Makhigul Maxudova [2] and Neilya Ussebayeva [2]

1 Department of Health Policy and Community Health, Jiann-Ping Hsu College of Public Health, Georgia Southern University, Statesboro, GA 30460, USA
2 Department of Nursing, Faculty of Medicine and Public Health, Al-Farabi Kazakh National University, Almaty 050038, Kazakhstan; bilibayeva@kaznu.kz (G.B.); iglikova-a@mail.ru (A.I.); yerzhanova.aya@kaznu.kz (A.Y.); alekesheva@kaznu.kz (R.A.); maksudova63@gmail.com (M.M.); usebaeva@mail.ru (N.U.)
* Correspondence: ik01379@georgiasouthern.edu

Abstract: *Background and Objectives*: Kazakhstan's unique geographic, dietary, and cultural factors contribute to the widespread occurrence of vitamin D deficiency across the entire country population, particularly among children. This study aims to assess the mean prevalence of vitamin D deficiency in children in Kazakhstan and determine whether it differs between healthy and non-healthy children, as well as between infants and older age groups. *Materials and Methods*: A comprehensive literature search was performed across five databases by two researchers. Studies were eligible if they were observational and provided the number of children with serum 25-hydroxyvitamin D levels below 20 ng/mL out of the total number of children assessed in Kazakhstan. *Results*: Eleven studies were included in the analysis, assessing 1396 children, of whom 714 had the outcome of interest. The pooled mean estimate of vitamin D deficiency among children was 56% (95% CI, 46–65%), with particularly concerning rates among infants at 65% (95% CI, 44–82%). No substantial differences were observed between healthy and non-healthy children. *Conclusions*: The prevalence of vitamin D deficiency among children is alarmingly high. These results highlight the urgent necessity of tackling vitamin D deficiency as a public health priority. Incorporating vitamin D deficiency prevention into Kazakhstan's national healthcare program is vital for improving child health outcomes and reducing the long-term burden of associated complications.

Keywords: vitamin D; vitamin D deficiency; children; infants; prevalence; Kazakhstan; national program; systematic review; meta-analysis

1. Introduction

Vitamin D plays a critical role in the growth and development of children, influencing skeletal health, immune function, and overall well-being [1]. Sufficient vitamin D levels are crucial for the absorption of calcium and the process of bone mineralization [2,3]. The most common impacts of vitamin D deficiency (VDD) involve bone and musculoskeletal health, leading to rickets in children and osteomalacia in adults. Beyond bone health, VDD has been associated with several health complications in pregnant women, including pre-eclampsia, pregnancy-induced diabetes, premature birth, and postpartum mood disorder [4]. In infants and children, it is linked to low birth weight, reduced bone density, respiratory tract infections, and worsening asthma symptoms [5,6]. VDD in infants and children is also linked to increased autoimmunity and allergies [7]. Given the vulnerability of children to VDD due to their physiological growth demands, understanding its prevalence is vital for developing effective prevention and management strategies.

Kazakhstan's unique geographical, dietary, and cultural characteristics may contribute significantly to VDD among its population, particularly children [8–10]. The country's vast territory experiences long winters and limited sunlight exposure during the colder months, which restricts the synthesis of vitamin D through the skin. Additionally, traditional dietary patterns in Kazakhstan often lack sufficient vitamin D intake sources, such as high-fat fish, and dairy products with added nutrients [11,12]. Cultural norms, including modest clothing styles in some communities, may further limit sun exposure, exacerbating the risk of deficiency [13]. A systematic review of VDD among adults in Kazakhstan reported alarmingly high rates of 57% [14]. These combined factors may contribute to the high prevalence of VDD, especially among vulnerable groups like infants and children.

Despite these known risk factors, there is a notable lack of comprehensive data on VDD among children in Kazakhstan. While several studies have examined vitamin D levels in the Kazakhstani population, data specific to children remain scarce and not systemic. Furthermore, no specific guidelines exist for the prevention and treatment of VDD in children in Kazakhstan, aside from those addressing rickets [15]. This gap in research and evidence is concerning, given the critical developmental window during childhood and the potential long-term health consequences of deficiency. Previous studies conducted in other countries have demonstrated the prevalence and determinants of VDD, but similar data specific to Kazakhstan's unique context is insufficiently explored [16–18]. This lack of evidence hinders the formulation of targeted public health interventions and policies.

Addressing this research gap is imperative to guide public health initiatives in Kazakhstan. The aim of this study is to evaluate the mean prevalence of VDD among children in Kazakhstan and examine whether it differs between healthy and non-healthy children, as well as between infants and older children.

2. Materials and Methods

2.1. Search Strategy Framework

An initial search of the PROSPERO international database for registered studies on similar topics identified a review protocol focusing on the mean vitamin D levels in Kazakhstan and another protocol examining VDD levels specifically among adults in Kazakhstan [19,20]. To assess the mean prevalence of VDD among children in Kazakhstan, this systematic review protocol was registered in the PROSPERO international database (PROSPERO ID: CRD42025635124). Subsequently, a comprehensive search was conducted across five databases: PubMed, ScienceDirect, Scopus, Web of Science, and Google Scholar. The search strategy employed the keywords "vitamin D" AND "Kazakhstan". No restrictions were applied regarding publication year, but the search was limited to studies published in English and Russian, focusing on humans. The search was performed between 1 November 2024 and 31 December 2024. Additional filters were applied, including the selection of research articles and the exclusion of other types of publications. In Google Scholar, the search was restricted to titles only.

2.2. Inclusion and Exclusion Criteria of Studies and Data Extraction

To determine the eligibility of the retrieved articles, pre-specified inclusion and exclusion criteria were applied, guided by the PICOS framework [21]. Population (P): Studies focusing on children aged 0 to 18 years in Kazakhstan. Intervention/Exposure (I): Serum 25-hydroxyvitamin D (25(OH)D) levels were measured to determine vitamin D status, with vitamin D deficiency (VDD) defined as a serum 25(OH)D level below 20 ng/mL.

Comparison (C): Studies focusing on healthy children or children with acute or chronic conditions. A secondary comparison was made based on different age groups. Outcomes (O): Studies reporting the prevalence or number of children with VDD, along with data on the total number of children assessed. Study Design (S): Observational studies, including cohort studies with cross-sectional data, cross-sectional studies, and case–control studies published in English or Russian. The exclusion criteria included studies that focused exclusively on children with VDD or those that included a matched number of vitamin D-deficient and non-deficient children; studies reporting only the mean serum 25(OH)D levels without additional relevant data; studies with duplicate results already included in the analysis; studies examining the adult population in Kazakhstan; reviews, conference proceedings, abstracts, case reports, editorials, and commentaries; and studies using different cut-off values to define VDD.

The review and synthesis of the literature were carried out in accordance with the Preferred Reporting Items for Systematic Reviews and Meta-Analyses (PRISMA) guidelines [22]. After removing duplicates, two authors autonomously assessed the eligibility of the studies based on the title and abstract of the search results. Full-text articles that satisfied the preliminary screening criteria were then evaluated against the established eligibility criteria for data extraction. Data extracted from the chosen studies included the last name of the first author, publication year, study city or district, characteristics of the study population (e.g., specific condition or healthy controls), sample size, number of boys, age in years or in months, 25(OH)D levels in blood if provided, 25(OH)D level assessment method, and the number of children diagnosed with VDD. The data extraction process was conducted autonomously by two researchers responsible for data extraction, and any disagreements were clarified through consultation with a third author to achieve consensus. This collaborative approach ensured accuracy and consistency in study selection and data extraction.

2.3. Risk of Bias Assessment

The risk of bias assessment was carried out using the Newcastle–Ottawa Scale (NOS), which is specifically designed for case–control studies, as well as its revised form for cross-sectional studies [23]. This scale evaluated each study based on eight criteria across three domains: selection, assessed with four criteria; comparability, assessed with one criterion; and exposure, assessed with three criteria. The adapted version for cross-sectional studies evaluated each study based on six criteria divided into three main domains: selection, assessed with three criteria; comparability, assessed with one criterion; and exposure, assessed with two criteria. Each criterion was given a score of up to one point, with the comparability criterion capable of earning two points. The overall score ranged from 0 to 9 for case–control studies and from 0 to 7 for cross-sectional studies, with higher scores indicating better study quality. Two authors (IK and GB) independently assessed the quality of the included studies, and a third author (NU) calculated the inter-rater agreement between them. Case–control studies that achieved a score of seven or higher, and cross-sectional studies with five points or more, were included in the review.

2.4. Statistical Strategy for Data Synthesis

The RStudio software (version 2024.12.0), along with the 'metafor' and 'meta' packages, was utilized to determine the pooled mean prevalence of VDD among children in Kazakhstan. This was performed employing a random-effects model for prevalence meta-analysis, with 95% confidence intervals [24,25]. Forest plots were produced to visually represent the pooled analysis results. A meta-regression analysis based on the year of publication and the number of boys in the study was applied to assess heterogeneity. To further explore the sources of heterogeneity, an influence analysis and leave-one-out analysis were performed [25]. The study's generalizability was examined through a publication bias assessment, which involved visually inspecting a drapery plot and conducting statistical analysis with Egger's test. A subgroup analysis was used to compare healthy children with those who had health conditions and to analyze differences between infants and older children [25].

3. Results

3.1. Included Study Characteristics

The applied search strategy resulted in 234 articles. After removing 67 duplicates, 167 non-duplicative search results were initially screened, and 124 titles were deemed ineligible for full-text review. Out of 43 remaining articles, 42 articles underwent full-text review, as one article's full text was not available. Upon full assessment, eleven studies met the inclusion criteria. Seven studies focused on adults, five studies were reviews, and five were excluded for other reasons. Seven studies were excluded because they either included only children with VDD or included a matched number of vitamin D-deficient children and non-deficient children [26–32]. Additionally, four studies presented the same results as studies already included in the review [33–36]. In three of the excluded studies, VDD was defined as serum 25(OH)D levels below 30 ng/mL or below 25 ng/mL [37–39]. Figure 1 displays the PRISMA flow diagram [22].

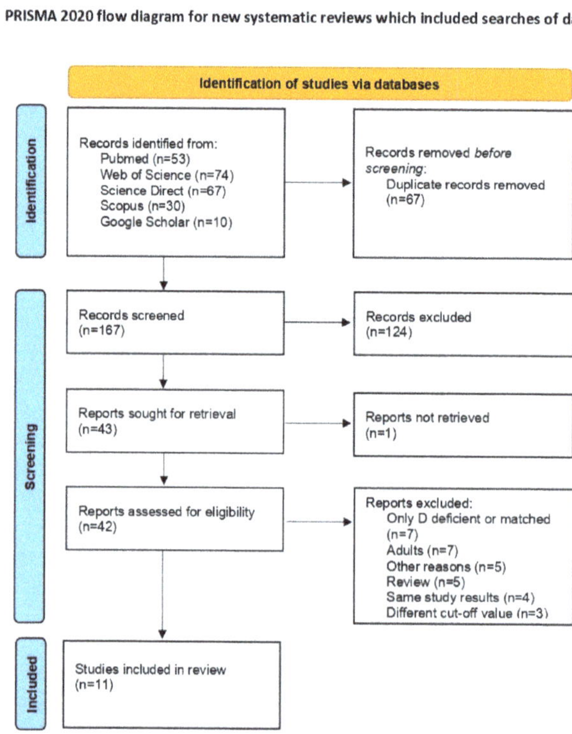

Figure 1. PRISMA Flow diagram of Study Selection.

The selected eleven studies were published between 2020 and 2024. Three studies were conducted in Aktobe, Karaganda, and Astana, respectively, while one study was conducted in Almaty and Semey. The methodological designs included five case–control studies, five cross-sectional studies, and one cohort study. Among these, three studies focused on patients with chronic kidney disease, while one study examined cancer patients, recurrent respiratory infection (RRI) patients, congenital pneumonia cases, diabetic nephropathy, and patients infected with *Helicobacter pylori* (*H. pylori*). Additionally, five studies included healthy patient groups. Three of the included studies focused exclusively on infants, while the remaining studies examined children across various age groups. In total, 1396 children were assessed across the eleven studies. Of these, 714 children were found to have serum 25(OH)D levels below 20 ng/mL, classifying them as vitamin D deficient. In seven out of eleven studies, the method for serum 25(OH)D level assessment was not provided. Further details regarding the selected and analyzed articles are presented in Table 1.

Table 1. Overview of the Included Studies.

First Author, Year	Region	Study Design	Groups	Total	Boys	Age (Mean ± SD) or Range	25(OH)D (ng/mL) (Mean ± SD)	25(OH)D Assessment	VDD (%)
Zhumalina, 2019 [40]	Aktobe	Case–control	Healthy, Kobda (a) Healthy, Kenkiyak (b)	52 (a) 80 (b)	n/a n/a	8–17 years (a) 8–17 years (b)	28 ± 11 (a) 24 ± 12 (b)	n/a	14 (27) (a) 26 (33) (b)
Balmukhanova, 2021 [41]	Almaty	Cross-sectional	CKD	73	38	2–18 years	Varied-based CKD stage	n/a	35 (48)
Dyussenova, 2021 [42]	Karaganda	Cross-sectional	CKD	40	16	1–17 years	n/a	ELISA	25 (62)
Zhamankulov, 2021 [43]	Astana	Cross-sectional	RRI	94	53	5.8 ± 3.3 years	31 ± 3	n/a	28 (30)
Nakipov, 2022 [44]	Astana	Cross-sectional data from cohort	Cancer, control (a) Cancer, nutritional intervention (b)	100 (a) 100 (b)	55 (a) 55 (b)	0–17 years	27 ± 12	n/a	60 (60) (a) 67 (67) (b)
Dyussenova, 2023 [45]	Karaganda	Case–control	CKD	90	34	1–17 years	n/a	n/a	36 (40)
Taiorazova, 2023 [46]	Semey	Case–control	Healthy (a) Congenital pneumonia (b)	152 (a) 76 (b)	67 (a) 44 (b)	newborn	21 ± 6 (a) 12 ± 7 (b)	Demeditec 25-OH Vitamin D total ELISA	63 (41) (a) 60 (79) (b)
Zeinebekova, 2023 [47]	Karaganda	Case–control	Diabetic nephropathy	109	n/a	0–17 years	n/a	n/a	75 (69)
Rysbekov, 2024 [48]	Astana	Case–control	Healthy (a) *H. pylori* present (b)	65 (a) 63 (b)	29 (a) 20 (b)	10–14 years (a) 11–15 years (b)	n/a	n/a	51 (78) (a) 35 (56) (b)
Zhumalina, 2024 [49]	Aktobe	Cross-sectional	Healthy	198	98	6.2 ± 2.4 months	n/a	LC-MS/MS methodology	58 (29)
Zhumalina, 2024 [50]	Aktobe	Cross-sectional	7–12 months (a) 1–6 months (b) 0–28 days (c) Healthy	32 (a) 27 (b) 45 (c)		7–12 months (a) 1–6 months (b) 0–28 days (c)	34 ± 6 (a) 21 ± 2 (b) 13 ± 5 (c)	ECLIA	19 (59) (a) 23 (85) (b) 39 (87) (c)

Abbreviations: 25(OH)D—25-hydroxyvitamin D; CKD—chronic kidney disease; ECLIA—electrochemiluminescent immunoassay; H—healthy; *H. pylori*—*Helicobacter pylori*; LC-MS/MS—Liquid Chromatography–Tandem Mass Spectrometry; n/a—not available; RRI—recurrent respiratory infection; SD—standard deviation; VDD—vitamin D deficient.

3.2. Meta-Analysis of Vitamin D Deficiency Prevalence

Eleven studies, with seventeen groups, presented data on the prevalence of VDD among children in Kazakhstan. Analysis of five studies with eight groups shows that the pooled mean estimate of VDD in healthy children was 55% (95% CI, 39–71%), with high heterogeneity: $I^2 = 92\%$, Q (df = 7) = 92, $p < 0.01$. Analysis of eight studies with nine groups shows that the pooled mean estimate of VDD in children with health conditions was 57% (95% CI, 46–67%), with high heterogeneity: $I^2 = 87\%$, Q (df = 8) = 63, $p < 0.01$ (Figure 2a).

Additionally, an analysis of eight studies with eleven groups shows that the pooled mean estimate of VDD in children of various ages was 52% (95% CI, 41–62%), with high heterogeneity: $I^2 = 89\%$, Q (df = 10) = 88, $p < 0.01$. Analysis of three studies with six groups shows that the pooled mean estimate of VDD in infants was 65% (95% CI, 44–82%), with high heterogeneity: $I^2 = 94\%$, Q (df = 5) = 86, $p < 0.01$. The total pooled mean estimate of VDD in children was 56% (95% CI, 46–65%), $I^2 = 91\%$, Q (df = 16) = 177, $p < 0.01$ (Figure 2b).

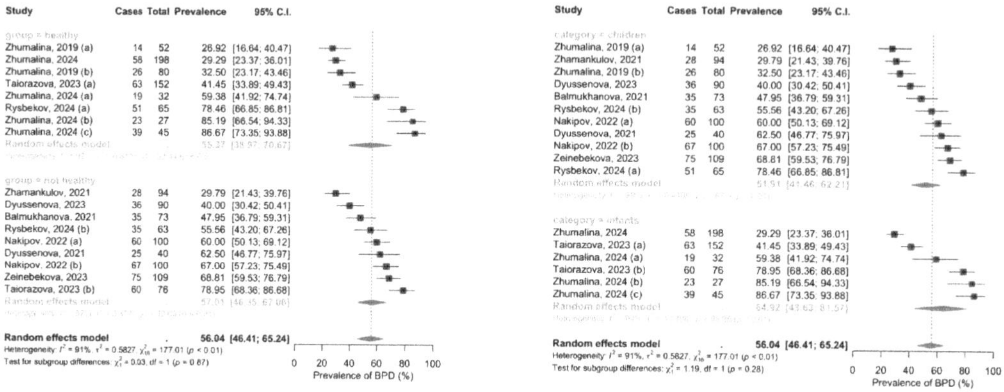

(**a**) (**b**)

Figure 2. Vitamin D Deficiency Rates Among Kazakhstani Children: (**a**) based on health conditions; (**b**) based on age groups. Abbreviations: CI—confidence interval; Zhumalina, 2019 (a) [40]—environmentally friendly region; Zhumalina, 2019 (b) [40]—oil and gas producing region; Nakipov, 2022 (a) [44]—children with oncology, no nutritional support; Nakipov, 2022 (b) [44]—children with oncology, with nutritional support; Taiorazova, 2023 (a) [46]—healthy; Taiorazova, 2023 (b) [46]—diabetic nephropathy; Rysbekov, 2024 (a) [48]—children with no *H. Pylori*; Rysbekov, 2024 (b) [48]—children with *H. Pylori*; Zhumalina, 2024 (a) [50]—7–12 months; Zhumalina, 2024 (b) [50]—1–6 months; Zhumalina, 2024 (c) [50]—0–28 days.

A meta-regression analysis demonstrated a significant positive association between publication year and the pooled mean estimate of VDD. Specifically, more recent studies reported a higher prevalence of VDD, a finding that was statistically significant ($p < 0.01$) (Figure 3a). A second meta-regression analysis explored the influence of gender on the pooled estimate of VDD. This analysis suggested that an increase in the proportion of male participants was associated with a decrease in the pooled mean prevalence of VDD. However, this relationship was not statistically significant ($p = 0.07$) (Figure 3b).

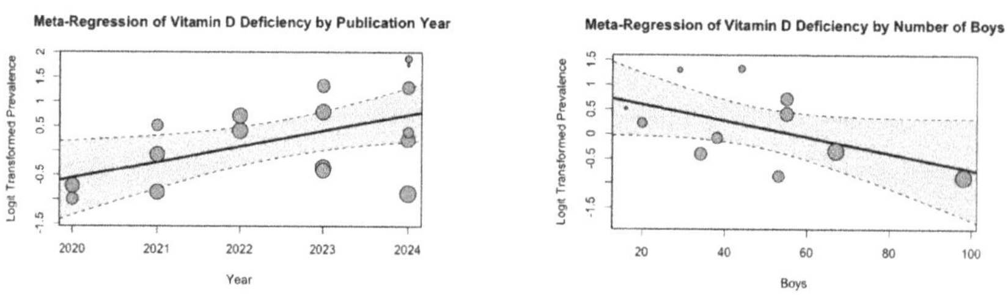

(**a**) (**b**)

Figure 3. Meta-Regression Analysis of the Pooled Mean VDD Estimate in Children: (**a**) by Year of Publication; (**b**) by Number of Boys.

An influence analysis and leave-one-out analysis did not identify any studies that significantly impacted the pooled estimate of the prevalence of VDD among children in Kazakhstan (Figure 4a,b).

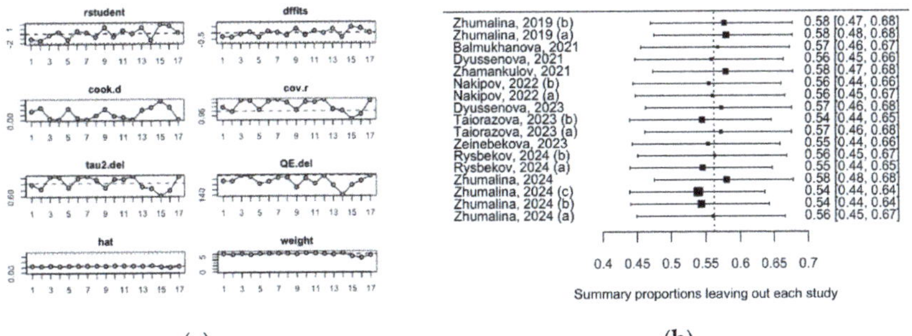

Figure 4. Heterogeneity Assessment of the Pooled Mean VDD Estimate in Children: (**a**) Influence Analysis; (**b**) Leave-One-Out Analysis.

Figure 5 presents the drapery plot of the publication bias assessment with no evident asymmetry. The lack of publication bias was additionally validated through the non-significant findings of Egger's test for publication bias ($p > 0.05$).

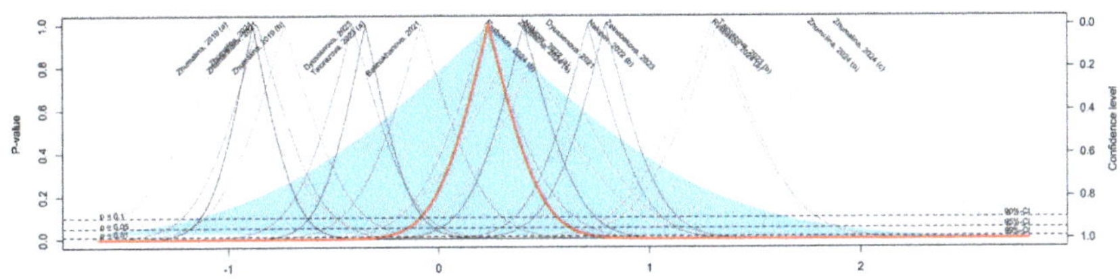

Figure 5. Drapery Plot of the Publication Bias Assessment.

3.3. Evaluation of Risk of Bias

The results of the risk of bias evaluation are outlined in Table 2, separately for case–control and cross-sectional studies, according to the NOS. All the included case–control studies achieved a NOS score of 7 or higher out of a possible 8, while all cross-sectional studies obtained a minimum score of 5 out of 7. These scores indicate that the included studies were of high quality with a low risk of bias. Consequently, they were included in the present systematic review and meta-analysis.

Table 2. Newcastle–Ottawa Scale Results for Risk of Bias Assessment.

First Author, Year	Selection	Comparability	Exposure	Total
		Study design: Case–control		
Zhumalina, 2019 [40]	3	1	3	7
Dyussenova, 2023 [45]	3	1	3	7
Taiorazova, 2023 [46]	4	1	3	8
Zeinebekova, 2023 [47]	4	1	3	8
Rysbekov, 2024 [48]	3	1	3	7
		Study design: Cross-sectional		
Balmukhanova, 2021 [41]	3	1	2	6
Dyussenova, 2021 [42]	3	1	2	6
Zhamankulov, 2021 [43]	2	1	2	5
Nakipov, 2022 [44]	2	1	2	5
Zhumalina, 2024 [49]	3	1	2	6
Zhumalina, 2024 [50]	2	1	2	5

4. Discussion

4.1. Main Findings of the Present Study and Their Practical Implications

This systematic review and meta-analysis sought to evaluate the prevalence of VDD, defined as a serum 25(OH)D level below 20 ng/mL, among children in Kazakhstan. The findings reveal an alarmingly high prevalence, with the total pooled mean estimate of VDD in children in Kazakhstan at 56% (95% CI, 46–65%). Notably, the prevalence did not significantly differ based on health status; VDD rates were nearly identical among healthy and non-healthy children, at 55% (95% CI, 39–71%) and 57% (95% CI, 46–67%), respectively. However, age emerged as a critical determinant of VDD. Infants demonstrated a substantially higher prevalence, with almost two-thirds being vitamin D deficient at 65% (95% CI, 44–82%) compared to children of various older age groups, where the prevalence was 52% (95% CI, 41–62%).

These findings are consistent with trends observed in the global literature. For instance, a recent meta-analysis on VDD among healthy children in Iran, using the same deficiency threshold, reported a prevalence of 31% (95% CI, 30–31%), markedly lower than that observed in Kazakhstan [16]. By contrast, a meta-analysis examining VDD among neonates in Turkey revealed even higher rates of 87% (95% CI, 70–95%) [18]. Similarly, a meta-analysis conducted in Africa, utilizing a higher cutoff for deficiency (serum 25(OH)D level below 30 ng/mL), reported a prevalence of 64% (95% CI, 9–100%) among newborns [17]. Importantly, these studies underscore the significant correlation between maternal and neonatal vitamin D levels, a finding corroborated by our prior meta-analysis on adults in Kazakhstan, which reported a similarly high prevalence of VDD (57%; 95% CI, 45–69%) [14]. These consistent patterns highlight the widespread nature of VDD across different demographic groups and emphasize the need for targeted interventions.

The high prevalence of VDD, particularly among infants, underscores the urgent need for targeted interventions to address this public health challenge in Kazakhstan. While the national healthcare development program outlines a comprehensive strategy to prevent and manage non-communicable diseases by addressing key risk factors such as hypertension, obesity, diabetes, and unhealthy lifestyle behaviors, the omission of VDD prevention is a significant gap [51]. Given the critical role of vitamin D in bone health, immune function, and overall well-being, particularly for children and pregnant women, this omission warrants immediate attention [2,3]. Moreover, recent evidence links VDD to an increased risk of respiratory tract infections, impaired growth, and poor dental health in children, emphasizing the broader health implications of the deficiency [52–54]. Furthermore, emerging evidence highlights the broader implications of maternal VDD, including its impact on neurocognitive development in offspring. For example, Melough et al. (2020) demonstrated that maternal plasma 25(OH)D levels during gestation are positively associated with neurocognitive development in children, underscoring the importance of addressing VDD in pregnant women to mitigate long-term developmental risks [55].

To address this gap, Kazakhstan should integrate strategies for the prevention and management of VDD into its national healthcare development program. Successful examples from other countries provide actionable models. Finland, for instance, implemented mandatory food fortification policies that significantly reduced population-level VDD [56]. In Poland, updated guidelines on the prevention and treatment of VDD emphasize daily supplementation of cholecalciferol for high-risk populations and provide recommendations for sun exposure [57]. In the United States, the Office of Dietary Supplements successfully led the National Vitamin D Initiative from 2004 to 2018, promoting awareness and prevention efforts [58,59]. Additionally, a national supplementation program for vitamin D in Iran demonstrated efficacy in reducing the prevalence of VDD and highlighted the importance of a prevention-based approach over a treatment-focused one [60–62]. Similarly, Canada has established robust supplementation programs targeting high-risk populations, such as infants, pregnant women, and older adults, achieving measurable reductions in deficiency rates and associated health complications [63,64].

Screening programs for pregnant women should also be prioritized in Kazakhstan, as maternal vitamin D status directly impacts neonatal and infant outcomes [4,5]. Public health campaigns promoting awareness of vitamin D's importance, along with educational initiatives about adequate sunlight exposure and dietary intake, are essential. Collaborative efforts between healthcare providers, policymakers, and researchers are necessary to design evidence-based guidelines that address VDD comprehensively. Such initiatives will not only improve child health outcomes but also mitigate the long-term burden of health complications associated with this preventable condition.

4.2. Limitations

First, we were unable to analyze region-specific data or stratify the findings based on participants' specific health conditions due to the limited number of studies included in this analysis. Consequently, the heterogeneity in selected article populations and settings may have influenced the pooled estimates. Second, limitations inherent in our previous meta-analysis on adults, such as the absence of analyses accounting for metabolic conditions, the seasonality of vitamin D measurements, and the amount of sun exposure among participants, also apply to the present meta-analysis [14]. Finally, most studies did not specify the assay method used to measure serum 25(OH)D. Among those that did, there was considerable variability in the techniques employed. Differences in reagents, assay sensitivity, and specificity are essential in the interpretation of the accuracy and comparability of vitamin D measurements [65,66].

To mitigate potential biases and ensure methodological rigor, we adhered to a standardized protocol throughout the study. We used pre-defined eligibility criteria and a structured data extraction table to minimize subjectivity during study selection, data extraction, and interpretation. Furthermore, we followed the PRISMA guidelines for conducting systematic reviews at every step of the process and transparently reported the methods used [22]. These measures strengthen the reliability of our findings, despite the inherent limitations of the available data.

4.3. Future Research Directions

To address the limitations of this study and build a more comprehensive understanding of VDD in Kazakhstan, future research should focus on:

- Investigating the role of metabolic disorders, seasonality, and sun exposure on vitamin D levels in children of varying ages.
- Assessing the prevalence of maternal VDD in Kazakhstan.
- Evaluating the efficacy of maternal interventions, such as screening and supplementation, on reducing VDD in newborns.
- Assessing the sensitivity and specificity of assays used

5. Conclusions

This meta-analysis highlights an alarmingly high prevalence of VDD among children in Kazakhstan at 56% (95% CI, 46–65%), with particularly concerning rates among infants at 65% (95% CI, 44–82%). These findings align with global evidence and underscore the critical need to address VDD as a public health priority. Incorporating VDD prevention into Kazakhstan's national healthcare program is vital to improving child health outcomes and reducing the long-term burden of associated complications. A comprehensive upstream approach that combines supplementation with broader public health initiatives will be key to reducing VDD prevalence and protecting future generations.

Author Contributions: Conceptualization, I.K.; methodology, I.K.; software, I.K.; validation, I.K., G.B. and A.Y.; formal analysis, I.K.; investigation, I.K., G.B. and A.Y.; resources, I.K., G.B., R.A., A.I., M.M. and N.U.; data curation, I.K., G.B. and A.Y.; writing—original draft preparation, I.K. and G.B.; writing—review and editing, I.K., G.B., A.I., A.Y., R.A., M.M. and N.U.; visualization, I.K.; supervision, I.K., A.Y., M.M. and N.U.; project administration, R.A., A.I., M.M. and N.U.; funding acquisition, G.B. All authors have read and agreed to the published version of the manuscript.

Funding: This research received no external funding.

Institutional Review Board Statement: Ethical review and approval were waived for this study as this is a systematic review of the published literature. Study protocol registration: PROSPERO ID: CRD42025635124.

Informed Consent Statement: Not applicable.

Data Availability Statement: The original contributions presented in this study are included in the article. Further inquiries can be directed to the corresponding author.

Conflicts of Interest: The authors declare no conflicts of interest.

References

1. Roth, D.E.; Abrams, S.A.; Aloia, J.; Bergeron, G.; Bourassa, M.W.; Brown, K.H.; Calvo, M.S.; Cashman, K.D.; Combs, G.; De-Regil, L.M.; et al. Global Prevalence and Disease Burden of Vitamin D Deficiency: A Roadmap for Action in Low- and Middle-Income Countries. *Ann. N. Y. Acad. Sci.* **2018**, *1430*, 44–79. [CrossRef] [PubMed]
2. Bouillon, R.; Marcocci, C.; Carmeliet, G.; Bikle, D.; White, J.H.; Dawson-Hughes, B.; Lips, P.; Munns, C.F.; Lazaretti-Castro, M.; Giustina, A.; et al. Skeletal and Extraskeletal Actions of Vitamin D: Current Evidence and Outstanding Questions. *Endocr. Rev.* **2019**, *40*, 1109–1151. [CrossRef] [PubMed]
3. Minich, D.M.; Henning, M.; Darley, C.; Fahoum, M.; Schuler, C.B.; Frame, J. Is Melatonin the "Next Vitamin D"?: A Review of Emerging Science, Clinical Uses, Safety, and Dietary Supplements. *Nutrients* **2022**, *14*, 3934. [CrossRef]
4. van der Pligt, P.; Willcox, J.; Szymlek-Gay, E.A.; Murray, E.; Worsley, A.; Daly, R.M. Associations of Maternal Vitamin D Deficiency with Pregnancy and Neonatal Complications in Developing Countries: A Systematic Review. *Nutrients* **2018**, *10*, 640. [CrossRef]
5. Ni, M.; Zhang, Q.; Zhao, J.; Shen, Q.; Yao, D.; Wang, T.; Liu, Z. Relationship between Maternal Vitamin D Status in the First Trimester of Pregnancy and Maternal and Neonatal Outcomes: A Retrospective Single Center Study. *BMC Pediatr.* **2021**, *21*, 330. [CrossRef] [PubMed]
6. Stoica, A.B.; Mărginean, C. The Impact of Vitamin D Deficiency on Infants' Health. *Nutrients* **2023**, *15*, 4379. [CrossRef] [PubMed]
7. Mailhot, G.; White, J.H. Vitamin D and Immunity in Infants and Children. *Nutrients* **2020**, *12*, 1233. [CrossRef]
8. Ma, S.; Li, W.; Tojibaev, K.S.; Turginov, O.; Yang, W.; Ma, K. Regionwide and Nationwide Floristic Richness Reveal Vascular Plant Diversity in Central Asia. *Plants* **2024**, *13*, 2275. [CrossRef]
9. Gromova, O.; Doschanova, A.; Lokshin, V.; Tuletova, A.; Grebennikova, G.; Daniyarova, L.; Kaishibayeva, G.; Nurpeissov, T.; Khan, V.; Semenova, Y.; et al. Vitamin D Deficiency in Kazakhstan: Cross-Sectional Study. *J. Steroid Biochem. Mol. Biol.* **2020**, *199*, 105565. [CrossRef] [PubMed]
10. Yerezhepov, D.; Gabdulkayum, A.; Akhmetova, A.; Kozhamkulov, U.A.; Rakhimova, S.E.; Kairov, U.Y.; Zhunussova, G.; Kalendar, R.N.; Akilzhanova, A. Vitamin D Status, VDR, and TLR Polymorphisms and Pulmonary Tuberculosis Epidemiology in Kazakhstan. *Nutrients* **2024**, *16*, 558. [CrossRef]
11. Akhmetova, V.; Balji, Y.; Kandalina, Y.; Iskineyeva, A.; Mukhamejanova, A.; Baspakova, A.; Uzakov, Y.; Issayeva, K.; Zamaratskaia, G. Self-Reported Consumption Frequency of Meat and Fish Products among Young Adults in Kazakhstan. *Nutr. Health* **2024**, *30*, 309–318. [CrossRef] [PubMed]
12. Rebezov, M.; Nikitin, Y.; Temerbayeva, M.; Uryumtseva, T. Current State and Prospects of Fortified Food Production in Russia and Kazakhstan. *Bull. Innov. Univ. Eurasia* **2020**, *80*, 143–151. [CrossRef]
13. Karimova, G.Z.; Khaimah, A.; Aidana Rassilbay, U.; Sauers, D.A. Lingerie and Morality: Generation Y Kazakhstani Women's Attitude Toward Lingerie. *J. East. Eur. Cent. Asian Res.* **2017**, *4*, 1–10. [CrossRef]
14. Karibayeva, I.; Bilibayeva, G.; Yerzhanova, A.; Alekesheva, R.; Iglikova, A.; Maxudova, M.; Ussebayeva, N. Prevalence of Vitamin D Deficiency Among Adults in Kazakhstan: A Systematic Review and Meta-Analysis. *Medicina* **2024**, *60*, 2043. [CrossRef] [PubMed]

15. Клинические Протоколы МЗ РК Рахит. Available online: https://diseases.medelement.com/disease/%D1%80%D0%B0%D1%85%D0%B8%D1%82/14337 (accessed on 19 January 2025).
16. Jazayeri, M.; Moradi, Y.; Rasti, A.; Nakhjavani, M.; Kamali, M.; Baradaran, H.R. Prevalence of Vitamin D Deficiency in Healthy Iranian Children: A Systematic Review and Meta-Analysis. *Med. J. Islam. Repub. Iran* **2018**, *32*, 83–93. [CrossRef] [PubMed]
17. Mogire, R.M.; Mutua, A.; Kimita, W.; Kamau, A.; Bejon, P.; Pettifor, J.M.; Adeyemo, A.; Williams, T.N.; Atkinson, S.H. Prevalence of Vitamin D Deficiency in Africa: A Systematic Review and Meta-Analysis. *Lancet Glob. Health* **2020**, *8*, e134–e142. [CrossRef] [PubMed]
18. Alpdemir, M.; Analysis, M.; Fatih Alpdemir, M. Vitamin D Deficiency Status in Turkey: A Meta-Analysis. *Int. J. Med. Biochem.* **2019**, *2*, 118–149. [CrossRef]
19. Karibayeva, I.; Abydynova, A. Serum Vitamin D Level Among Adults, Adolescents, and Children in Kazakhstan: A Systematic Review and Meta-Analysis of Published Studies: CRD42024598871. Available online: https://www.crd.york.ac.uk/prospero/#recordDetails (accessed on 20 November 2024).
20. Karibayeva, I.; Bilibayeva, G. Prevalence of Vitamin D Deficiency Among Adults in Kazakhstan: A Systematic Review and Meta-Analysis: CRD42024610447. Available online: https://www.crd.york.ac.uk/prospero/#recordDetails (accessed on 15 January 2025).
21. Amir-Behghadami, M.; Janati, A. Population, Intervention, Comparison, Outcomes and Study (PICOS) Design as a Framework to Formulate Eligibility Criteria in Systematic Reviews. *Emerg. Med. J.* **2020**, *37*, 387. [CrossRef]
22. Page, M.J.; McKenzie, J.E.; Bossuyt, P.M.; Boutron, I.; Hoffmann, T.C.; Mulrow, C.D.; Shamseer, L.; Tetzlaff, J.M.; Akl, E.A.; Brennan, S.E. The PRISMA 2020 Statement: An Updated Guideline for Reporting Systematic Reviews. *BMJ* **2021**, *372*, n71. [CrossRef]
23. Wells, G.; Shea, B.; O'Connell, D.; Peterson, J.; Welch, V.; Losos, M.; Tugwell, P. Ottawa Hospital Research Institute. Available online: https://www.ohri.ca/programs/clinical_epidemiology/oxford.asp (accessed on 20 November 2024).
24. Posit Team RStudio: Integrated Development Environment for R. Available online: http://www.posit.co/ (accessed on 22 January 2024).
25. Harrer, M.; Cuijpers, P.; Furukawa, T.A.; Ebert, D.D. *Doing Meta-Analysis with R: A Hands-On Guide*; Chapman & Hall/CRC Press: Boca Raton, FL, USA; London, UK, 2021; Chapter 4, ISBN 978-0-367-61007-4.
26. Amanzholkyzy, A.; Nurgaliyeva, R.E.; Kaldybayeva, A.T.; Batyrova, T.Z.; Balmaganbetova, F.K.; Aibassova, Z.A. Biochemical Variability of Vitamin D Receptor (Vdr) Gene and Its Relationship with Bone Mineral Density in Children of the Western Region of the Republic of Kazakhstan. *Res. J. Pharm. Technol.* **2019**, *12*, 735–740. [CrossRef]
27. Amanzholkyzy, A.; Donayeva, A.; Kulzhanova, D.; Abdelazim, I.A.; Abilov, T.; Baubekov, Z.; Samaha, I.I. Relation between Vitamin D and Adolescents' Serum Prolactin. *Prz. Menopauzalny* **2023**, *22*, 202–206. [CrossRef]
28. Donayeva, A.; Amanzholkyzy, A.; Abdelazim, I.A.; Rakhyzhanova, S.; Mannapova, A.; Abilov, T.; Khamidullina, Z.; Bimagambetova, K.; Gubasheva, G.; Kulzhanova, D.; et al. The Relationship between Vitamin D and Adolescents' Parathyroid Hormone and Bone Mineral Density. *Prz. Menopauzalny* **2024**, *23*, 1–5. [CrossRef] [PubMed]
29. Donayeva, A.; Amanzholkyzy, A.; Abdelazim, I.; Kurmangazin, M.; Khamidullina, Z.; Kurmanalina, M.; Sumanova, A.; Shabanbayeva, Z.; Baubekov, Z.; Bissaliyev, B.; et al. The Effect of Vitamin D on Adolescents' Primary Dysmenorrhea. *J. Med. Life* **2023**, *16*, 1658–1662. [CrossRef]
30. Donayeva, A.; Kulzhanova, D.; Amanzholkyzy, A.; Abdelazim, I.A.; Abilov, T.; Baubekov, Z.; Samaha, I.I. Relationship between Vitamin D and Adolescents' Hypothyroidism—A Cross-Sectional Study. *Prz. Menopauzalny* **2023**, *22*, 186–190. [CrossRef]
31. Donayeva, A.; Amanzholkyzy, A.; Abdelazim, I.A.; Saparbayev, S.; Nurgaliyeva, R.; Kaldybayeva, A.; Zhexenova, A.; Stankevicius, E.; Khamidullina, Z.; Gubasheva, G.; et al. The Relation between Vitamin D and the Adolescents' Mid-Luteal Estradiol and Progesterone. *Eur. Rev. Med. Pharmacol. Sci.* **2023**, *27*, 6792–6799. [CrossRef]
32. Zhumalina, A.K.; Kim, I.S.; Delyagin, W.M. Vitamin D Level and Indicators of Bone Tissue Metabolism in Kazakh Infants. *Russ. Fam. Dr.* **2023**, *27*, 23–29. [CrossRef]
33. Myrzabekova, G.T.; Rabandiyarov, M.R.; Suleimanova, S.B.; Zhubanysheva, K.B.; Kalakova, A.A. Assessment of Vitamin D Status and Respiratory Disease Risk Factors in Children. *Interdiscip. Approaches Med.* **2021**, *2*, 43–49. [CrossRef]
34. Gordiyenko, M.; Dyussenova, S.B.; Kunts, E.A.; Sarmankulova, G.A.; Kurilova, V. Vitamin D Deficiency in Children with Chronic Renal Disease. *Med. Ecol.* **2020**, *4*, 65–71.
35. Taiorazova, G.; Alimbaeva, A.; Tanatarov, S.; Smailova, Z.; Lobanov, Y.; Ailbayeva, N.M.; Berikuly, D.; Akhmetzhanova, D.; Imanbayeva, D. Leading Antenatal Factors of Congenital Pneumonia in Premature Newborns with Vitamin D Deficiency. *Sci. Healthc.* **2022**, *24*, 71–77. [CrossRef]
36. Dyussenova, S.; Isayev, V.; Bukayev, E. Analysis of the Relationship between Vitamin D and CKD. *Med. Ecol.* **2022**, *2*, 40–41.
37. Zhamankulov, A.; Rozenson, R.; Morenko, M.; Meral, G.; Akhmetova, U. Recurrent Respiratoryinfections in Children. *Astana Med. J.* **2020**, *106*, 227–231.

38. Amanzholkyzy, A.; Nurgalieva, R.E.; Dosimov, A.Z.; Stankevicius, E.; Kaldybaeva, A.T. Ethnic Manifestations of Gene Polymorphisms of Vitamin D Receptor (VDR) in Adolescents of Western Kazakhstan Region. *J. Natl. Med. Assoc.* **2018**, *110*, 78–83. [CrossRef]
39. Hearst, M.O.; Himes, J.H.; Johnson, D.E.; Kroupina, M.; Syzdykova, A.; Aidjanov, M.; Sharmonov, T. Growth, Nutritional, and Developmental Status of Young Children Living in Orphanages in Kazakhstan. *Infant Ment. Health J.* **2014**, *35*, 94–101. [CrossRef] [PubMed]
40. Zhumalina, A.K.; Bekmukhambetov, E.Z.; Tusupkaliev, B.T.; Zharlikasinova, M.B. Development of Scientifically Justified Proposals on the Prevention and Treatment of Environmentally Determined Constitutional Growth Delay in Children in the West Kazakhstan Region. *Environ. Geochem. Health* **2019**, *41*, 1251–1265. [CrossRef]
41. Balmukhanova, A.; Kabulbayev, K.; Alpay, H.; Kanatbayeva, A.; Balmukhanova, A. FGF-23 and Phosphate in Children with Chronic Kidney Disease: A Cross-Sectional Study in Kazakhstan. *Medicina* **2020**, *57*, 15. [CrossRef] [PubMed]
42. Dyussenova, S.B.; Gordiyenko, M.Y.; Serikova, G.B.; Turlybekova, S.A.; Issayeva, A.A.; Yerimbetova, N.A.; Goroshko, V.O. Vitamin D Deficiency in Children with Chronic Renal Disease. *Open Access Maced. J. Med. Sci.* **2021**, *9*, 1751–1757. [CrossRef]
43. Zhamankulov, A.; Rozenson, R.; Morenko, M.; Shnayder, K.; Akhmetova, U.; Tyo, A. COVID-19 and Recurrent Respiratory Infections in Children of Kazakhstan. *Russ. Open Med. J.* **2021**, *10*, 104. [CrossRef]
44. Nakipov, Z.; Tursynbekova, A.; Dauletova, G.; Mussakhanova, A.; Dossybayeva, G.; Kerimbayeva, Z.; Saurbayeva, G.; Kaliyeva, A.; Turgambayeva, A.; Yen, M.; et al. A Pilot Study of Nutrition Management in the Department of Pediatric Oncology Department of a Hospital in Kazakhstan. *Open Access Maced. J. Med. Sci.* **2022**, *10*, 736–747. [CrossRef]
45. Dyussenova, S.B.; Sarmankulova, G.A.; Sabiyeva, M.M.; Tlegenova, K.S.; Kurilova, V. V The Role of Vitamine d in the Clinic of Chronic Kidney Disease in Children. *Sci. Healthc.* **2023**, *4*, 109–117. [CrossRef]
46. Taiorazova, G.; Alimbayeva, A.; Tanatarov, S. The Role of Vitamin D and Trace Elements in Premature Newborns with Congenital Pneumonia. *Bratisl. Med. J.* **2023**, *124*, 572–577. [CrossRef]
47. Zeinebekova, A.B.; Umarova, A.M.; Usmanova, D.U.; Turkara, A.M.; Kovalchuk, V.E.; Dyussenova, S.B. Early Predictors of Kidney Damage in Children and Adolescents with Type 1 Diabetes Mellitus. *Clin. Nephrol.* **2023**, *15*, 54–57. [CrossRef]
48. Rysbekov, K.; Abdrakhmanova, S.; Satybaeva, R.; Babenko, D.; Abdikadyr, Z. Connection of Vitamin D Levels in Blood Serum with Helicobacter Pylori Infection in Paediatric Patients. *Gastroenterol. Rev./Przegląd Gastroenterol.* **2024**, *19*, 1–8. [CrossRef]
49. Zhumalina, A.; Tusupkaliev, B.; Mania, A.; Kim, I.; Zharlykasinova, M. The Importance of Determining the Level of Bone Metabolism Markers and Vitamin D in the First Year of Life in the Kazakh Population. *J. Pediatr. Pharmacol. Ther.* **2024**, *29*, 410–416. [CrossRef]
50. Zhumalina, A.; Kim, I.; Tusupkaliev, B.; Zharlykasinova, M.; Zhekeyeva, B. Features of D-Vitamin Status in Young Children in the Kazakh Population. *Pol. Merkur. Lek.* **2024**, *52*, 161–170. [CrossRef]
51. Resolution of the Government of the Republic of Kazakhstan No. 945 On the Approval of the Concept for the Development of Healthcare in the Republic of Kazakhstan Until 2026. Available online: https://adilet.zan.kz/rus/docs/P2200000945 (accessed on 16 January 2025).
52. Durá-Travé, T.; Gallinas-Victoriano, F. Dental Caries in Children and Vitamin D Deficiency: A Narrative Review. *Eur. J. Pediatr.* **2024**, *183*, 523–528. [CrossRef]
53. Xiao, P.; Cheng, H.; Wang, L.; Hou, D.; Li, H.; Zhao, X.; Xie, X.; Mi, J. Relationships for Vitamin D with Childhood Height Growth Velocity and Low Bone Mineral Density Risk. *Front. Nutr.* **2023**, *10*, 1081896. [CrossRef]
54. Zisi, D.; Challa, A.; Makis, A. The Association between Vitamin D Status and Infectious Diseases of the Respiratory System in Infancy and Childhood. *Hormones* **2019**, *18*, 353–363. [CrossRef]
55. Melough, M.M.; Murphy, L.E.; Graff, J.C.; Derefinko, K.J.; Lewinn, K.Z.; Bush, N.R.; Enquobahrie, D.A.; Loftus, C.T.; Kocak, M.; Sathyanarayana, S.; et al. Maternal Plasma 25-Hydroxyvitamin D during Gestation Is Positively Associated with Neurocognitive Development in Offspring at Age 4–6 Years. *J. Nutr.* **2021**, *151*, 132–139. [CrossRef]
56. Raulio, S.; Erlund, I.; Männistö, S.; Sarlio-Lähteenkorva, S.; Sundvall, J.; Tapanainen, H.; Vartiainen, E.; Virtanen, S.M. Successful Nutrition Policy: Improvement of Vitamin D Intake and Status in Finnish Adults over the Last Decade. *Eur. J. Public Health* **2017**, *27*, 268–273. [CrossRef]
57. Płudowski, P.; Kos-Kudła, B.; Walczak, M.; Fal, A.; Zozulińska-Ziółkiewicz, D.; Sieroszewski, P.; Peregud-Pogorzelski, J.; Lauterbach, R.; Targowski, T.; Lewiński, A.; et al. Guidelines for Preventing and Treating Vitamin D Deficiency: A 2023 Update in Poland. *Nutrients* **2023**, *15*, 695. [CrossRef]
58. Office of Dietary Supplements Vitamin D Initiative. Available online: https://ods.od.nih.gov/Research/VitaminD.aspx (accessed on 16 January 2025).
59. Brown, L.L.; Cohen, B.; Tabor, D.; Zappalà, G.; Maruvada, P.; Coates, P.M. The Vitamin D Paradox in Black Americans: A Systems-Based Approach to Investigating Clinical Practice, Research, and Public Health—Expert Panel Meeting Report. *BMC Proc.* **2018**, *12*, 6. [CrossRef] [PubMed]

60. Saberi-Karimian, M.; Ghazizadeh, H.; Zanganeh Baygi, M.; Minaie, M.; Sadeghi, F.; Pouraram, H.; Elmadfa, I.; Esmaily, H.; Khadem Rezaian, M.; Tavallaei, S.; et al. The National Health Program for Vitamin D Supplementation in a Developing Country. *Clin. Nutr. ESPEN* **2023**, *54*, 52–59. [CrossRef] [PubMed]
61. Aghapour, B.; Kheirouri, S.; Alizadeh, M.; Khodayari-Zarnaq, R. Vitamin D Deficiency Prevention Policies in Iran: A Retrospective Policy Analysis. *Front. Nutr.* **2023**, *10*, 1249402–1249412. [CrossRef]
62. Rostami, M.; Tehrani, F.R.; Simbar, M.; Yarandi, R.B.; Minooee, S.; Hollis, B.W.; Hosseinpanah, F. Effectiveness of Prenatal Vitamin D Deficiency Screening and Treatment Program: A Stratified Randomized Field Trial. *J. Clin. Endocrinol. Metab.* **2018**, *103*, 2936–2948. [CrossRef] [PubMed]
63. Canadian Paediatric Society Preventing Symptomatic Vitamin D Deficiency and Rickets Among Indigenous Infants and Children in Canada. Available online: https://cps.ca/documents/position/vitamin-d-deficiency-and-rickets-among-indigenous-infants-and-children (accessed on 16 January 2025).
64. Slater, J.; Larcombe, L.; Green, C.; Slivinski, C.; Singer, M.; Denechezhe, L.; Whaley, C.; Nickerson, P.; Orr, P. Dietary Intake of Vitamin D in a Northern Canadian Dené First Nation Community. *Int. J. Circumpolar Health* **2013**, *72*, 20723. [CrossRef]
65. Altieri, B.; Cavalier, E.; Bhattoa, H.P.; Perez-Lopez, F.R.; Lopez-Baena, M.T.; Perez-Roncero, G.R.; Chedraui, P.; Annweiler, C.; Della Casa, S.; Zelzer, S. Vitamin D Testing: Advantages and Limits of the Current Assays. *Eur. J. Clin. Nutr.* **2020**, *74*, 231–247. [CrossRef]
66. Fraser, W.D.; Milan, A.M. Vitamin D Assays: Past and Present Debates, Difficulties, and Developments. *Calcif. Tissue Int.* **2013**, *92*, 118–127. [CrossRef]

medicina

MDPI

Systematic Review

Prevalence of Vitamin D Deficiency Among Adults in Kazakhstan: A Systematic Review and Meta-Analysis

Indira Karibayeva [1,*], Galiya Bilibayeva [2], Aya Yerzhanova [2], Roza Alekesheva [2], Assiya Iglikova [2], Makhigul Maxudova [2] and Neilya Ussebayeva [2]

1 Department of Health Policy and Community Health, Jiann-Ping Hsu College of Public Health, Georgia Southern University, Statesboro, GA 30460, USA

2 Department of Nursing, Faculty of Medicine and Public Health, Al-Farabi Kazakh National University, Almaty 050038, Kazakhstan; bilibayeva@kaznu.kz (G.B.); yerzhanova.aya@kaznu.kz (A.Y.); alekesheva@kaznu.kz (R.A.); iglikova-a@mail.ru (A.I.); maksudova63@gmail.com (M.M.); usebaeva@mail.ru (N.U.)

* Correspondence: ik01379@georgiasouthern.edu

Abstract: *Background and Objectives*: Despite frequent references to the high prevalence of vitamin D deficiency in Kazakhstan, a comprehensive synthesis of existing research on this issue among adults is lacking. This systematic review and meta-analysis aim to address this gap by determining the mean prevalence of vitamin D deficiency among adults in Kazakhstan. A secondary objective is to evaluate whether the prevalence differs between healthy adults and those with chronic conditions. *Materials and Methods*: A systematic search was conducted in PubMed, Scopus, ScienceDirect, Web of Science, and Google Scholar by two independent researchers using the keywords: "vitamin D" AND "Kazakhstan", following the Preferred Reporting Items for Systematic Reviews and Meta-Analyses guidelines. Studies were included if they reported the prevalence of vitamin D in adults in Kazakhstan, defined as a blood level of 25-hydroxyvitamin D 25(OH)D below 20 ng/mL. *Results*: Seven studies were included in this review, encompassing 3616 individuals, of whom 2239 had vitamin D deficiency. Using a random-effects model, the pooled mean prevalence of vitamin D deficiency among adults with chronic conditions was 60% (95% CI, 38–79%), with high heterogeneity. Similarly, the analysis of five studies involving healthy adults revealed a pooled mean prevalence of 55% (95% CI, 38–70%), also with high heterogeneity. Overall, the pooled mean prevalence of vitamin D deficiency in the adult population was 57% (95% CI, 45–69%). *Conclusions*: This analysis indicates a high prevalence of vitamin D deficiency among adults in Kazakhstan, with 57% of the population affected. Addressing this issue requires a multifaceted approach, including policy reforms that consider the impact of time zone changes on sunlight exposure and the active involvement of nurse practitioners in preventive strategies.

Keywords: vitamin D; vitamin D deficiency; adults; prevalence; Kazakhstan; systematic review; meta-analysis

1. Introduction

Vitamin D is integral to the regulation of calcium and phosphate metabolism and is involved in melatonin synthesis and mitochondrial regulation, thereby playing a pivotal role in maintaining bone integrity, mineral balance, and immune system function [1,2]. Primarily synthesized in the skin through the ultraviolet-B radiation-induced conversion of 7-dehydrocholesterol, vitamin D can also be obtained from dietary sources, notably fatty fish [3]. However, factors such as limited sun exposure, sedentary indoor lifestyles, inadequate dietary intake, higher latitudes, obesity-related sequestration of vitamin D metabolites in adipose tissue, and certain medical conditions impairing absorption contribute to the widespread prevalence of vitamin D deficiency globally [4,5].

Kazakhstan, a landlocked nation spanning approximately 2,724,900 square kilometers, is frequently noted for its high prevalence of vitamin D deficiency [6–8]. Geographically, the country extends from the 40th parallel north at its southernmost point to the 56th parallel north at its northernmost reaches, placing it well above the Equator. This northern latitude results in prolonged winters with reduced ultraviolet B exposure, significantly limiting endogenous vitamin D synthesis. Furthermore, traditional dietary patterns in this landlocked region are deficient in key vitamin D sources such as fish [9]. Modern indoor lifestyles further reduce sun exposure, even during warmer seasons, compounding the risk of deficiency.

Despite frequent references to the high prevalence of vitamin D deficiency in Kazakhstan, a comprehensive synthesis of existing research on this issue among adults is lacking. This systematic review and meta-analysis aim to address this gap by estimating the mean prevalence of vitamin D deficiency among adults in Kazakhstan. A secondary objective is to evaluate whether the prevalence varies between healthy adults and those with chronic conditions.

2. Materials and Methods

The study protocol is registered with the National Institute for Health Research's PROSPERO International Prospective Register of Systematic Reviews [10] (ID: CRD42024610447).

2.1. Search Strategy

An initial search of the PROSPERO database to identify registrations of comparable studies revealed one study protocol that assessed the mean vitamin D levels among the Kazakhstani population [11]. Since the objective of the present study was to evaluate the mean prevalence of vitamin D deficiency among adult population in Kazakhstan, the authors proceeded with registering the current study protocol in the PROSPERO database. Following this, a systematic search was conducted across five electronic databases: PubMed, Scopus, ScienceDirect, Web of Science, and Google Scholar. The search commenced on 2 July 2024, and concluded on 1 November 2024. The search strategy utilized the keywords: "vitamin D" AND "Kazakhstan". No restrictions were placed on publication date; however, the results were limited to English- and Russian-language publications and studies conducted on humans. Where applicable, filters were applied to include only research articles and exclude other publication types.

2.2. Eligibility Criteria

The types of studies to be included were determined using the following eligibility criteria: The inclusion criteria were as follows: 1. Studies reporting the number of adults in the population in Kazakhstan with vitamin D deficiency, defined as a blood level of 25-hydroxyvitamin D 25(OH)D below 20 ng/mL. 2. Observational studies including cohort studies, cross-sectional studies, and case–control studies. 3. Studies on the adult population in Kazakhstan. 4. Studies published in English or Russian languages. The exclusion criteria were as follows: 1. Studies reporting the mean value of 25-hydroxyvitamin D in serum or lacking required information. 2. Studies with duplicative results. 3. Case reports, reviews, editorials, and conference abstracts. 4. Studies published in languages other than English or Russian.

2.3. Selection of Studies and Data Extraction

The literature review and synthesis were conducted according with the Preferred Reporting Items for Systematic Reviews and Meta-Analyses (PRISMA) guidelines [12]. Two authors independently screened the titles and abstracts of the search results, following duplicate removal, to assess their relevance. Full texts of studies that met the initial criteria were retrieved and evaluated against the pre-defined inclusion and exclusion criteria. Data extracted from eligible studies included the first author's last name, year of publication, region where the study was conducted, description of the included population (e.g., disease name, if applicable, or healthy), sample size, number of male participants, mean age, mean serum 25(OH)D levels and number of adults with confirmed vitamin D deficiency. Two authors independently performed data extraction from the selected studies. Any discrepancies were resolved through consultation with a third author to ensure consensus among all three authors responsible for the study selection and data extraction process.

2.4. Risk of Bias (Quality) Assessment

The studies included in this review were evaluated for risk of bias (quality) using the Newcastle–Ottawa Scale (NOS) for case–control studies and its adapted version for cross-sectional studies, as recommended by the Cochrane Non-Randomized Studies Methods Working Group [13]. The NOS for case–control studies assesses each study based on eight criteria divided into three main categories: selection of study groups (four questions), comparability of these groups (one question), and exposure (three questions). Each criterion is assigned up to one point, while the comparability criterion can receive a maximum of two points. The total score ranges from 0 to 9, with higher scores indicating better study quality. The adapted NOS for cross-sectional studies evaluates each study across six criteria divided into three main categories: selection (three questions), comparability (one question), and outcome (two questions). Each criterion is assigned up to one point, and the comparability criterion can receive a maximum of two points, yielding a total score ranging from 0 to 7, with higher scores reflecting better study quality. Quality assessments were conducted independently by two authors (IK and GB) after agreeing on the assessment procedures. A third author (AY) calculated the inter-rater agreement between the two assessors. In this review, studies scoring seven points or higher were classified as high-quality, while those scoring four points or less were deemed low-quality.

We conducted a self-assessment of the potential risk of bias (quality) assessment in our systematic review using A Measurement Tool to Assess Systematic Reviews-2 (AMSTAR-2), which evaluates the methodological quality of systematic reviews, including those with randomized and non-randomized clinical studies [14]. AMSTAR-2 comprises 16 domains that assess various aspects such as protocol registration, thoroughness of the literature search, study selection, data extraction, risk of bias evaluation, heterogeneity, and reporting of results. Each domain is rated to identify potential biases or methodological weaknesses, culminating in an overall quality rating of low, moderate, or high.

2.5. Statistical Strategy for Data Synthesis

We utilized RStudio software (version 4.3.2) with the 'meta' and 'metafor' packages to calculate the pooled mean prevalence of vitamin D deficiency among adults in Kazakhstan, using a random-effects model for the meta-analysis [15,16]. Forest plots were generated to display the pooled estimates. A meta-regression analysis was conducted with age and population size as covariates. To explore sources of heterogeneity, we performed an influence analysis. The generalizability of the study findings was assessed through a publication bias evaluation, which included visual inspection of a funnel plot and statistical analysis using Egger's test. Additionally, to further investigate sources of heterogeneity, we conducted a subgroup analysis comparing healthy adults to those with chronic conditions [16].

3. Results

3.1. Included Study Characteristics

The initial database search yielded 226 articles. After removing 61 duplicates, 165 unique articles remained for screening. Of these, 33 were retrieved for full-text review following the exclusion of 132 non-relevant titles. Upon further assessment, seven articles met the inclusion criteria. Ten studies lacked data on vitamin D deficiency, six focused on children [17–22], five were excluded for other reasons, and four were reviews. A PRISMA flow diagram detailing the study selection process is presented in Figure 1 [12].

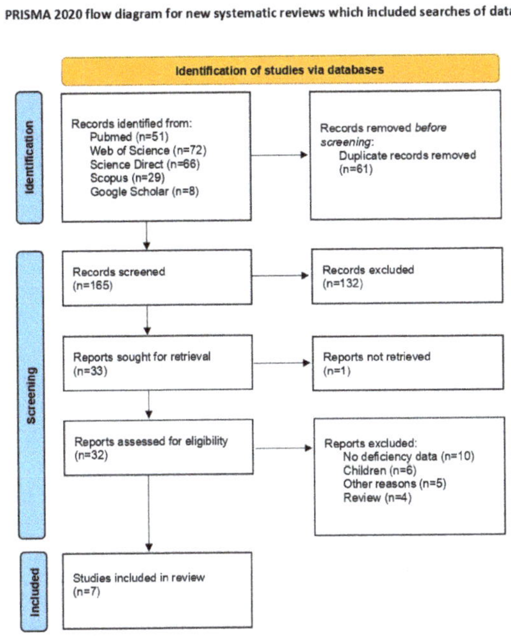

Figure 1. PRISMA flow diagram of study selection process.

The included studies were published between 2015 and 2024. Two studies were conducted across multiple regions, two in Karaganda, two in Astana, and one in Almaty city. Among these, two studies did not include healthy controls, one was conducted among a healthy population only, and the remaining studies involved both patients with chronic diseases and healthy controls. Collectively, the seven studies assessed a total of 3616 individuals, identifying vitamin D deficiency in 2239 participants. Detailed information on the included articles is provided in Table 1.

Table 1. Description of the included studies.

First Author, Year	Region/City	Study Design	Disease Name/Healthy	Sample	Male	Age (Mean ± SD)	25(OH)D (ng/mL) (Mean ± SD)	Numberwith VDD
Nugmanova, 2015 [23]	Almaty	Case–control	HIV undet. (a) HIV det. (b)	304 (a) 260 (b)	168 (a) 143 (b)	38.2 ± 9.0 (a) 35.9 ± 8.7 (b)	25.90 ± 13.20 (a) 26.40 ± 11.40 (b)	120 (a) 82 (b)
Algazina, 2019 [24]	Astana	Case–control	Psoriasis Healthy	20 (NH) 26 (H)	10 (NH) 13 (H)	41.38 ± 4.2 (NH) 41.57 ± 5.67 (H)	NA	7 (NH) 0 (H)
Gromova, 2020 [7]	Multiple	Cross-sectional	Healthy	1347	528	44 ± 14	NA	943
Safi, 2020 [25]	Astana	Case–control	PCOS Healthy	51 (NH) 30 (H)	0 0	18–44	16.25 17.52	22 (NH) 17 (H)
Zhumina, 2020 [26]	Karaganda	Case–control	Leukemia Healthy	31 (NH) 34 (H)	14 (NH) 17 (H)	57.71 ± 13.7 (NH) 54.73 ± 15.1 (H)	10.85 ± 7.00 (NH) 21.61 ± 7.78 (H)	28 (NH) 22 (H)
Izmailovich, 2022 [27]	Karaganda	Cross-sectional	Allergic Rhinitis	416	149	39 ± 8	16.10 ± 6.90	312
Yerezhepov, 2024 [8]	Multiple	Case–control	Tuberculosis Healthy	411 (NH) 686 (H)	224 (NH) 303 (H)	35 ± 13.1 (NH) 40.5 ± 13.9 (H)	12.90 ± 3.80 (NH) 24.80 ± 3.10 (H)	360 (NH) 326 (H)

Abbreviations: 25(OH)D—25-hydroxyvitamin D; H—healthy; HIV—Human Immunodeficiency Virus; NA—not available; NH—not healthy; PCOS—polycystic ovarian syndrome; SD—standard deviation.

3.2. Prevalence of Vitamin D Deficiency

Six studies, covering seven groups, reported on the prevalence of vitamin D deficiency among patients with various health conditions. Using a random-effects model, the pooled mean prevalence of vitamin D deficiency in adults with chronic conditions was 60% (95% CI, 38–79%), with high heterogeneity. In contrast, analysis of five studies on healthy adults using a random-effects model yielded a pooled mean prevalence of 55% (95% CI, 38–70%), also showing high heterogeneity. The overall pooled mean prevalence of vitamin D deficiency in the adult population was 57% (95% CI, 45–69%) (Figure 2).

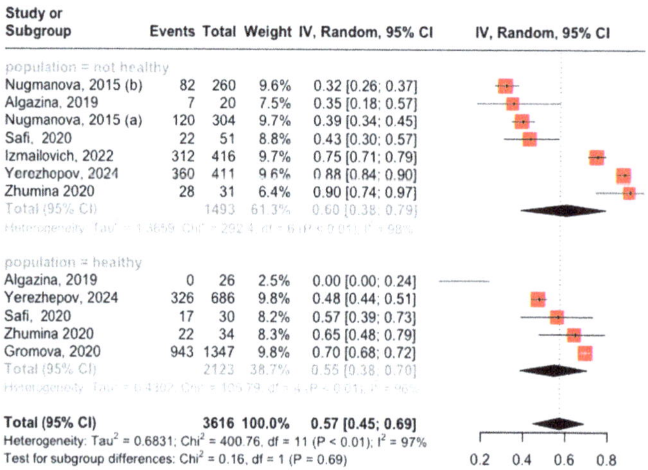

Figure 2. Forest plot of vitamin D deficiency among adults in Kazakhstan. Abbreviations: CI—confidence interval; HIV—Human Immunodeficiency Virus; Nugmanova, 2015: (a) HIV viral load undetectable; Nugmanova, 2015 (b): HIV viral load detectable.

3.3. Meta-Regression Analysis

A meta-regression analysis revealed a negative impact of age on the pooled mean prevalence of vitamin D deficiency. The analysis indicates that as age increases, the prevalence of vitamin D deficiency also rises, although the finding was not statistically significant ($p > 0.05$). (Figure 3).

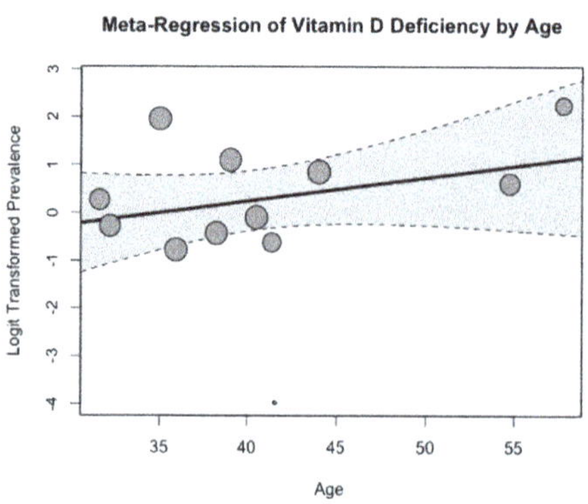

Figure 3. Meta-regression analysis of vitamin D deficiency by age.

3.4. Heterogeneity Assessment

An influence analysis was conducted to identify the studies with the greatest impact on the pooled estimate. The pooled mean estimate was primarily influenced by study #2, by Nugmanova 2015 (b), which included patients with a detectable HIV viral load [23] (Figure 4a). The leave-one-out analysis confirmed these results, showing that when the Nugmanova 2015 (b) study was excluded, the pooled estimate reached its highest value at 53% (Figure 4b). The AMSTAR-2 evaluation, detailed in the Supplementary Materials (Table S1), indicates that this systematic review has a moderate level of methodological quality.

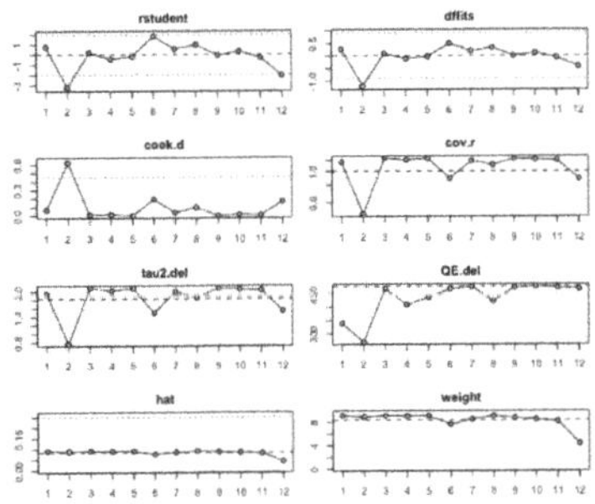

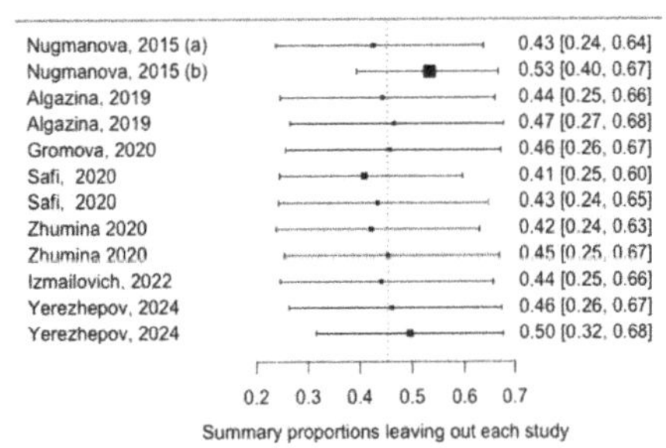

(a) (b)

Figure 4. Influence analysis of vitamin D deficiency: (**a**) influence analysis; (**b**) leave-one-out analysis. Abbreviations: Nugmanova, 2015: (**a**) HIV viral load undetectable; Nugmanova, 2015 (**b**): HIV viral load detectable.

3.5. Publication Bias Assessment

Upon visual inspection of the funnel plot, no asymmetry was evident (Figure 5). The absence of publication bias was further confirmed by non-significant results from Egger's test for publication bias ($p > 0.05$).

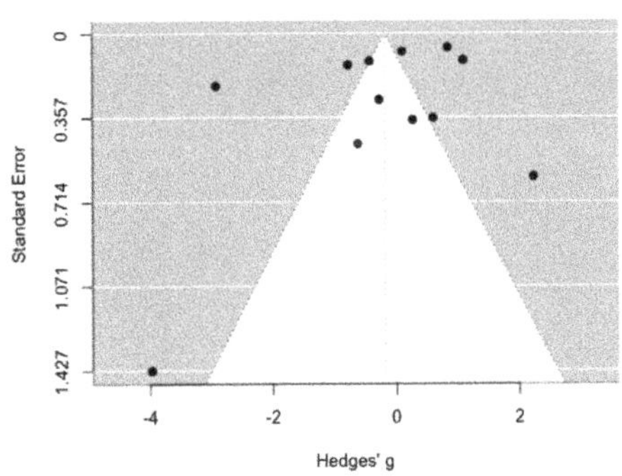

Figure 5. Publication bias assessment.

3.6. Risk of Bias (Quality) Assessment Results

All included case–control studies had a NOS score of 7 or higher out of 8, and all cross-sectional studies had a NOS score of 6 out of 7, indicating the high quality and a low risk of bias of the included studies, as presented in Table 2.

The AMSTAR-2 evaluation, detailed in the Supplementary Materials (Table S1), indicates that this systematic review has a moderate level of methodological quality.

Table 2. Newcastle–Ottawa risk of bias (quality) assessment results.

Study	Selection	Comparability	Exposure	Total
		Case–control studies		
Nugmanova, 2015 [23]	4	1	3	8
Algazina, 2019 [24]	3	1	3	7
Safi, 2020 [25]	4	1	3	8
Zhumina, 2020 [26]	4	1	2	7
Yerezhepov, 2024 [8]	4	1	3	8
		Cross-sectional studies		
Gromova, 2020 [7]	3	1	2	6
Izmailovich, 2022 [27]	3	1	2	6

4. Discussion

Our systematic review and meta-analysis reveals a significant prevalence of vitamin D deficiency among adults in Kazakhstan, with an overall rate of 57% (95% CI, 45–69%). Notably, the prevalence is slightly lower among healthy adults (55%, 95% CI, 38–70%) and higher among those with chronic conditions (60%, 95% CI, 38–79%). Additionally, mean serum 25(OH)D levels were below 20 ng/mL in four out of five studies that reported them, particularly among adults with chronic conditions. These findings align with the existing literature, which indicates high rates of vitamin D deficiency in northern-hemisphere countries, especially those with limited fish consumption, underscoring a pressing public health concern.

Addressing this widespread deficiency requires a comprehensive, multi-tiered strategy at both the policy and primary healthcare levels. This approach aligns with the World Health Organization's framework for the global monitoring of non-communicable diseases [28], given the limited fish consumption and sunlight exposure in the region.

Undoubtedly, policy-level interventions should focus on addressing social determinants of health and ensuring an accessible, high-quality health system capable of delivering essential preventive services. Kazakhstan has made significant progress in increasing healthcare system financing through the introduction of the Compulsory Social Health Insurance System in January 2020, which aims to improve healthcare service delivery [29]. Nevertheless, policy interventions should also encourage outdoor physical activities to enhance sun exposure and decrease the risk of cardiovascular diseases and diabetes, the leading causes of mortality among adults in Kazakhstan [30]. A policy change in March 2024, which unified the country under a single time zone (UTC + 5) [31], may have inadvertently reduced sunlight exposure and negatively impacted public health. This shift resulted in earlier winter sunsets, around 4 PM, limiting daylight hours for outdoor activities, especially for those engaging in such activities for work. Given Kazakhstan's vast expanse of approximately 2700 km from west to east, naturally spanning time zones from UTC + 3 to UTC + 6, the adoption of a single time zone may not align with the country's geographical and solar realities [31].

The second implication of our study is the need for educational initiatives targeting the general population. An Endocrine Society Clinical Practice Guideline on vitamin D does not recommend empirical vitamin D supplementation beyond the current Dietary Reference Intake or advocate routine screening for 25(OH)D levels in the general population [32]. Empirical supplementation of vitamin D can be achieved through a combination of fortified foods [33] and daily food supplements, rather than through intermittent high doses to reduce the risk of disease in healthy adults under the age of 75 [32]. Thus, primary healthcare providers and nurse practitioners, in particular, play a crucial role in implementing these preventive strategies at the community level [34]. The ongoing interactions of nurse practitioners with both healthy individuals and patients with chronic conditions position them uniquely to educate on the importance of vitamin D, its dietary sources, and lifestyle modifications to improve vitamin D levels. Moreover, a study by Gregor and Sebach showed the high effectiveness of a nurse-practitioner-led vitamin D intervention program in a primary care setting [35]. In Kazakhstan, as in other post-Soviet countries, the practice of dispanserization—regular monitoring of patients with chronic diseases—facilitates frequent interactions between nurse practitioners and patients [36]. This framework enables nurse practitioners to deliver personalized guidance and raise awareness about effective, evidence-based interventions for vitamin D supplementation.

Limitations

This study has certain limitations. The lack of region-specific data prevents an analysis of potential geographical variations in vitamin D deficiency across Kazakhstan. Additionally, we did not assess the presence of metabolic conditions, such as obesity, diabetes, and hypertension, in the patient group. This omission is significant, as these conditions are known to influence vitamin D metabolism and status [37]. Furthermore, the absence of information regarding the timing of vitamin D measurements is a constraint, as vitamin D levels are known to fluctuate seasonally. We also did not evaluate the extent of sun exposure among participants, a factor that directly affects vitamin D synthesis [38]. Finally, subjectivity in study selection, data extraction, and interpretation could introduce reviewer bias. To mitigate this, the authors employed recommended strategies, such as utilizing a standardized protocol, conducting assessments in duplicate, and resolving discrepancies through consensus and third-party adjudication [14].

5. Conclusions

Our analysis reveals a high prevalence of vitamin D deficiency among Kazakhstan's adult population, with 57% affected. The deficiency rate remains concerning among healthy adults at 55%, and even higher in adults with chronic conditions at 60%. Addressing this issue requires a multifaceted approach, which includes policy reforms that take into account the effects of time zone changes on sunlight exposure, as well as the active involvement of nurse practitioners in implementing preventive educational strategies.

Future Research Directions

To build upon our findings and address the limitations of the current study, future research should focus on the following: (1) investigating the impact of metabolic disorders on serum vitamin D levels in the general population; (2) assessing variations in serum vitamin D levels relative to sunlight exposure, considering factors such as seasonality and regional differences; (3) conducting meta-analyses to evaluate mean vitamin D levels across different demographics, including both adults and children, to inform targeted interventions. By pursuing these research avenues, we can develop a more comprehensive understanding of vitamin D deficiency in Kazakhstan, ultimately leading to more effective public health strategies and policies.

Supplementary Materials: The following supporting information can be downloaded at: https://www.mdpi.com/article/10.3390/medicina60122043/s1, Table S1: AMSTAR 2 Results.

Author Contributions: Conceptualization, I.K. and G.B.; methodology, I.K.; software, I.K.; validation, I.K., G.B. and A.Y.; formal analysis, I.K.; investigation, I.K., G.B. and A.Y.; resources, R.A., A.I., M.M. and N.U.; data curation, I.K., G.B. and A.Y.; writing—original draft preparation, I.K., G.B. and A.Y.; writing—review and editing, I.K., G.B., A.Y., R.A., A.I., M.M. and N.U.; visualization, I.K.; supervision, M.M. and N.U.; project administration, R.A., A.I., M.M. and N.U.; funding acquisition, G.B. All authors have read and agreed to the published version of the manuscript.

Funding: This research received no external funding.

Institutional Review Board Statement: Ethical review and approval were waived for this study as this is a systematic review of the published literature.

Informed Consent Statement: Not applicable.

Data Availability Statement: The raw data supporting the conclusions of this article will be made available by the authors on request.

Conflicts of Interest: The authors declare no conflicts of interest.

References

1. Bouillon, R.; Marcocci, C.; Carmeliet, G.; Bikle, D.; White, J.H.; Dawson-Hughes, B.; Lips, P.; Munns, C.F.; Lazaretti-Castro, M.; Giustina, A.; et al. Skeletal and Extraskeletal Actions of Vitamin D: Current Evidence and Outstanding Questions. *Endocr. Rev.* **2019**, *40*, 1109–1151. [CrossRef] [PubMed]
2. Minich, D.M.; Henning, M.; Darley, C.; Fahoum, M.; Schuler, C.B.; Frame, J. Is Melatonin the "Next Vitamin D"?: A Review of Emerging Science, Clinical Uses, Safety, and Dietary Supplements. *Nutrients* **2022**, *14*, 3934. [CrossRef] [PubMed]
3. Crowe, F.L.; Steur, M.; Allen, N.E.; Appleby, P.N.; Travis, R.C.; Key, T.J. Plasma Concentrations of 25-Hydroxyvitamin D in Meat Eaters, Fish Eaters, Vegetarians and Vegans: Results from the EPIC-Oxford Study. *Public Health Nutr.* **2011**, *14*, 340–346. [CrossRef] [PubMed]
4. Pludowski, P.; Grant, W.B.; Karras, S.N.; Zittermann, A.; Pilz, S. Vitamin D Supplementation: A Review of the Evidence Arguing for a Daily Dose of 2000 International Units (50 Mg) of Vitamin D for Adults in the General Population. *Nutrients* **2024**, *16*, 391. [CrossRef]
5. van Schoor, N.; de Jongh, R.; Lips, P. Worldwide Vitamin D Status. *Feldman Pike's Vitam. D* **2024**, *2*, 47–75. [CrossRef]
6. Ma, S.; Li, W.; Tojibaev, K.S.; Turginov, O.; Yang, W.; Ma, K. Regionwide and Nationwide Floristic Richness Reveal Vascular Plant Diversity in Central Asia. *Plants* **2024**, *13*, 2275. [CrossRef]
7. Gromova, O.; Doschanova, A.; Lokshin, V.; Tuletova, A.; Grebennikova, G.; Daniyarova, L.; Kaishibayeva, G.; Nurpeissov, T.; Khan, V.; Semenova, Y.; et al. Vitamin D Deficiency in Kazakhstan: Cross-Sectional Study. *J. Steroid Biochem. Mol. Biol.* **2020**, *199*, 105565. [CrossRef]
8. Yerezhepov, D.; Gabdulkayum, A.; Akhmetova, A.; Kozhamkulov, U.A.; Rakhimova, S.E.; Kairov, U.Y.; Zhunussova, G.; Kalendar, R.N.; Akilzhanova, A. Vitamin D Status, VDR, and TLR Polymorphisms and Pulmonary Tuberculosis Epidemiology in Kazakhstan. *Nutrients* **2024**, *16*, 558. [CrossRef]
9. Akhmetova, V.; Balji, Y.; Kandalina, Y.; Iskineyeva, A.; Mukhamejanova, A.; Baspakova, A.; Uzakov, Y.; Issayeva, K.; Zamaratskaia, G. Self-Reported Consumption Frequency of Meat and Fish Products among Young Adults in Kazakhstan. *Nutr. Health* **2024**, *30*, 309–318. [CrossRef]
10. National Institute for Health and Care Research PROSPERO. International Prospective Register of Systematic Reviews. Available online: https://www.crd.york.ac.uk/prospero/ (accessed on 27 March 2024).
11. Karibayeva, I.; Abydynova, A. PROSPERO. Available online: https://www.crd.york.ac.uk/prospero/#recordDetails (accessed on 20 November 2024).
12. Page, M.J.; McKenzie, J.E.; Bossuyt, P.M.; Boutron, I.; Hoffmann, T.C.; Mulrow, C.D.; Shamseer, L.; Tetzlaff, J.M.; Akl, E.A.; Brennan, S.E. The PRISMA 2020 Statement: An Updated Guideline for Reporting Systematic Reviews. *BMJ* **2021**, *372*, n71. [CrossRef]
13. Wells, G.; Shea, B.; O'Connell, D.; Peterson, J.; Welch, V.; Losos, M.; Tugwell, P. Ottawa Hospital Research Institute. Available online: https://www.ohri.ca/programs/clinical_epidemiology/oxford.asp (accessed on 20 November 2024).
14. Shea, B.J.; Reeves, B.C.; Wells, G.; Thuku, M.; Hamel, C.; Moran, J.; Moher, D.; Tugwell, P.; Welch, V.; Kristjansson, E.; et al. AMSTAR 2: A Critical Appraisal Tool for Systematic Reviews That Include Randomised or Non-Randomised Studies of Healthcare Interventions, or Both. *BMJ* **2017**, *358*, 1–9. [CrossRef] [PubMed]
15. Posit team RStudio: Integrated Development Environment for R. Available online: http://www.posit.co/ (accessed on 22 January 2024).
16. Harrer, M.; Cuijpers, P.; Furukawa, T.A.; Ebert, D.D. *Doing Meta-Analysis with R: A Hands-On Guide*; Chapman & Hall/CRC Press: Boca Raton, FL, USA; London, UK, 2021; Volume Chapter 4, ISBN 978-0-367-61007-4.
17. Zhumalina, A.K.; Kim, I.S.; Delyagin, W.M. Vitamin D Level and Indicators of Bone Tissue Metabolism in Kazakh Infants. *Russ. Fam. Dr.* **2023**, *27*, 23–29. [CrossRef]
18. Zhumalina, A.; Tusupkaliev, B.; Mania, A.; Kim, I.; Zharlykasinova, M. The Importance of Determining the Level of Bone Metabolism Markers and Vitamin D in the First Year of Life in the Kazakh Population. *J. Pediatr. Pharmacol. Ther.* **2024**, *29*, 410–416. [CrossRef] [PubMed]
19. Donayeva, A.; Amanzholkyzy, A.; Abdelazim, I.A.; Rakhyzhanova, S.; Mannapova, A.; Abilov, T.; Khamidullina, Z.; Bimagambetova, K.; Gubasheva, G.; Kulzhanova, D.; et al. The Relationship between Vitamin D and Adolescents' Parathyroid Hormone and Bone Mineral Density. *Prz. Menopauzalny* **2024**, *23*, 1–5. [CrossRef]
20. Amanzholkyzy, A.; Donayeva, A.; Kulzhanova, D.; Abdelazim, I.A.; Abilov, T.; Baubekov, Z.; Samaha, I.I. Relation between Vitamin D and Adolescents' Serum Prolactin. *Prz. Menopauzalny* **2023**, *22*, 202–206. [CrossRef]
21. Donayeva, A.; Amanzholkyzy, A.; Abdelazim, I.A.; Saparbayev, S.; Nurgaliyeva, R.; Kaldybayeva, A.; Zhexenova, A.; Stankevicius, E.; Khamidullina, Z.; Gubasheva, G.; et al. The Relation between Vitamin D and the Adolescents' Mid-Luteal Estradiol and Progesterone. *Eur. Rev. Med. Pharmacol. Sci.* **2023**, *27*, 6792–6799. [CrossRef]

22. Donayeva, A.; Kulzhanova, D.; Amanzholkyzy, A.; Abdelazim, I.A.; Abilov, T.; Baubekov, Z.; Samaha, I.I. Relationship between Vitamin D and Adolescents' Hypothyroidism—A Cross-Sectional Study. *Prz. Menopauzalny* **2023**, *22*, 186–190. [CrossRef]
23. Nugmanova, Z.S.; Patel, N.; Akhmetova, G.M.; Kurmangalieva, G.S.; Abdumananova, M.K.; Akanov, A.A.; Kovtunenko, N.G.; McNutt, L.A. Relationship between Vitamin D and Human Immunodeficiency Virus (HIV) Viral Load among HIV-Infected Patients in Kazakhstan. *J. Infect. Dev. Ctries.* **2015**, *9*, 1277–1283. [CrossRef]
24. Algazina, T.; Touir, G.; Pshembayeva, S.; Jetpisbayeva, Z.; Batpenova, G. The Role of Vitamin D in the Development of Psoriasis and Acne. *Georgian Med. News* **2019**, *290*, 96–100.
25. Safi, A.; Orazov, M.; Kalinchenko, S. The Role of Cholecalciferol Deficiency in the Pathogenesis of Polycystic Ovary Syndrome. *Women's Health* **2020**, *16*, 1745506520969606–1745506520969616. [CrossRef]
26. Zhumina, A.G.; Li, K.; Konovalova, A.A.; Li, Y.A.; Ishmuratova, M.Y.; Pogossyan, G.P.; Danilenko, M. Plasma 25-Hydroxyvitamin D Levels and VDR Gene Expression in Peripheral Blood Mononuclear Cells of Leukemia Patients and Healthy Subjects in Central Kazakhstan. *Nutrients* **2020**, *12*, 1229. [CrossRef] [PubMed]
27. Izmailovich, M.; Gazaliyeva, M.; Glushkova, N.; Semenova, Y.; Burankulova, S.; Shaydarova, S.; Bayazitova, M.; Kuznetsova, I. Association between Serum 25-Hydroxyvitamin D Concentration and Severity of Seasonal Allergic Rhinitis in Karaganda Region (Kazakhstan). *J. Clin. Med. Kazakhstan* **2022**, *19*, 46–50. [CrossRef] [PubMed]
28. World Health Organization Noncommunicable Disease Surveillance, Monitoring and Reporting. Available online: https://www.who.int/teams/ncds/surveillance/monitoring-capacity/gmf (accessed on 20 November 2024).
29. Karibayeva, I.; Moiynbayeva, S.; Akhmetov, V.; Yerkenova, S.; Shaikova, K.; Moshkalova, G.; Mussayeva, D.; Tarakova, B.; Semenova, Y.; Ivankov, A.; et al. Interrupted Time Series Analysis of the Impact of the COVID-19 Pandemic and Compulsory Social Health Insurance System on Fertility Rates: A Study of Live Births in Kazakhstan, 2019–2023. *Front. Public Health* **2024**, *12*, 1454420–1454430. [CrossRef] [PubMed]
30. Tochieva, Z.U.; Iskakova, F.A.; Abzaliev, K. Dynamics of Deaths and Mortality Rate in Kazakhstan Population. *Heart Vessel. Transplant.* **2023**, *7*, 1–10. [CrossRef]
31. Kornberg, S.; Gundersen, M. Kazakhstan to Move to Single Time Zone in March. Available online: https://www.timeanddate.com/news/time/kazakhstan-single-time-zone.html (accessed on 20 November 2024).
32. Demay, M.B.; Pittas, A.G.; Bikle, D.D.; Diab, D.L.; Kiely, M.E.; Lazaretti-Castro, M.; Lips, P.; Mitchell, D.M.; Murad, M.H.; Powers, S.; et al. Vitamin D for the Prevention of Disease: An Endocrine Society Clinical Practice Guideline. *J. Clin. Endocrinol. Metab.* **2024**, *109*, 1907–1947. [CrossRef]
33. Marwaha, R.K.; Dabas, A. Interventions for Prevention and Control of Epidemic of Vitamin D Deficiency. *Indian. J. Pediatr.* **2019**, *86*, 532–537. [CrossRef]
34. Cooper, A. The Role of Advanced Nursing Practitioners in Improving Chronic Disease Management: A Quantitative Analysis. *Res. Rev. J. Nurs. Health Sci.* **2023**, *9*, 1–2. [CrossRef]
35. Gregor, R.A.; Sebach, A.M. Nurse Practitioner–Led Vitamin D Screening and Supplementation Program in Rural Primary Care. *J. Nurse Pract.* **2022**, *18*, 155–158. [CrossRef]
36. Shepin, O.; Petruchuk, O.; Korotkih, R.; Davletshin, F. The Dispanserization and Public Health. Report 2: The Population Health and the Organization of Preventive Medical Examinations. *Probl. Sotsialnoi Gig. Zdr. Istor. Med.* **2011**, *3*, 3–7.
37. Al-Oanzi, Z.H.; Alenazy, F.O.; Alhassan, H.H.; Alruwaili, Y.; Alessa, A.I.; Alfarm, N.B.; Alanazi, M.O.; Alghofaili, S.I. The Role of Vitamin D in Reducing the Risk of Metabolic Disturbances That Cause Cardiovascular Diseases. *J. Cardiovasc. Dev. Dis.* **2023**, *10*, 209. [CrossRef]
38. Rebelos, E.; Tentolouris, N.; Jude, E. The Role of Vitamin D in Health and Disease: A Narrative Review on the Mechanisms Linking Vitamin D with Disease and the Effects of Supplementation. *Drugs* **2023**, *83*, 665–685. [CrossRef]

MDPI AG
Grosspeteranlage 5
4052 Basel
Switzerland
Tel.: +41 61 683 77 34

Medicina Editorial Office
E-mail: medicina@mdpi.com
www.mdpi.com/journal/medicina

www.ingramcontent.com/pod-product-compliance
Lightning Source LLC
Chambersburg PA
CBHW061628210926
51850CB00009B/2477